Complete Review for the Pharmacy Technician

Fourth Edition

T0321285

Fourth Edition

Complete Review for the Pharmacy Technician

Kristin Wiisanen, PharmD, FAPhA, FCCP
Clinical Professor
University of Florida College of Pharmacy
Gainesville, Florida

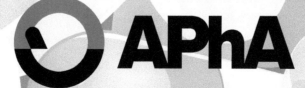

American Pharmacists Association
Washington, D.C.

Senior Director, Books and Digital Publishing: Janan Sarwar
Editorial Director: Jesse Vineyard
Acquisitions Editor: Jesse Vineyard
Production Editor: Brittany Williams
Editorial Services: Absolute Service, Inc.
Cover Design: Michelle I. Powell, APhA Integrated Design and Production

©2021 by the American Pharmacists Association
APhA was founded in 1852 as the American Pharmaceutical Association.

Published by the American Pharmacists Association
2215 Constitution Avenue, NW
Washington, DC 20037-2985
www.pharmacist.com
www.pharmacylibrary.com

To comment on this book by e-mail, send your message to the publisher at aphabooks@aphanet.org.

Library of Congress Cataloging-in-Publication Data

Names: Wiisanen, Kristin, author. | Posey, L. Michael. Complete review for
  the pharmacy technician. | American Pharmacists Association, issuing body.
Title: Complete review for the pharmacy technician / Kristin Wiisanen.
Description: 4th edition. | Washington, D.C. : American Pharmacists
  Association, [2021] | Preceded by Complete review for the pharmacy
  technician / L. Michael Posey, Kristin W. Weitzel. 3rd ed. 2014. |
  Includes bibliographical references and index. | Summary: "Complete
  Review for the Pharmacy Technician is the ideal manual for students
  entering formal technician training programs, for community and hospital
  pharmacy technicians beginning in-house training, and for candidates
  preparing for the Pharmacy Technician Certification Examination"--
  Provided by publisher.
Identifiers: LCCN 2021018950 | ISBN 9781582123691 (paperback)
Subjects: MESH: Pharmacy Technicians | Pharmaceutical Preparations |
  Pharmaceutical Services | Pharmacy
Classification: LCC RM301.13 | NLM QV 21.5 | DDC 615.1076--dc23
LC record available at https://lccn.loc.gov/2021018950

How to Order This Book
Online: www.pharmacist.com/shop
By phone: 800-878-0729 (770-280-0085 from outside the United States)
VISA®, MasterCard®, and American Express® cards accepted.

Dedication

*This book is dedicated to John Titus Presley and Myrtle Perkins Presley.
Thank you for all that you did to make this and many other books possible.*

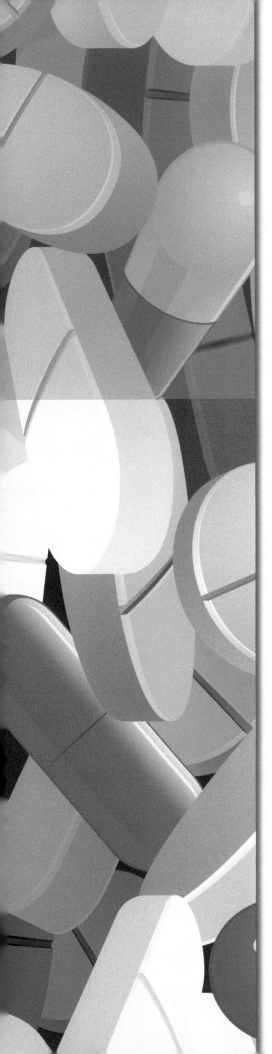

Table of Contents

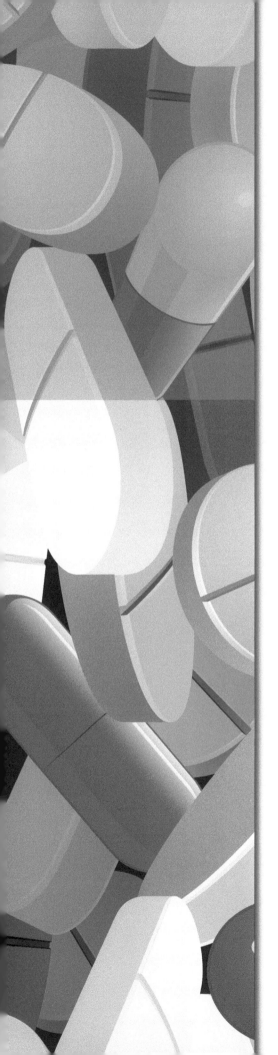

Preface to the Fourth Edition

The earliest mentions of people who specialized in the use of plants and herbal products in recorded history were in ancient Babylon and China, both at about BC 2000. For most of the time since then, pharmacists, and more recently pharmacy technicians, have focused on preparing and dispensing medications for specific patients. Whether making herbal poultices and decoctions in earlier centuries or dispensing injectable medicines and biosimilars today, pharmacy has been concentrated for centuries almost solely on delivering a physical product—the drug.

In recent decades, we have seen rapid advances in drug discovery and significant professional and legislative progress, including pharmacist-specific provisions of the Medicare Modernization and Affordable Care Acts and value-based care, and a growing number of advanced clinical roles and responsibilities for both pharmacists and pharmacy technicians. More recently, the COVID-19 pandemic has created an unprecedented need for all health care professionals to expand their roles to ensure that patients have access to much-needed care, medications, and vaccines. Today, these and many other factors have led us to a new professional landscape for pharmacy technicians. This landscape includes increasing technician responsibilities in the medication preparation and dispensing process and opportunities for supportive or direct patient care roles in tech-check-tech, medication reconciliation, medication history, immunization administration, and other innovative services.

This changing health care landscape has been matched by novel opportunities for pharmacy technicians to grow and develop professionally. In March 2019, the Pharmacy Technician Certification Board (PTCB) launched the first of its new certificate programs to provide opportunities for advanced formal training and recognition for technicians in the areas of product verification, medication histories, hazardous drug management, controlled substances, third-party billing, and immunizations. For the first time ever, PTCB-certified pharmacy technicians who meet certain requirements are eligible to earn an Advanced Certified Pharmacy Technician (CPhT-Adv) credential. These certificate programs and advanced credentialing opportunities join PTCB's Compounded Sterile Product Technician certification exam that launched in 2017.

The fourth edition of this book has been updated to reflect the needs of this changing landscape for pharmacy technicians. The content has been revised throughout to include information that technicians need to know in these advanced roles and is now aligned with the 4 domains of the PTCB certification exam to make preparation for the exam simpler. A new chapter has been added to describe these professional growth and development opportunities. And there is an increased emphasis on patient safety and the pharmacy technician's role in patient-centered care activities throughout the text, consistent with current and emerging practice.

With these increasing opportunities, the profession has moved beyond an era in which a single textbook can meet all of the pharmacy technician's educational needs. This is a landmark achievement for pharmacy technicians. We hope this revised edition of the *Complete Review for the Pharmacy Technician* provides a starting point for many current and potential pharmacy technicians to explore new horizons in this profession.

Kristin Wiisanen
June 2021

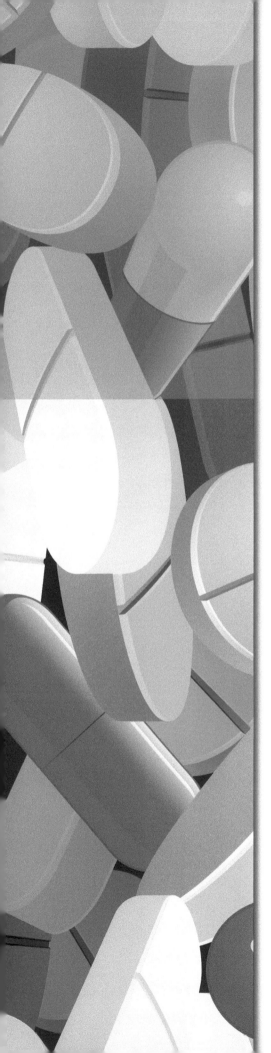

Acknowledgments

APhA would like to acknowledge the following authors who contributed to chapters in this book.

Katherine Vogel Anderson, PharmD, BCACP
Clinical Associate Professor
University of Florida College of Pharmacy
Department of Pharmacotherapy and Translational Research
Gainesville, FL

Kimberly Atkinson, PharmD
PGY-1 Pharmacy Resident
Pharmacotherapy and Translational Research
University of Florida College of Pharmacy
Gainesville, FL

Adonice Khoury, PharmD, BCPS
Clinical Assistant Professor
University of Florida College of Pharmacy
Department of Pharmacotherapy and Translational Research
Gainesville, FL

Janet Schmittgen, PharmD
Clinical Lecturer
Department of Pharmacotherapy and Research
University of Florida College of Pharmacy
Gainesville, FL

APhA would like to acknowledge the following individuals who reviewed the content in this book.

Loyd V. Allen, Jr., PhD, RPh
Editor-in-Chief
International Journal of Pharmaceutical
Compounding

Zahirah Ahmed, PharmD
Clinical Staff Pharmacist
TriStar Centennial Medical Center

Ashley Anthony, CPhT
Overlook Medical Center

Zubin Austin, PhD, FCAHS
Professor and Murray Koffler Chair in
Management and Leslie Dan Faculty of
Pharmacy and the Institute for Health
Policy, Management, and Evaluation–
Faculty of Medicine
University of Toronto

Kenneth Hohmeier, PharmD
Associate Professor of Clinical Pharmacy
and Translational Science
University of Tennessee Health Science
Center

Daniel Hooper PharmD, BCSCP
Sterile Products Supervisor
TriStar Centennial Medical Center

Laly Havern, PharmD
Manager, Office of Clinical Integrity
Walgreens

Lizbeth Limon, CPhT
Senior Business Analyst, Patient
Outcomes Performance
Walgreens

Jonathan Little, PharmD
Project Management Specialist, Research
and Innovation
American Pharmacists Association
Foundation

Cynthia Robertson, CPhT
Three Rivers Medical Center Pharmacy

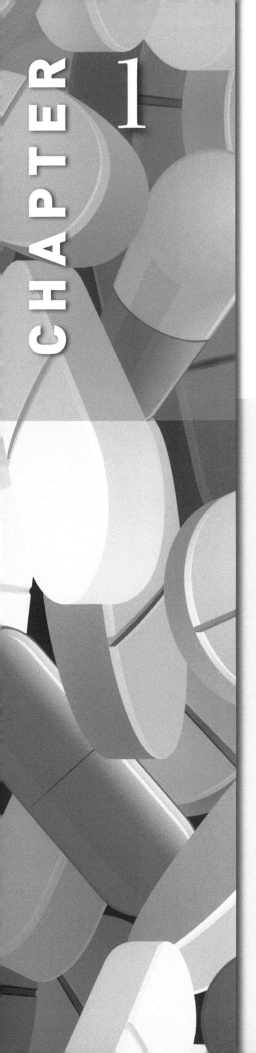

CHAPTER 1

Drug Classifications and Formulations

This chapter introduces anatomy, physiology, diseases, pathophysiology, and epidemiology and presents the most common prescription and nonprescription drugs in a large table, including uses, dosage limits, and common adverse effects. Chapter 1 also briefly describes the most common formulations for drugs and presents routes of drug administration.

Introduction

Medications are powerful substances that can have profound—even lethal (producing death)—effects on the human body. In this chapter, we begin to appreciate how drugs work, what diseases can be prevented or treated with common agents, what adverse effects can be expected from these drugs, and what other adverse outcomes can be expected when medication therapy goes awry.

As with most chapters in an introductory text, you will need to consult other books for detailed information on medications and their effects. This is a complicated field, one that pharmacists study every semester during their 4 professional years of pharmacy school. While you do not need to know many of the details that pharmacists learn, your goal as a technician should be to attain the following level of knowledge:

- Given a generic or trade name of a commonly used drug, state the other name, drug category, available dosage forms, common adverse effects (also called side effects), common or serious drug interactions, and storage considerations (products that need to be refrigerated or kept in special containers).
- For a common disease, state nonprescription and prescription drug options used in its treatment.
- Given a patient's drug regimen, identify possible problems involving drug interactions, drugs that should not be taken together (contraindications), and common adverse effects the patient should watch for.

With these objectives in mind, let's take a look at pharmacotherapy—the use of medications to treat human disease.

Normal Human Anatomy and Body Function

To appreciate the effects of medications on disease, you must first have some idea of how the human body works under normal circumstances. For this reason, students of pharmacy and other health care professions

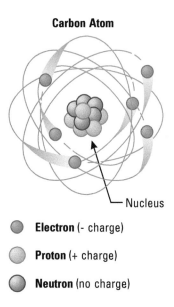

Figure 1-1 Structure of a Carbon Atom

Carbon Atom

Nucleus

Electron (- charge)

Proton (+ charge)

Neutron (no charge)

spend a substantial amount of time studying **human anatomy** and normal body function, or **physiology**.

Chemical and Cellular Physiology

An atom is the most basic structure of matter. It is composed of a nucleus and electrons that revolve around the nucleus, much like the planets travel around the sun. The nucleus is composed of positively charged protons as well as uncharged neutrons.

Atoms are defined by the number of protons in their nuclei. As shown in Figure 1-1, carbon has 6 protons. (One proton is not visible in the figure.) If that atom has 7 protons, it would no longer be carbon. Instead, it would be nitrogen (Table 1-1). The number of protons in the nucleus is also referred to as the atomic number. An element is made up of only one type of atom and cannot be further broken down by ordinary chemical means. Ninety-six percent of the body is composed of just 4 elements—oxygen, carbon, hydrogen, and nitrogen.

In addition to an atomic number, each element has an atomic mass number, which is the sum of its protons and neutrons. For example, carbon (abbreviated as "C") has a mass number of 12, meaning that each

Table 1-1 Common Elements Found in the Human Body

Elements (Abbreviation)	Atomic Numbers (number of protons in nucleus)	Most Common Stable Atomic Masses (number of protons plus neutrons in nucleus)	Mass of Element Found in 70-kg Person (kg)
Hydrogen (H)	1	1	7
Carbon (C)	6	12	16
Nitrogen (N)	7	14	1.8
Oxygen (O)	8	16	43
Sodium (Na)	11	23	0.1
Phosphorus (P)	15	31	0.780
Sulfur (S)	16	32	0.14
Chlorine (Cl)	17	35 or 37	0.095
Potassium (K)	19	39	0.14
Calcium (Ca)	20	40	1
Iron (Fe)	26	56	4.2
Iodine (I)	53	127	0.02

atom in the element has a total of 12 neutrons and protons in its nucleus.

While elements generally have an equal number of protons and neutrons, not all do. In fact, the presence of 1 or more extra neutrons can result in an unstable configuration. These unstable atoms break down by emitting, or sending out, radioactive particles that over time transform the atom to the more stable configuration. Chapter 13 includes more information on medications that contain radioactive elements.

A **molecule** is produced when 2 or more atoms share electrons or combine with each other through a type of magnetic attraction. For example, a molecule of water is designated H_2O, meaning that 2 atoms of hydrogen (H) share electrons with 1 atom of oxygen (O).

Biological systems are made up largely of molecules that can be classified as sugars (carbohydrates), fats (lipids), and proteins (which often help make chemical reactions occur and are therefore called enzymes). Carbohydrates, fats, and proteins make up most of the human diet, along with vitamins and minerals such as calcium and iron.

Amino acids—20 of them—are the building blocks of proteins. Proteins can be relatively simple molecules, such as insulin, or can be very complex structures, and their effects on cells are often striking.

A **cell** is a living structural and functional unit surrounded by a membrane that has many substructures, as illustrated in Figure 1-2. At the center of each cell is the nucleus, which contains genetic material. As cells divide, each cell contains the same genetic material. Chromosomes are long strands of DNA, an abbreviation for deoxyribonucleic acid. In DNA, the sugar deoxyribose forms a kind of backbone in combination with phosphate (phosphorus plus oxygen), and this backbone supports paired nucleotide bases composed of either adenine–thymine or cytosine–guanine. Each person has 46 chromosomes in each cell, 23 contributed from each parent.

Sections of these 46 chromosomes that code for proteins are called **genes**. Genes are characterized by the specific order and pairing of 4 nucleotide bases. Genes essentially code for the production of proteins within the cell, but some genes also turn on and off the activity of other genes.

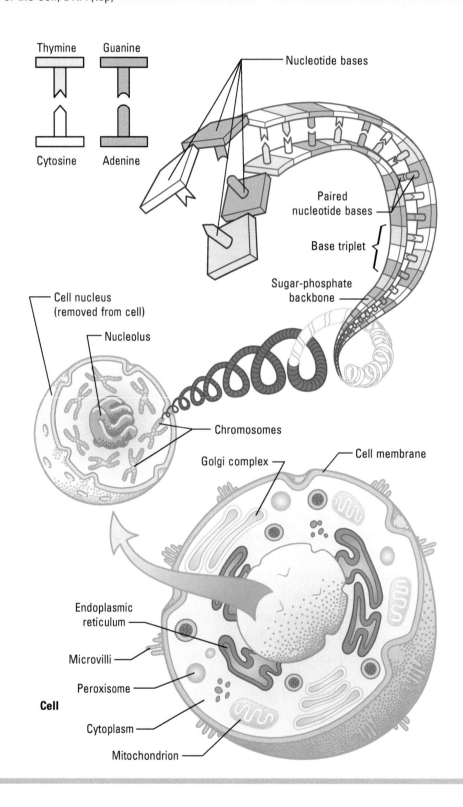

Anatomy and Organ Systems

As you may remember from biology or health courses in high school, the human body is made up of many highly specialized tissues, including bones, muscles, and nerves. Specialized cells are grouped together in organs of the body, such as the lungs or stomach. Organs that interrelate to one another in function are termed **organ systems**. The body has 11 organ systems, as outlined below.

Many diseases result from disruptions in 1 or more of these organ systems. Drugs and drug products that are primarily used to treat these diseases are often grouped together, and you should be able to name several agents useful in treating the most common diseases affecting people. The organ system approach is generally used for making these drug categorizations, as shown at the end of this chapter in Table 1-3.

Integumentary System

As shown in Figure 1-3, the integumentary system includes the skin, hair, nails, and sweat glands. This system is responsible for protection, body temperature regulation, conservation of water, and production of vitamin D precursors. The integumentary system literally holds the body together and helps it stay cool and interact with its environment.

The skin is composed of a thin, outermost area called the epidermis, under which lies the thicker dermis. Just beneath the skin is the subcutaneous tissue, which contains fat cells, blood vessels, and nerves to supply the skin. Sebaceous glands are usually connected to hair follicles and secrete an oily substance called sebum, which keeps the skin and hair from drying out. Sweat glands produce around 600 mL of sweat per day, which serves to cool the body as it evaporates. Vitamin D, needed for the absorption of calcium, is made when sunlight activates a precursor located in the skin. The skin is the site of administration for many drugs—those injected into the subcutaneous tissue and those administered by transdermal patch. In both cases, the drug generally reaches the blood and is carried throughout the body.

Skeletal System

As shown in Figure 1-4, the skeletal system consists of bones, cartilage, and joints. Without the skeletal system, people would be like jellyfish—incapable of initiating movement or picking up items.

Adults have 206 bones, including 106 just in the hands and feet! Bones protect internal organs, allow body movement, and provide attachment for skeletal muscle.

Bones are richly supplied with blood vessels and nerves. The bone marrow, located in the ends of long bones in the arms and legs and in the pelvis, ribs, sternum (breastbone), and skull, produces blood cells. Bone also stores calcium, phosphorus, and triglycerides.

Joints—formed when 2 bones meet—allow movement. They contain synovial fluid that lubricates the joint.

Cartilage is similar in function to bone but very different in many other ways. Cartilage, which you can feel in your ears and nose, consists of collagen fibers and does not contain blood vessels or nerves. It provides support but allows flexibility.

Muscular System

Muscles attach to bones and coordinate body movements, maintain posture, produce body heat, and control outflow of certain liquids (Figure 1-5). Without the

| Figure 1-3 | Structure of the Skin |

Labels: Stratum lucidum, Stratum spinosum, Stratum germinativum, Stratum corneum, Stratum granulosum, Meissner corpuscle, Pore, Apocrine sweat gland, Sebaceous gland, Hairshaft, Pacinian corpuscle, Apocrine sweat gland, Nerves, Blood vessels, Skin Level, Epidermis, Nerves (around hair), Dermis, Hair muscle, Hair follicle, Subcutaneous tissue, Muscle, without hair, with hair

Figure 1-4 Skeletal System of the Human Body

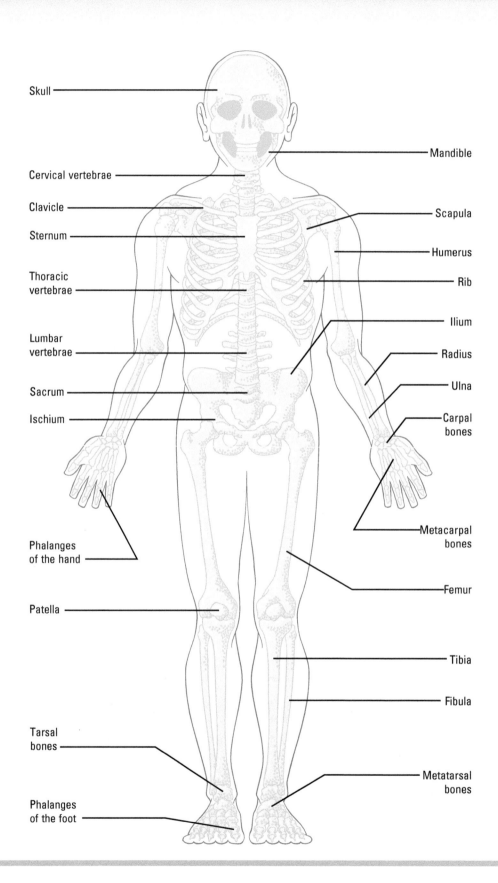

Skull

Cervical vertebrae

Clavicle

Sternum

Thoracic vertebrae

Lumbar vertebrae

Sacrum

Ischium

Phalanges of the hand

Patella

Tarsal bones

Phalanges of the foot

Mandible

Scapula

Humerus

Rib

Ilium

Radius

Ulna

Carpal bones

Metacarpal bones

Femur

Tibia

Fibula

Metatarsal bones

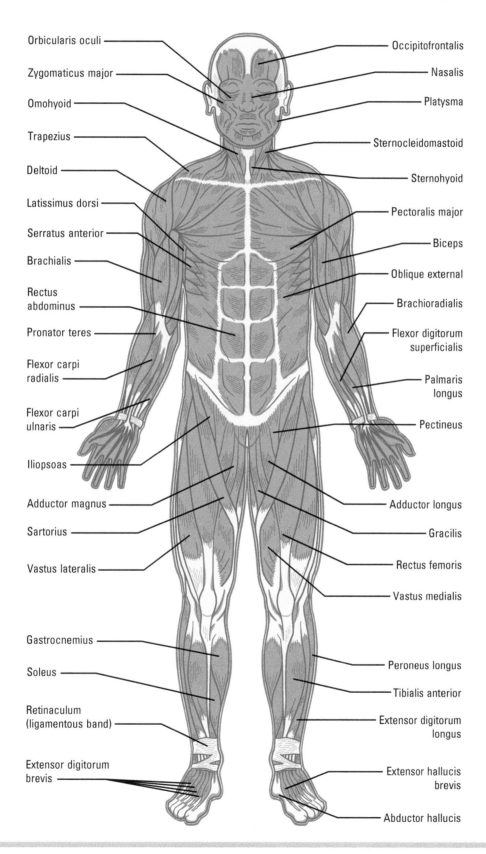

Orbicularis oculi

Zygomaticus major

Omohyoid

Trapezius

Deltoid

Latissimus dorsi

Serratus anterior

Brachialis

Rectus abdominus

Pronator teres

Flexor carpi radialis

Flexor carpi ulnaris

Iliopsoas

Adductor magnus

Sartorius

Vastus lateralis

Gastrocnemius

Soleus

Retinaculum (ligamentous band)

Extensor digitorum brevis

Occipitofrontalis

Nasalis

Platysma

Sternocleidomastoid

Sternohyoid

Pectoralis major

Biceps

Oblique external

Brachioradialis

Flexor digitorum superficialis

Palmaris longus

Pectineus

Adductor longus

Gracilis

Rectus femoris

Vastus medialis

Peroneus longus

Tibialis anterior

Extensor digitorum longus

Extensor hallucis brevis

Abductor hallucis

(figure continues on next page)

Figure 1-5 (continued)

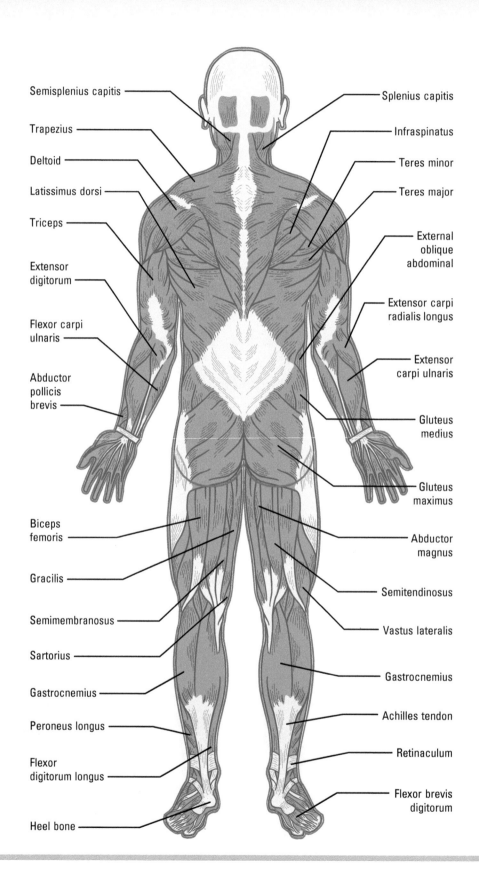

Semisplenius capitis

Trapezius

Deltoid

Latissimus dorsi

Triceps

Extensor digitorum

Flexor carpi ulnaris

Abductor pollicis brevis

Biceps femoris

Gracilis

Semimembranosus

Sartorius

Gastrocnemius

Peroneus longus

Flexor digitorum longus

Heel bone

Splenius capitis

Infraspinatus

Teres minor

Teres major

External oblique abdominal

Extensor carpi radialis longus

Extensor carpi ulnaris

Gluteus medius

Gluteus maximus

Abductor magnus

Semitendinosus

Vastus lateralis

Gastrocnemius

Achilles tendon

Retinaculum

Flexor brevis digitorum

muscles and associated tissues (ligaments and tendons), the body would collapse like a floppy puppet.

Three types of muscles are found in the human body:

- **Skeletal muscle**—connects to and moves bones. Impulses from nerves allow voluntary movement. Since the nerve and muscle don't directly touch, a chemical called a neurotransmitter (acetylcholine, in this case) is released from a nerve ending at the junction of the nerve and muscle to direct muscle movement.
- **Cardiac muscle**—contained in the walls of the heart and causes the heart to contract (beat). Unlike skeletal muscle, contraction is not dependent on neurotransmitters and is autoregulated.
- **Smooth muscle**—found in blood vessels, airways, the iris of the eye, and in other hollow organs such as the bladder. Like cardiac muscle, smooth muscle is not voluntarily controlled.

Nervous System

The nervous system, depicted in Figure 1-6, is responsible for gathering information from in and around the body (whether it be a pinprick on the skin or a noise heard or the acidity of the blood), processing this information in the brain and determining how to react, and lastly, conveying the brain's "decision" back to the muscles, glands, and organs responsible for performing the function. In addition, nerves go to the internal organs of the body to monitor and, in some cases, direct activity.

Nerves that send information to the brain are called afferent nerves, and those that send information from the brain to the tissue are called efferent nerves. The nervous system is composed of the central nervous system (CNS), the brain (including the cerebellum, shown in Figure 1-6) and spinal cord, and the peripheral nervous system (PNS)—all of the nerves outside of the CNS. The PNS can be further subdivided as follows:

- **Somatic nervous system**—afferent nerves gather information from the 5 senses (sight, smell, touch, taste, and sound) and efferent nerves return information to skeletal muscles (Figure 1-7). This system is under voluntary control.

- **Autonomic nervous system**—afferent nerves gather information from various organs such as the stomach and lungs. Efferent nerves are classified as sympathetic and parasympathetic and generally have opposing actions, like increasing versus decreasing the heart rate. This system is generally involuntary. That is, it operates without the person being aware of or in control of its actions.

Endocrine System

This system includes glands that secrete hormones and related substances that control functions such as metabolism, reproduction, and growth. Hormones are chemicals that act as messengers and are excreted in response to signals originating in the "master" glands—the hypothalamus, a part of the brain, and pituitary glands, located at the base of the brain and connected to the hypothalamus (Figure 1-8).

For example, if blood glucose (sugar) levels are low, the hypothalamus will excrete a hormone to tell the pituitary to secrete a second hormone that tells the pancreas to secrete glucagon and the liver to produce glucose. If blood glucose becomes too high, the hypothalamus secretes an inhibiting hormone that ultimately stops the production of glucose and causes the release of insulin from the pancreas. Thus, hormones are excreted via a chemical feedback mechanism.

The pineal gland in the brain secretes melatonin, which induces sleep. Melatonin is sold in pharmacies and other retail outlets as a dietary supplement that helps people get to sleep.

As shown in Figure 1-8, other glands in the human body include the following:

- **Thyroid gland**—produces thyroid hormone, which controls cellular metabolism and regulates body temperature.
- **Parathyroid gland**—regulates body levels of calcium, phosphate, and magnesium.
- **Thymus gland**—produces hormones that promote immunity (the body's defense system against infection).
- **Adrenal glands**—produce glucocorticoids (cortisol), mineralocorticoids (aldosterone), small amounts of androgens, and epinephrine

Figure 1-6   Nervous System of the Human Body

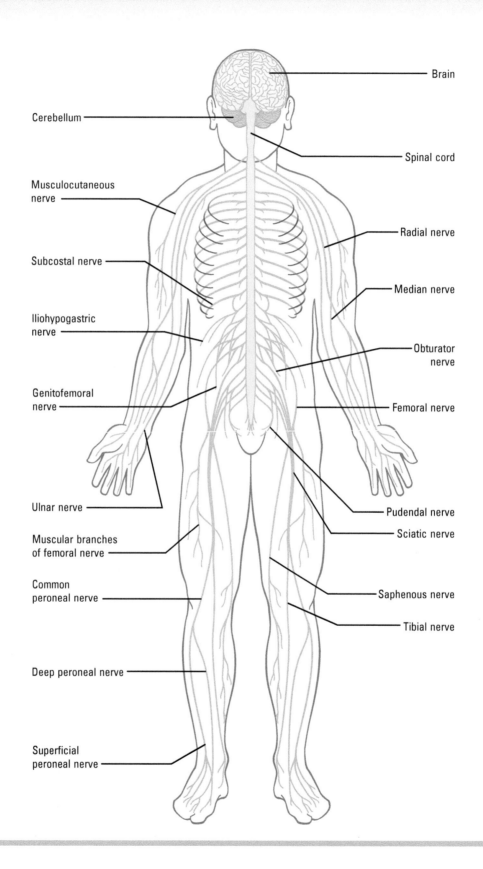

Brain

Cerebellum

Spinal cord

Musculocutaneous nerve

Radial nerve

Subcostal nerve

Median nerve

Iliohypogastric nerve

Obturator nerve

Genitofemoral nerve

Femoral nerve

Ulnar nerve

Pudendal nerve

Muscular branches of femoral nerve

Sciatic nerve

Common peroneal nerve

Saphenous nerve

Tibial nerve

Deep peroneal nerve

Superficial peroneal nerve

Figure 1-7 The 5 Senses

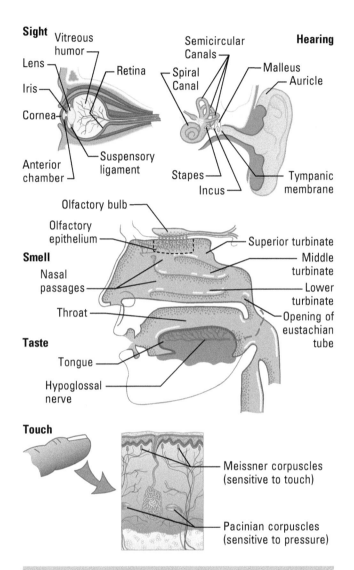

Figure 1-8 Endocrine System of the Human Body

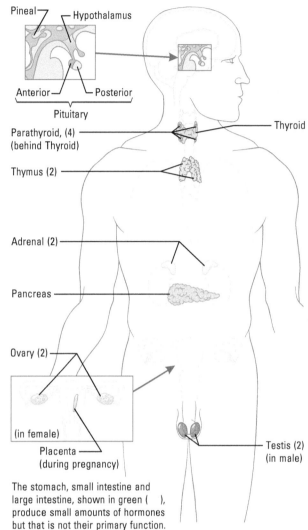

The stomach, small intestine and large intestine, shown in green (   ), produce small amounts of hormones but that is not their primary function.

and norepinephrine. Glucocorticoids regulate metabolism and resistance to stress and have anti-inflammatory effects. Mineralocorticoids regulate blood pressure by affecting the amount of fluid retained in the circulation. Epinephrine and norepinephrine, also known as adrenaline and noradrenaline, respectively, are neurotransmitters that are excreted during exercise or in stressful situations to increase heart rate and blood flow to various organs and to dilate the airways.

- **Pancreas**—secretes insulin, which lowers blood glucose levels, and glucagon, which raises blood glucose levels.

- **Ovaries (females)**—produce estrogen and progesterone, which regulate the menstrual cycle, maintain pregnancy and lactation, and promote development of female sexual characteristics.
- **Testes (males)**—produce testosterone, needed for sperm production and male sexual characteristics.

Cardiovascular System

The cardiovascular system consists of the heart, blood vessels, and blood (Figure 1-9). This system is

Figure 1-9 Cardiovascular System of the Human Body

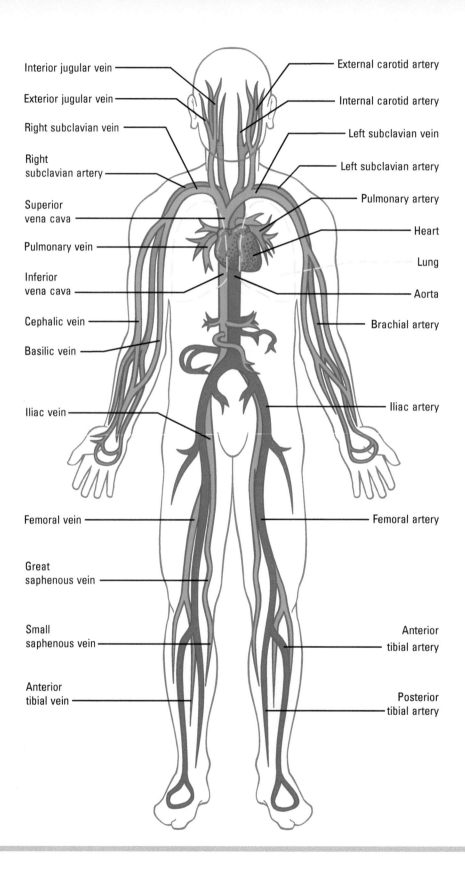

Interior jugular vein

Exterior jugular vein

Right subclavian vein

Right subclavian artery

Superior vena cava

Pulmonary vein

Inferior vena cava

Cephalic vein

Basilic vein

Iliac vein

Femoral vein

Great saphenous vein

Small saphenous vein

Anterior tibial vein

External carotid artery

Internal carotid artery

Left subclavian vein

Left subclavian artery

Pulmonary artery

Heart

Lung

Aorta

Brachial artery

Iliac artery

Femoral artery

Anterior tibial artery

Posterior tibial artery

responsible for transporting oxygenated blood throughout the body and deoxygenated blood back to the heart. Blood carries nutrients, waste products, gases, and hormones to different tissues. This system is also responsible for some immune functions and regulation of temperature. This system has many parts, including the following:

- **Heart**—The heart contains 4 chambers and 4 valves. The right atrium receives deoxygenated blood from the body through the superior and inferior venae cavae. It is then pumped through the tricuspid valve into the right ventricle, which pumps blood to the lungs through the pulmonary valve into the right and left pulmonary arteries where it picks up oxygen. From the lungs, the now oxygenated blood is received back into the heart through the pulmonary veins, into the left atrium. Blood passes through the bicuspid valve into the left ventricle. The left ventricle pumps blood through the aortic valve and into the aorta, which then pushes the blood throughout the body.
- **Blood vessels**—Blood vessels that carry blood from the heart are called arteries. Arterial blood contains oxygen. Capillaries are very small blood vessels that connect arteries and veins, and this is where nutrients and gases (like oxygen) are exchanged within the tissues. Since the oxygen has been released into the tissues, veins carry deoxygenated blood back to the heart. The heart muscle itself is also fed by coronary arteries and veins.
- **Blood**—Blood contains a liquid portion called plasma. Plasma is mostly water but also contains proteins and other solutes. Plasma without the clotting proteins is called serum. In addition to plasma, blood contains many cells, including red blood cells (erythrocytes), which carry oxygen; white blood cells (leukocytes), which are of many types but generally fight infections and aid in immune responses; and platelets (thrombocytes), which aid in blood clotting.

Lymphatic System

The lymphatic system is made up of lymphatic tissue, lymphatic vessels, and lymph fluid (Figure 1-10). This system is crucial in fighting infection and maintaining immune response to foreign substances. It also plays a role in draining excess fluid and transporting fat. T cells and B cells, which are important in providing an immune response to a foreign substance, are produced in lymphatic tissue. Lymphatic tissue is found in the bone marrow, thymus gland, lymph nodes, spleen, adenoids, and tonsils.

Lymph is a clear fluid that bathes cells, and it flows through lymphatic vessels to rid the body of excess fluid.

Respiratory System

The respiratory system includes the nasal cavity, pharynx (throat), larynx (voice box), trachea (windpipe), bronchi, and lungs (Figure 1-11). The primary function of this system is the exchange of gases that occurs between the alveoli and the capillaries.

Oxygen (O_2) from the air is absorbed into lung tissue, where it is then passed through vessels into the blood. Carbon dioxide (CO_2), a by-product of cellular metabolism, is released from the blood and exhaled through the respiratory system.

If CO_2 builds up, the blood becomes too acidic (the pH is too low), and this is toxic to cells. The pH value represents the hydrogen ion content of the blood. Similarly, if the pH of the blood is too high, the blood becomes too basic, and this, too, can damage cells throughout the body. Thus, the respiratory system is essential to maintaining the right concentration of hydrogen ions in the body. This is referred to as acid–base balance.

The respiratory system also permits the sense of smell, filters air that is breathed in, and produces sound (voice) as exhaled air interacts with the larynx in the throat.

Digestive System

The digestive, or gastrointestinal, system consists of the gastrointestinal tract, which runs from the mouth to the anus, and accessory digestive organs such as the

Figure 1-10 Lymphatic System of the Human Body

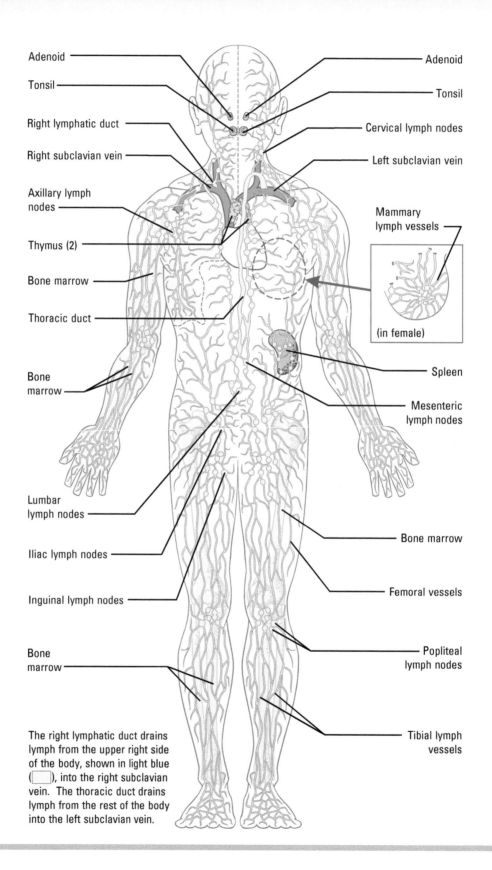

Adenoid

Tonsil

Right lymphatic duct

Right subclavian vein

Axillary lymph nodes

Thymus (2)

Bone marrow

Thoracic duct

Bone marrow

Lumbar lymph nodes

Iliac lymph nodes

Inguinal lymph nodes

Bone marrow

Adenoid

Tonsil

Cervical lymph nodes

Left subclavian vein

Mammary lymph vessels

(in female)

Spleen

Mesenteric lymph nodes

Bone marrow

Femoral vessels

Popliteal lymph nodes

Tibial lymph vessels

The right lymphatic duct drains lymph from the upper right side of the body, shown in light blue (☐), into the right subclavian vein. The thoracic duct drains lymph from the rest of the body into the left subclavian vein.

Figure 1-11	Respiratory System of the Human Body

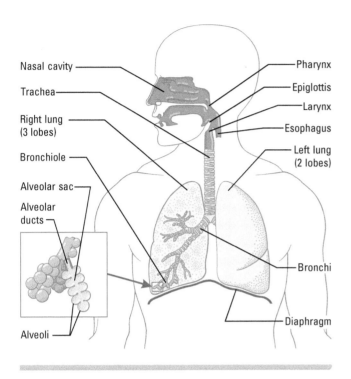

Figure 1-12	Gastrointestinal System of the Human Body

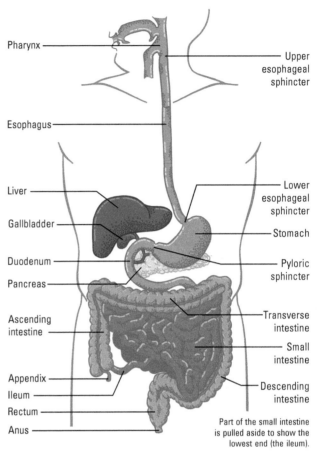

Part of the small intestine is pulled aside to show the lowest end (the ileum).

pancreas, gallbladder, and liver (Figure 1-12). These structures have the following functions:

- **Gastrointestinal tract**—comprises the pharynx, esophagus, stomach, small intestine (duodenum, jejunum, and ileum), large intestine or colon, and rectum. Its job is to process food from the time it is eaten until it is digested, or broken down into small subunits, and then absorbed or eliminated. The degree of acidity changes along the gastrointestinal tract, and this affects the absorption and breakdown of food and drugs. In the stomach, the pH is low (very acidic), causing ingested substances to be broken down, but little absorption occurs for most nutrients and drugs. One notable exception is ethanol—the alcohol in beverages—which is absorbed from the stomach. This accounts for its rapid onset of effects. Nutrients, water, and drugs are primarily absorbed in the small intestine, where the pH is higher (more basic). In fact, drugs are designed to take advantage of this digestive processing that occurs in the stomach, so that by the time the drug reaches the small intestine it is small enough for absorption.

- **Pancreas**—produces and secretes pancreatic enzymes that aid in breaking down food. The pancreas also produces hormones such as insulin and glucagon. These enzymes were mentioned earlier under the discussion of the endocrine system, and they are important in patients who have diabetes.

- **Liver**—detoxifies or breaks down ingested substances. The liver secretes bile, which is needed for fat absorption and is important in the breakdown or metabolism of carbohydrates and proteins. It also helps maintain the proper blood glucose level, stores some vitamins and minerals, and produces compounds that allow the blood to clot when needed.

Figure 1-13   Drug Metabolism in the Liver

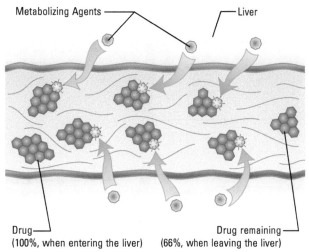

Metabolizing Agents —⟍   ⎰— Liver

Drug —⎤
(100%, when entering the liver)   Drug remaining —⎤
(66%, when leaving the liver)

Low first-pass metabolism

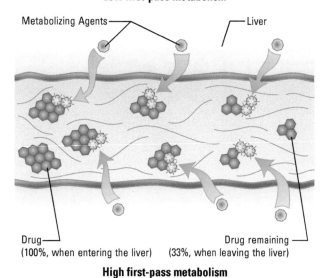

Metabolizing Agents —⟍   ⎰— Liver

Drug —⎤
(100%, when entering the liver)   Drug remaining —⎤
(33%, when leaving the liver)

High first-pass metabolism

As shown in Figure 1-13, drugs are often metabolized (broken down) in the liver by various hepatic (liver) enzymes (specialized proteins that facilitate chemical changes) and the cytochrome P450 (CYP 450) enzymes. These enzymes are involved in many drug interactions when 2 drugs are metabolized by the same enzyme or when one drug alters the function of an enzyme responsible for metabolizing a second drug. Also, drugs absorbed from the intestines are carried directly to the liver, where

they undergo first-pass metabolism. As shown in the lower part of Figure 1-13, some drugs are extensively metabolized at this point, meaning that only a small part of an oral dose actually reaches the general circulation of the body (low bioavailability). This is called high, or extensive, first-pass metabolism. Drugs that undergo little transformation are said to undergo low first-pass metabolism. Metabolism is discussed further later in this chapter in the section on pharmacokinetics.

■ **Gallbladder**—stores bile, a yellowish-green substance that, when secreted through bile ducts into the small intestine, helps the body emulsify fats so that they can be absorbed into the blood.

Urinary System

The urinary system consists of 2 kidneys, 2 ureters, a bladder, and a urethra (Figure 1-14). The kidneys filter blood and remove unnecessary substances and excess water. Regulation of electrolyte levels (eg, sodium, potassium, calcium, chloride) is maintained by the kidneys. The kidneys help maintain acid–base balance (which is also regulated by the respiratory system, as described earlier) by regulating the amount of hydrogen ions (acid) and bicarbonate ions (base) that are excreted.

Figure 1-14   Urinary System of the Human Body

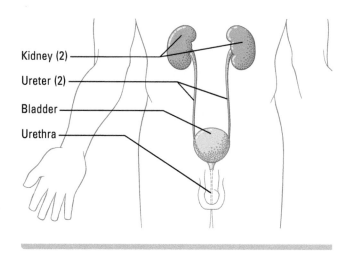

Kidney (2)

Ureter (2)

Bladder

Urethra

The kidneys also control blood pressure by regulating the amount of water excreted and by releasing enzymes that constrict or dilate the blood vessels. Urine produced by the kidneys is transported through the ureters to the bladder, a storage container, until released through the urethra, which terminates in the penis in males and at the vaginal opening in females. In males, the urethra travels through a doughnut-shaped organ, the prostate gland (Figure 1-15). Men with benign prostatic hypertrophy (BPH) have problems with urination because of the associated inflammation.

Reproductive System

The male and female reproductive systems, depicted in Figure 1-15, are responsible for propagation of the human species (reproduction). Men produce sperm that when united with an egg from the woman, form a zygote. The zygote implants in the lining of the uterus, where it develops into a fetus and then a baby, which is normally delivered 36-40 weeks later.

Female reproductive organs include the following:

- **Ovaries**—produce and release eggs and hormones (estrogen and progesterone).
- **Fallopian tubes**—connect the ovaries to the uterus and are the site of fertilization.
- **Uterus**—where a fertilized egg implants to grow into a fetus.
- **Vagina**—a passageway for sperm, menstrual flow, and childbirth.
- **Vulva**—collective term for external female genitals.
- **Mammary tissue (breasts)**—produce milk for infants.

Male reproductive organs include the following:

- **Testes**—produce sperm and secrete the hormone testosterone.
- **Scrotum**—a sac containing the testes.
- **Prostate gland**—helps produce semen.
- **Penis**—contains the urethra and is a passageway for semen and urine.

Physiology: Body Function

If anatomy provides a picture of the human body, physiology is a movie. In other words, anatomy describes the body at rest, but the living body is never at rest. The heart is beating, blood is moving through veins and arteries, sensory nerves are detecting changes in the environment, brain cells are interpreting input and returning instructions, the intestines are processing nutrients, and the kidneys are eliminating wastes. The study of the ways in which the body and its organ systems work is **physiology**.

Just as drugs can be described as affecting certain organs or organ systems, the actions of many agents are known to be specific to the physiologic processes of 1 or more organs. Because our knowledge of medical science is so much more complete than in the past (and rapidly increasing each year), medications have been developed that target cell defects and disrupted physiologic processes more specifically. These medicines then work more effectively and with fewer adverse effects than many older drugs.

Pathophysiology: When Something Is Wrong

When the body is working as it normally does, a state of **homeostasis** is said to exist. The body is able to perform all the functions expected of it; the organs and organ systems work in concert with each other; nutrients and oxygen are distributed to cells throughout the body; and wastes are processed and eliminated by the lungs, kidneys, and intestines.

When something disrupts this homeostasis, an abnormal state ensues—one we call **disease**. Some diseases cause or are the result of problems at the cell level, including adaptation, injury, growth, or death. This disruption may be caused by many different factors:

- Poisons or harmful substances that have entered the body
- Microorganisms such as bacteria, viruses, or fungi
- Lack of nutrients or oxygen
- Genetic abnormalities
- Aging of the body
- Unknown factors

Figure 1-15   Male and Female Reproductive Systems of the Human Body

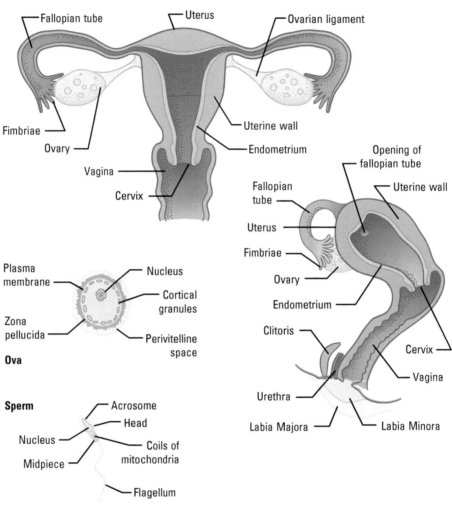

Female Reproductive System

Fallopian tube
Uterus
Ovarian ligament
Fimbriae
Ovary
Vagina
Cervix
Uterine wall
Endometrium

Opening of fallopian tube
Uterine wall
Fallopian tube
Uterus
Fimbriae
Ovary
Endometrium
Clitoris
Cervix
Vagina
Urethra
Labia Majora
Labia Minora

Plasma membrane
Nucleus
Cortical granules
Zona pellucida
Perivitelline space

Ova

Sperm
Acrosome
Head
Nucleus
Coils of mitochondria
Midpiece
Flagellum

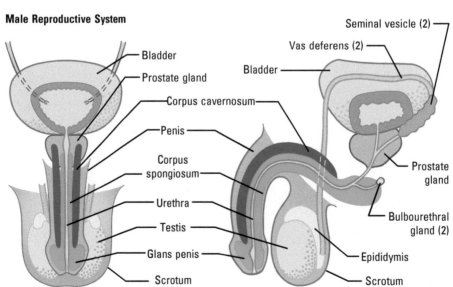

Male Reproductive System

Bladder
Prostate gland
Corpus cavernosum
Penis
Corpus spongiosum
Urethra
Testis
Glans penis
Scrotum

Seminal vesicle (2)
Vas deferens (2)
Bladder
Prostate gland
Bulbourethral gland (2)
Epididymis
Scrotum

The study of what goes wrong in diseases is called **pathophysiology**. By understanding the pathophysiology of diseases and knowing what drugs are available that affect those abnormal processes, you can readily understand which drugs are used for which diseases.

The physician or other prescriber will usually determine the patient's **diagnosis** before selecting the appropriate treatment. In making a diagnosis, the physician considers the patient and his or her race, age, sex, family and medical histories, and genetic makeup; how the patient feels; the results of the physical examination and laboratory tests; and therapies that have worked in other people with similar clinical presentations. With this knowledge, the physician can generally make a definitive diagnosis and outline a reasonable treatment plan that will provide the best chance of compensating for or correcting the disease.

Pharmacists do not usually make diagnoses, as their expertise lies more in knowing about treatments. However, patients routinely ask pharmacists for assistance with nonprescription medications and dietary supplements, all sold without a prescription, and this can involve determining what is causing the bothersome symptoms. As a pharmacy technician, it is important for you to work closely with the pharmacist in helping to answer patients' questions. Appropriately referring an inquiry about a treatment or nonprescription medication to the pharmacist helps to ensure that patients receive needed assessment and care.

Risk Factors for Disease

Simply put, **risk factors** are those characteristics unique to a given patient that increase his or her odds of having a particular disease. Examples of the relationships between disease and risk factors include the following:

- Hypertension, or high blood pressure, is more common among blacks than whites, and it tends to occur in families, indicating a **genetic predisposition**.
- Depression is more common among women than men, and depression and suicide are more likely to occur in a patient when 1 or more first-degree relatives (father, mother, brother, or sister) also have had depression or attempted or committed suicide.
- Diabetes is more common among blacks, Hispanics, American Indians, and Asian Americans. Sedentary lifestyles (not getting much exercise) increase the risk of type 2 diabetes.
- For many diseases, including type 2 diabetes and Alzheimer disease, older patients are at greater risk than are younger patients.

Thus, risk factors are an important part of the clinical evaluation of patients and provide valuable evidence for reaching a decision about diagnosis. In addition, patients should be aware of their own risk factors so that they can make appropriate adjustments in their lifestyle. For instance, improving diet, getting more exercise, and reducing or eliminating the use of tobacco and alcohol can decrease the risk of getting certain diseases.

An area of increasing importance to genetic risk factors in the early 21st century is gene therapy and pharmacogenomics. The Human Genome Project, an effort supported by the National Institutes of Health, has mapped the location of every human gene on the 23 chromosome pairs. Pharmaceutical companies are increasingly using this information to produce therapies targeted to patients based on their genetic makeup. Through genetic testing, people may be able to learn early in their lives which diseases are likely to cause them problems later in life and how they will respond to certain drugs. They can then use this information to reduce their risks of getting the disease or to improve their treatment options.

Some medications are more likely to cause serious side effects in patients with a certain genetic variant that alters the metabolism of that drug. If, before taking the medication, the patient undergoes genetic testing that reveals he or she possesses this variant, the dose of the medication can be altered or another drug chosen to avoid adverse effects. For example, if the patient has less CYP 450 enzymes than expected, then they might break down a drug more slowly than expected and therefore need a lower dose than normal. This is already taking place with some medications, particularly in the treatment of heart disease and some cancers.

Signs and Symptoms of Disease

In addition to risk factors, 2 other types of evidence help the clinician reach a diagnosis:

- **Subjective clues**, or how the patient describes the condition, referred to as **signs** of the disease.
- **Objective clues**, or what the physician or other health professionals find during physical examination and laboratory or other tests, called **symptoms** of the disease.

Working the clues through a diagnostic framework, the physician rules out various possibilities until 1 or more diseases remain. At times, physicians cannot determine for sure which disease is present and must try therapy for one of the possibilities empirically (without knowing for sure) to see whether the patient's condition improves. If it does, then that disease is assumed to be present. If it does not, therapy can then be tried for a second possibility, and so on, until the correct diagnosis is determined.

Epidemiology: Studying Large Numbers of People

Epidemiology provides valuable knowledge by analyzing populations of people, rather than just individuals. A good example of the application of epidemiology is when food poisoning occurs at a school or other large gathering of people. By combining information about which people with food poisoning ate which foods, the dish that caused the food poisoning can be identified. If each patient were analyzed individually, and the clues from one person were not applied to the next, investigators could never figure out which dish was the culprit.

Likewise, many important ideas about disease and pharmacotherapy have been identified based on epidemiology. Researchers have been able to figure out,

for example, which drugs cause which adverse effects, and that high cholesterol levels are associated with heart disease.

Pharmacotherapy: Treating Disease With Drugs

Several different options are available for treating most diseases:

- **Lifestyle modifications**—changing the patient's diet, exercise level, or physical surroundings (for example, removing a pet from a home if the patient is allergic to the pet).
- **Decreasing risk factors**—eliminating tobacco, alcohol, illicit drugs, or other modifiable factors.
- **Surgery**—performing medical interventions that eliminate the cause or correct a problem.
- **Pharmacotherapy**—treating with prescription or nonprescription medications or dietary supplements such as vitamins and minerals or herbal products.

Our focus in this chapter is on pharmacotherapy, especially treatment with prescription drugs. To understand what drugs do in the body, you must understand basic principles of pharmacokinetics and pharmacodynamics.

Pharmacokinetics: How Drugs Move Through the Body

Pharmacokinetics is the study of the movement of drugs through the body. Complicated mathematical models and equations are used by pharmacists to calculate doses of drugs. For some agents, the **therapeutic doses**, or doses that produce the desired effects in people, vary from person to person. Some medications may be **toxic** in some patients, even at doses that do not produce excessive effects in other people. The value of pharmacokinetics lies in the prevention of drug-related toxicity in patients by increasing the chances that the right dose will be used in each patient.

When a drug is placed into the human body, 4 processes describe its movement: **absorption**,

distribution, **metabolism**, and **excretion**. By understanding the processes for each drug, pharmacists and other health professionals are able to predict doses and blood levels of drugs using pharmacokinetic equations. Let's look at each of these areas.

Absorption

Absorption is the process through which the drug enters the blood. Whether injected into tissues, absorbed through the skin from a transdermal patch, inhaled into the nose or lungs, or taken by mouth, drugs must generally reach the blood to be transported to active sites, where they exert their therapeutic, adverse, and toxic effects. Only intravenous administration of drugs skips the process of absorption, because the drugs are injected directly into the blood. Even in this case, the drugs usually move from the blood into 1 or more cells or tissues to exert a therapeutic effect. This movement is explained more fully in the discussion of distribution.

To understand the process of absorption, suppose a 1-g dose is administered by mouth in the form of a tablet. It might break apart in the gastric fluids of the stomach and pass to the small intestine in little particles. This process is called disintegration. As the pH (hydrogen ion concentration) rises in the small intestine, the drug might move from the particles and into the gastrointestinal fluids in a process called dissolution (Figure 1-16). Once a drug dissolves in the gastrointestinal fluids, it is available to be absorbed through the wall of the intestine and into the blood.

Bioavailability is the term used to describe the ratio between the amount of drug that reaches the blood and the amount of drug placed into the body. A drug with high bioavailability means that most of the drug taken ends up getting into systemic circulation via the blood. A drug with low bioavailability means that a relatively small amount of the drug taken actually reaches systemic circulation via the blood. For instance, of the 1-g dose administered in the earlier example, only 0.9 g reaches the blood. This ratio, 0.9/1, represents the oral bioavailability of the drug. It is usually expressed as a decimal fraction (0.9) or percentage (90%).

As mentioned earlier in the digestive system section, absorbed materials from the gastrointestinal tract go directly to the liver so that the body can check them

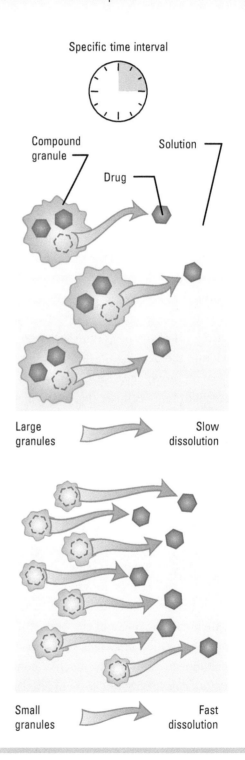

Figure 1-16 Dissolution: Making Drugs Available for Absorption

Specific time interval

Compound granule

Drug

Solution

Large granules — Slow dissolution

Small granules — Fast dissolution

for foreign or unwanted substances. The liver, the main metabolizing organ in the body, might detect this drug and convert some of it to inactive metabolites before it ever leaves the liver. Conversely, the liver might metabolize an inactive drug to an active drug. In this case, that drug is referred to as a prodrug.

Distribution

Distribution is the movement of the drug through the blood and into various cells or tissues where it exerts its effect. Again, pharmacokineticists have developed various models and equations that can be used to describe this movement mathematically. The models use the concept of "compartments" to reflect the amounts of drugs in various fluids, tissues, and organs. For instance, the drug concentration might be 3 mcg/mL in the blood compartment, 3 ng/mL in the brain compartment, and 30 mcg/g in a fat tissue compartment. The high amount of drug that has distributed into fat tissue in this example means the drug would likely stay in the body for a long time because fat tissue has no way of getting rid of the drug until it moves, or partitions, back into the blood.

The extent to which a drug distributes through various compartments is described mathematically as its volume of distribution. In the example of this drug that distributes into fat tissue, the drug would be said to have a large volume of distribution.

Metabolism

Metabolism describes the chemical changes made to the drug by the body. These changes are often made by the liver but can sometimes be made by the gastrointestinal tract wall, kidneys, lungs, or blood. As noted in the earlier discussion of bioavailability, the liver is the main metabolizing organ of the body. It has many special proteins, called enzymes, that can change—that is, metabolize—drugs into inactive compounds, or metabolites. These enzymes are contained in special structures of the liver, the CYP 450 system, which are depicted in Figure 1-13.

As mentioned under the preceding discussion of the liver, many drugs interact with one another because they both have effects on or are metabolized by specific enzymes in this system. These enzymes are categorized by their function and structure and given names such as CYP 1A2 and CYP 3A4.

Metabolism usually changes the drug from an active entity, capable of producing effects in the body, to an inactive chemical that has no effect on the body. Some drugs are metabolized into compounds that exert actions in the body (active metabolites). Other times, the body converts an inactive chemical, called a prodrug, into an active drug. Prodrugs are usually designed by pharmaceutical scientists to be absorbed or distributed better, and the body's metabolism apparatus is then used to convert the prodrug into the active drug after it has cleared this hurdle or barrier.

Excretion

Excretion or elimination is the process through which the drug or its metabolites leave the body, usually in the urine or feces, or sometimes through the lungs (Figure 1-17). Drugs can be excreted as either active drugs or inactive metabolites. Often, the changes made by the liver during metabolism convert the drug into a form that is easier for the kidneys or intestines to

Figure 1-17 Elimination of Medications

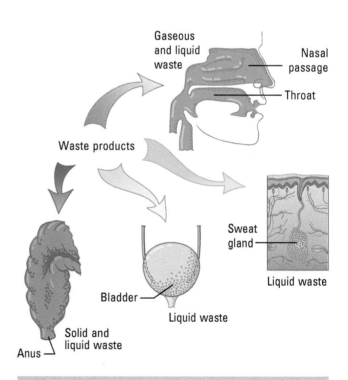

Gaseous and liquid waste

Nasal passage

Throat

Waste products

Sweat gland

Liquid waste

Bladder

Liquid waste

Solid and liquid waste

Anus

eliminate. The amount of drug excreted or metabolized to inactive compounds in a given organ or tissue over a certain amount of time is expressed mathematically as its clearance for that organ or tissue. The time it takes for the serum drug concentration to decline by one-half is called the drug's half-life.

Alcohol: The Perfect Example

An interesting example of absorption, distribution, metabolism, and excretion is alcohol, one of the most commonly used—and abused—drugs in our society. Alcohol, administered in the form of a liquid, is absorbed in the stomach and the first part of the small intestine, which is why people feel the effects of alcohol so quickly when it is consumed on an empty stomach. Once absorbed, alcohol moves through the blood and into the brain, where it acts as a CNS depressant. Basically, it slows down the transmission of impulses among the nerves in the brain. Alcohol does this in a dose-dependent fashion—the higher the alcohol concentration, the more effect it exerts on the brain.

Alcohol is metabolized in the liver, lungs, urine, and sweat to inactive compounds, including acetaldehyde. The amount of acetaldehyde and other metabolites produced is predictably proportional to the amount of alcohol in the blood, and a predictable amount of acetaldehyde is excreted through the lungs and into the breath (expired air). This relationship is the basis for the breath test used by police to estimate the blood alcohol concentrations in drivers of automobiles. So, as you can see, pharmacokinetics has practical applications, even outside medicine.

Pharmacodynamics: What Drugs Do in the Body

The previous section on pharmacokinetics focuses on the concentration of drug in the blood. But most drugs do not exert any effect on the blood, so in these cases, blood concentration is irrelevant. As a result, we need to also study pharmacodynamics—the relationship between serum or tissue drug levels and drug effects.

For most medications, a relationship between drug levels and therapeutic or toxic effects can be described mathematically using pharmacodynamics. For instance, higher concentrations of blood pressure drugs have more antihypertensive effects than do lower concentrations. In the alcohol example mentioned in the last section, the effects of alcohol can be related to the blood concentration. At low concentrations, about 50 mg/dL, a feeling of well-being (euphoria) is produced. As the blood alcohol rises to 100 mg/dL, impairment of motor functions (speech, reaction time, balance) begins, and this worsens to severe motor impairment as the concentration rises to 150 mg/dL. Between 150 mg/dL and 250 mg/dL, nausea and dysphoria replace the earlier euphoria, and consciousness is lost at about 300 mg/dL. If the person continues to drink before passing out, alcohol will continue to be absorbed from the gastrointestinal tract, and the blood alcohol level will keep rising. At about 400 mg/dL, the person will enter a coma, and if breathing stops, the person will die.

Strengths and Dosage Forms: How Drugs Are Administered

Drugs are commercially available in various strengths and dosage forms. The strength of a drug is the amount contained in a unit of the product, whether a tablet or a teaspoonful of a liquid (for example, diazepam 5-mg tablets or amoxicillin suspension 150 mg/5 mL). When preparing a prescription, you must be very careful to select the correct strength of the drug. Some drugs, such as digoxin and warfarin, have doses that can be therapeutic in one patient but toxic in another. Such medicines are said to have narrow therapeutic ranges or indexes. In the pharmacy, you may find that the various strengths of such drugs are placed on shelves away from each other. These drugs are separated to decrease the chances of someone accidentally picking up the wrong strength.

Many drugs also come in various dosage forms. Table 1-2 defines the most common dosage forms and provides considerations about the use of each. While giving a patient the wrong dosage form may not be as serious an error as the wrong drug or strength, it can still be problematic. For instance, an elderly patient may not be able to swallow tablets or capsules and therefore may require liquid preparations. Or a patient who is vomiting may require a rectal suppository rather than oral dosage forms. Be sure you have the correct dosage form—don't assume anything!

Table 1-2 Dosage Forms Commonly Used in Pharmaceutical Preparations

DOSAGE FORMS	DESCRIPTION	CONSIDERATIONS
Solid Dosage Forms		
Pills	Solid oral dosage forms that are made from a paste, rolled between the first finger and thumb, and then dried.	Common when pharmacists made pills in this manner in years past, but hardly any true pills are on the commercial market. Solid oral dosage forms are now tablets or capsules, and they should be referred to by these more correct names.
Tablets	Powders that are compressed with enough force that they stay together during shipping and handling but not enough force to prevent them from dissolving in the body.	May be swallowed, chewed and then swallowed, dissolved under the tongue or in the buccal pouch (the space in the mouth between the teeth and the cheek), or sometimes ground up for patients who cannot swallow the whole tablet. Dosage forms that contain timed-release, controlled-release, or delayed-release features should not be crushed (unless otherwise indicated on package labeling) as it disrupts these processes.
Capsules	Gelatin containers with loose powders or timed-release beads inside. These are easily made commercially or in the pharmacy when a prescription must be compounded.	Capsules are cheapest and easiest solid oral dosage form to make. They typically present no bioavailability problems since they dissolve easily in the fluids of the stomach and small intestine.
Liquid Dosage Forms		
Solutions	Liquids in which the drug is completely dissolved in the vehicle, making the product clear (but not necessarily colorless).	Because most drugs taste bitter, few oral solutions are used (suspensions mask the taste better). Rather, solutions are more often used for topical preparations, such as antibiotic solutions used for acne or sterile solutions that are used in the eyes.
Suspensions	A common liquid oral dosage form in which the drug is present in small particles in a flavored vehicle. Suspensions are never clear and must be shaken well to disperse the drug before a dose is measured.	Examples include liquid antibiotics used orally, anti-infective products used in the ears, and other agents prepared for pediatric or elderly patients, such as antipsychotic agents that can be given to those who will not or cannot swallow.
Syrups and elixirs	Also used to mask the bitter taste of medicines. Syrups are sweetened vehicles, whereas elixirs contain alcohol.	Examples include most cough syrups and elixirs such as phenobarbital.
Topical and Other Dosage Forms		
Creams and ointments	Semisolid preparations used to deliver drugs to the skin or mucous membranes (nose, vagina). Creams are water based and therefore easily washed off, while ointments are fat based and resistant to removal with water.	Examples include hydrocortisone cream and ointment. It should be noted that creams and ointments are not always interchangeable. In fact, when dealing with a prescription product, selection must be exactly what the prescriber intended.
Lotions (also called emulsions)	Lotions, or products used to soften or deliver drugs to the skin, are liquid preparations that contain 2 "phases." Similar to how drugs can be dissolved in a solution, a water phase can be dispersed in a fat (lipid) phase, or small lipid globules can be dispersed in a water phase.	Examples include Calamine lotion and the many lotions, such as Curel and Vaseline Intensive Care, that are used to rehydrate or soften the skin.

Table 1-2   (continued)

DOSAGE FORMS	DESCRIPTION	CONSIDERATIONS
Transdermal patches and subdermal inserts	Drugs can be delivered through the skin using patches that control the rate of drug administration and through the use of inserts that are surgically implanted under the skin.	Examples include Nitroderm patches and Implanon contraceptive inserts. A commonly asked question by patients regarding patches is whether or not they can be cut. Be careful not to advise the patient either way without consulting the pharmacist, as each patch has specific instructions for use that are specified in the product labeling.
Vaginal, Urethral, and Rectal Dosage Forms		
Suppositories	Dosage forms designed to remain solid at room or refrigerator temperature and to melt and release the drug when inserted into an orifice (or opening) of the body. The 2 most commonly used suppositories are inserted into the rectum or vagina, and a few suppositories are used in the urethra of men.	Numerous agents are formulated as rectal suppositories, including Phenergan, which is used when patients' nausea and vomiting are so severe that they cannot keep down the oral form of this drug. Vaginal suppositories include antifungal agents such as Monistat. Vaginal contraceptives are marketed as gels, foams, and jellies.
Injectable Dosage Forms		
Injectable solutions	Most injectable drugs are formulated as sterile solutions. Depending on the specific drug in the solution, these can be injected into arteries, veins, or tissues or can be used to make large-volume solutions that are then infused into the body through a vein, artery, or the peritoneal cavity (the space around the stomach, intestines, liver, and other nearby organs).	Because of the high concentrations of drugs in most injectable products, be extremely careful that you use the right drug and strength. Also, remember that some drugs cannot be given intravenously, while others cannot be injected into the muscle.
Injectable suspensions	A few injectable products are formulated as suspensions. These are always injected in muscle, where they are absorbed into the blood. Suspensions should never be injected into veins or arteries, since the particles in them can get stuck in the lungs and capillaries, causing serious injury or death.	Most injectable suspensions are antibiotics; these are absorbed from intramuscular injections fairly quickly. Other products, including antipsychotic agents, are made to be absorbed over a 3- or 4-week period. Since patients with schizophrenia and other psychoses are often afraid to take their medicines (they think the doctors are trying to kill them), these "depot" injections provide a way to give these patients their needed medications.
Injectable emulsions	When patients are unable to take food by mouth, they must be fed through the veins and arteries ("parenterally"). Lipid emulsions provide the fat that people normally get from their diets.	Examples include Liposyn, Intralipid, and Nutrilipid.

Commonly Used Drugs and Drug Categories

Table 1-3 (located at the end of this chapter) presents the basic facts about many of the drugs most commonly used in the United States. As you work in pharmacy, the generic and trade names of these agents will become very familiar to you. To speed this process along, you should memorize those drugs on this list that you encounter most often in your own workplace. Depending on the kind of pharmacy where you work, you may need to add other drugs to the list that are used frequently in your setting.

The column headings used in Table 1-3 and other commonly used terms deserve special mention, as detailed below.

Generic Name

The generic name is the name given to each drug by the United States Adopted Names (USAN) program, a joint project of the American Medical Association, the United States Pharmacopeial Convention, and American Pharmacists Association (APhA). Any company that markets this drug is required by the Food and Drug Administration (FDA) to place its generic name on the package label in at least half the size of the company's own brand name. Notice that related drugs have similar suffixes to their generic names. For instance, many lipid-lowering agents end in –*statin* (for example, lovastatin, pravastatin, simvastatin). This clue will help you remember which drugs are similar.

Brand Name

The brand name, also called the proprietary or trade name, is given to the product by the company that first created or marketed it. For instance, lovastatin is Mevacor, pravastatin is Pravachol, and simvastatin is Zocor. While some names relate to a fact about the drug (for instance, Premarin reflects the fact that the drug is obtained from *pre*gnant *mare*'s ur*ine*), many trade names are generated by marketing departments because people react well to them or relate to something about the drug name (for instance, the male drug for erectile dysfunction, Viagra, rhymes with Niagara, the waterfalls in upstate New York).

Dosage Forms

As discussed earlier and detailed in Table 1-2, drugs are marketed in various dosage forms according to the intended route of administration. Oral (by mouth) is the most familiar route of administration, but this method is impractical sometimes. For example, if the drug cannot be absorbed into the blood from the gastrointestinal tract or is immediately broken down after absorption (ie, insulin) or if a person is too sick to be able to swallow a drug, then another route of administration becomes necessary. "Injectable" means that the drug is intended for injection, which could mean into a muscle (intramuscular), vein (intravenous), skin (subcutaneous), or other tissue, so it is important to know precisely how and where the drug should be injected. Intranasal refers to nasal sprays that are typically, but not always, for local site of action in the nose itself. Topical administration implies that the drug is absorbed into the skin, and at least some of the dose may reach the circulation and produce systemic (whole-body) effects.

Common Uses

Drugs are officially approved for treatment or prevention of certain diseases by FDA. These uses are called the "approved indications" for that drug. However, once a drug is released into the US market, prescribers can use it for any indication they believe is medically appropriate. When such uses become widespread or confirmed in clinical studies, these uses of the drug are listed in pharmacy reference books as "unapproved indications" or commonly referred to as "off label."

Adverse Effects

Drugs have both good and bad effects on the body. The adverse effects are important considerations when choosing a drug. Adverse effects, sometimes called side effects, are drug actions that occur at normal doses of a drug (when the right amount of a drug has been given). The terms *toxicities* and *toxic effects* generally refer to those effects that are produced when too much of a drug is used. Listed in the adverse effects column of Table 1-3 are the common and serious adverse effects of medications. Common adverse effects are those

Table 1-3 Organ-Specific Listing of Commonly Used Medications

GENERIC NAME (BRAND NAME)	DOSAGE FORM	COMMON USES	COMMON/SEVERE ADVERSE EFFECTS	COMMENTS
CENTRAL NERVOUS SYSTEM (neurology and psychiatry)				
Antianxiety and Sleep Agents (anxiolytics and hypnotics)				
Benzodiazepines				
alprazolam (Xanax) (CS)	PO	Anxiety, panic disorder (attacks)	*Most common:* dizziness, sleepiness, delirium, N, V, D, C, HA, slow heart rate, slow breathing, confusion *Rare but serious:* blood problems	Prolonged use can lead to dependence and withdrawal syndrome when drugs are stopped.
clonazepam (Klonopin) (CS)	PO	Panic disorder, epilepsy		
diazepam (Valium) (CS)	PO, INJ	Anxiety, epilepsy, alcohol withdrawal		
lorazepam (Ativan) (CS)	PO, INJ	Anxiety, status epilepticus		
temazepam (Restoril) (CS)	PO	Insomnia		
Nonbenzodiazepines				
buspirone (BuSpar)	PO	Anxiety	Dizziness, drowsiness, N, HA, nervousness	Dependence is less likely than for benzodiazepines.
eszopiclone (Lunesta) (CS)	PO	Insomnia	Dry mouth, dizziness, hallucinations	
suvorexant (Belsomra) (CS)	PO	Insomnia	Drowsiness, HA	
zaleplon (Sonata) (CS)	PO	Insomnia	Memory loss	
zolpidem (Ambien, others) (CS)	PO, SL	Insomnia	Dizziness, lethargy	
Antidepressant Agents (for depression, also used in mania and bipolar disorder)				
Selective Serotonin Reuptake Inhibitors (SSRIs)				
citalopram (Celexa)	PO	Depression	Insomnia, N, tremor, nervousness, sweating, dry mouth, somnolence, weight loss	Discontinue therapy by gradually decreasing dose to avoid side effects. It can take 4-6 weeks to see beneficial effects.
escitalopram (Lexapro)	PO	Depression, anxiety		
fluoxetine (Prozac, others)	PO	Depression, OCD, panic disorder, bulimia		
paroxetine (Paxil, others)	PO	Depression, OCD, anxiety, panic disorder		
sertraline (Zoloft)	PO	Depression, OCD, panic disorder, anxiety		
Tricyclic Antidepressants				
amitriptyline (Elavil)	PO	Depression, pain of nerve origin (neuropathic pain)	AC, OH, sedation, confusion, weight gain, dizziness, heart problems	Dangerous in overdose.
doxepin (Sinequan)	PO	Depression, insomnia		
imipramine (Tofranil)	PO	Depression, childhood bedwetting		

(table continues on next page)

Table 1-3 (continued)

Generic Name (Brand Name)	Dosage Form	Common Uses	Common/Severe Adverse Effects	Comments
Other Antidepressants				
bupropion (Wellbutrin, others)	PO	Depression, smoking cessation	*Most common:* tremors, agitation, confusion, AC, dizziness *Rare but serious:* seizures	Zyban is trade name of smoking cessation product. This drug comes in many different time-release products that are not interchangeable; be very careful to select the right product.
desvenlafaxine (Pristiq, others)	PO	Depression	N, sedation, dizziness, anxiety, insomnia, anorexia, dry mouth	
duloxetine (Cymbalta)	PO	Depression, nerve pain, incontinence	Insomnia, somnolence, dizziness, N, C, dry mouth, anorexia	
trazodone (Desyrel, others)	PO	Depression, insomnia	*Most common:* drowsiness, dizziness, weight gain, blurred vision, OH *Rare but serious:* heart problems, painful erection	More commonly used for insomnia than depression due to sedation.
venlafaxine (Effexor, Effexor XR, others)	PO	Depression, anxiety	N, sedation, dizziness, anxiety, insomnia, anorexia, dry mouth	Do not abruptly discontinue.
Antipsychotic Agents (for schizophrenia and other psychotic disorders)				
aripiprazole (Abilify)	PO, INJ	Schizophrenia, bipolar mania	Sedation, weight gain	
chlorpromazine (Thorazine)	PO, INJ	Schizophrenia, bipolar disorder, vomiting	Sedation, EPS, AC, OH	
clozapine (Clozaril)	PO	Schizophrenia	*Most common:* sedation, dizziness, AC, heart problems, salivation *Rare but serious:* blood problems, seizures	Reserved for patients not responding to other therapy. Frequent blood tests are required.
haloperidol (Haldol)	PO, INJ	Schizophrenia, hyperactivity	*Most common:* EPS *Rare but serious:* heart problems	
olanzapine (Zyprexa, others)	PO, INJ	Schizophrenia, agitation, bipolar disorder	Sedation, AC, dizziness, weight gain	
quetiapine (Seroquel, Seroquel XR)	PO	Schizophrenia, bipolar mania	Sedation, OH, weight gain	

Table 1-3 (continued)

Generic Name (Brand Name)	Dosage Form	Common Uses	Common/Severe Adverse Effects	Comments
risperidone (Risperdal, others)	PO, INJ	Schizophrenia, bipolar mania	Agitation, AC, insomnia, nervousness, heart palpitations, weight gain	
ziprasidone (Geodon)	PO, INJ	Schizophrenia, bipolar mania, acute agitation	*Most common:* sedation, EPS, OH *Rare but serious:* heart problems	
Antiparkinsonian Agents (for Parkinson disease)				
benztropine (Cogentin)	PO, INJ	EPS induced by drugs for Parkinson disease	AC, heart problems	
levodopa/carbidopa (Sinemet, others)	PO	Parkinson disease	N, V, anorexia, OH, abnormal movements	Avoid abruptly discontinuing.
pramipexole (Mirapex, Mirapex ER)	PO	Parkinson disease, restless legs syndrome	OH, hallucinations, dizziness, sedation, N	
ropinirole (Requip, Requip XL)	PO	Parkinson disease, restless legs syndrome	OH, hallucinations, dizziness, sedation, N	
Drugs for Alzheimer Disease				
donepezil (Aricept)	PO	Alzheimer disease	*Most common:* N, V, D, anorexia, dizziness	Initiate therapy at low doses and slowly increase dose to lessen GI effects.
galantamine (Razadyne, Razadyne ER)	PO	Alzheimer disease	*Rare but serious:* slow heart rate, heart problems	
rivastigmine (Exelon)	PO, transdermal	Alzheimer disease		
memantine (Namenda, Namenda XR)	PO	Alzheimer disease	Dizziness, HA	
Centrally Acting Pain Medications (mostly narcotic analgesics)				
fentanyl (example: Duragesic) (CS)	Transdermal, SL, buccal, IV	Moderate to severe pain	*Most common:* C, N, hypokalemia, tolerance	Physical dependence and withdrawal can occur with all opiates (in the same drug class as heroin).
hydrocodone +/- acetaminophen (example: Norco, Vicodin, Zohydro ER) (CS)	PO	Analgesic (pain relief)	*Most common:* sedation, dizziness, N, C *Occurs with higher doses:* slowed breathing, slowed heart rate	
hydromorphone (example: Dilaudid) (CS)	PO, INJ, SUPP	Analgesic		
morphine (example: MS Contin) (CS)	PO, INJ, SUPP	Analgesic		

(table continues on next page)

Table 1-3 (continued)

Generic Name (Brand Name)	Dosage Form	Common Uses	Common/Severe Adverse Effects	Comments
oxycodone +/– acetaminophen (example: Percocet) (CS)	PO	Analgesic		
acetaminophen with codeine (example: Tylenol #3) (CS)	PO	Analgesic	N, C, allergic and skin reactions, drowsiness	
tramadol (Ultram, others) (CS)	PO	Analgesic	N, C, dizziness, sedation, restlessness	Not an opiate.
Opioid Reversal Agent				
naloxone (Narcan)	Nasal spray	For acute opioid overdose		Administer 1 spray into 1 nostril of the unconscious person, and call 911 immediately. May administer a second spray into the other nostril if the patient does not respond.
Opioid Dependence/Detoxification Medications				
buprenorphine (example: Subutex) (CS)	SL, INJ, transdermal, implant	Pain, opiate agonist dependence or withdrawal	C, HA, erythema, withdrawal, drowsiness	
buprenorphine with naloxone (example: Suboxone) (CS)	Oral dissolving film, SL	Opiate agonist dependence	C, anxiety, depression, abdominal pain, dependence, withdrawal	
Drugs for Migraines				
erenumab (Aimovig)	INJ	Migraine prophylaxis	Alopecia, constipation	
fremanezumab (Ajovy)	INJ		Injection site reaction	
galcanezumab (Emgality)	INJ	Cluster headache, migraine prophylaxis	Antibody formation, injection site reaction	
rizatriptan (Maxalt)	PO, ODT	Migraine	*Most common:* dizziness, flushing, tingling *Rare but serious:* heart attack	
sumatriptan (Imitrex, others)	PO, INJ, nasal spray	Migraine		
Antiepileptic Medications (to prevent seizures [also used for other purposes])				
carbamazepine (Tegretol, others)	PO	Epilepsy (seizures), nerve pain, mood disorder	*Most common:* N, drowsiness, dizziness *Rare but serious:* blood problems, liver problems, severe rash	Do not use in patients with histories of bone marrow suppression and related blood disorders.

Table 1-3 (continued)

GENERIC NAME (BRAND NAME)	DOSAGE FORM	COMMON USES	COMMON/SEVERE ADVERSE EFFECTS	COMMENTS
gabapentin (Neurontin, others)	PO	Adjuvant (add-on) therapy for seizures, nerve pain, restless legs syndrome	Sleepiness, dizziness, dry mouth, blurred vision	Commonly abused medication. Caution should be used if taken with other medication causing drowsiness.
lamotrigine (example: Lamictal)	PO, ODT	Partial seizures, tonic-clonic seizures, bipolar disorder, Lennox-Gastaut syndrome	Blurred vision, drowsiness, vomiting, abdominal pain	
levetiracetam (example: Keppra)	PO, ODT, INJ	Myoclonic seizures, partial seizures, tonic-clonic seizures	Drowsiness, fatigue, headache, irritability, vomiting	
oxcarbazepine (example: Trileptal)	PO	Partial seizures	Dizziness, drowsiness, fatigue, nausea, vomiting, visual impairment	
phenytoin (Dilantin)	PO, INJ	Epilepsy	*Most common but dose related:* nystagmus (eye deviations), abnormal movements, dizziness *Rare but serious:* severe rash; blood, liver, heart problems	Blood levels must be monitored to avoid toxicities. Do not interchange tablets and capsules or change brands without prescriber's knowledge.
pregabalin (Lyrica) (C)	PO	Seizures, nerve pain, fibromyalgia	Dizziness, somnolence, edema, dry mouth, blurred vision, weight gain	
topiramate (Topamax)	PO	Seizures, migraine prevention	Dizziness, drowsiness, balance issues, depression, anxiety, memory impairment *Rare but serious:* liver and blood problems	Can cause significant weight loss.
valproic acid (Depakote)	PO, INJ	Seizures, mania, migraine prevention	*Most common:* somnolence, dizziness, N, D, hair loss *Rare but serious:* liver, pancreas, and blood problems	Avoid in pregnancy.

(table continues on next page)

Table 1-3 (continued)

Generic Name (Brand Name)	Dosage Form	Common Uses	Common/Severe Adverse Effects	Comments
Drugs for Attention-Deficit/Hyperactivity Disorder (ADHD)				
amphetamine mixture (Adderall, others) (CS)	PO	ADHD	Decreased appetite, fast heart rate, restlessness, high blood pressure, insomnia	High abuse potential. May slow growth in children.
dexmethylphenidate (Focalin, Focalin XR) (CS)	PO	ADHD		
guanfacine (Tenex)	PO	ADHD		
lisdexamfetamine (Vyvanse) (CS)	PO	ADHD		
methylphenidate (Ritalin, Concerta, others) (CS)	PO	ADHD, narcolepsy		
atomoxetine (Strattera)	PO	ADHD	Decreased appetite, dizziness	May slow growth in children.
Antiemetics (to stop vomiting)				
granisetron (Kytril)	PO, INJ, TOP	N and V due to chemotherapy, radiation, surgery	HA, C	
metoclopramide (Reglan)	PO, INJ	N and V due to chemotherapy, diabetic gastroparesis	*Most common:* EPS, drowsiness, dizziness *Rare but serious:* neuroleptic malignant syndrome	
ondansetron (Zofran)	PO, INJ	N and V due to chemotherapy, radiation, surgery	Sedation, HA	
prochlorperazine (Compazine)	PO, INJ, SUPP	N, V	EPS, sedation	
promethazine (Phenergan)	PO, INJ, SUPP	N, V, motion sickness	Sedation, dizziness, abnormal movements	
EYE, EAR, NOSE, AND THROAT AGENTS (ophthalmology and otolaryngology)				
Antihistamines				
cetirizine (example: Zyrtec)	PO	Allergic rhinitis, chronic urticaria (hives)	Sedation	Available OTC.
desloratadine (Clarinex)	PO	Allergic rhinitis, chronic urticaria		
fexofenadine (Allegra)	PO	Allergic rhinitis, chronic urticaria		Available OTC.
loratadine (Claritin)	PO	Allergic rhinitis		Available OTC.

Table 1-3 (continued)

GENERIC NAME (BRAND NAME)	DOSAGE FORM	COMMON USES	COMMON/SEVERE ADVERSE EFFECTS	COMMENTS
Leukotriene Antagonist				
montelukast (Singulair)	PO	Asthma, allergic rhinitis	Indigestion	Can also be used for asthma.
Nasal Corticosteroids				
budesonide (example: Rhinocort)	Nasal spray	Allergic rhinitis	Sore throat, nosebleed, cough	Available OTC.
fluticasone (Flonase)	Nasal spray	Allergic rhinitis		
mometasone (Nasonex)	Nasal spray	Allergic rhinitis		
triamcinolone (Nasacort, Nasacort AQ)	Nasal spray	Allergic rhinitis		Available OTC.
Ophthalmics (for the eye)				
cyclosporine (Restasis)	Eye drop	Dry eyes	Eye irritation	
dorzolamide (Trusopt)	Eye drop	Elevated intraocular pressure (glaucoma)	Eye irritation, bitter taste	
ketotifen (example: Zaditor)	Eye drop	Allergic conjunctivitis, ocular pruritis	Headache, rhinitis	
latanoprost (Xalatan)	Eye drop	Elevated intraocular pressure (glaucoma)	Eye irritation, brown pigmentation of the iris	
timolol (Timoptic)	Eye drop	Elevated intraocular pressure	Eye redness, slow heart rate, low blood pressure	Can worsen existing breathing problems.
RESPIRATORY AGENTS (for the lungs and airways)				
Inhaled Corticosteroids				
budesonide (Rhinocort)	Oral inhalation	Asthma	Sore throat, nasal congestion, oral candidiasis (thrush, fungal infection of mouth)	
fluticasone (Flovent, others)	Oral inhalation	Asthma		
triamcinolone (Azmacort, others)	Oral inhalation	Asthma		
Beta-Agonists				
albuterol	PO, oral inhalation	Asthma	Fast heart rate, tremor, throat irritation	
salmeterol (Serevent, others)	Oral inhalation	Asthma, COPD		
formoterol (Foradil)	Oral inhalation	Asthma, COPD		

(table continues on next page)

Table 1-3   (continued)

GENERIC NAME (BRAND NAME)	DOSAGE FORM	COMMON USES	COMMON/SEVERE ADVERSE EFFECTS	COMMENTS
Muscarinic Antagonists				
ipratropium (Atrovent)	Oral inhalation, nasal spray	COPD (bronchitis, emphysema)	Cough, mouth/nose dryness, nervousness, nosebleed	
tiotropium (Spiriva)	Oral inhalation	COPD	Dry mouth	
GASTROENTEROLOGIC AGENTS (for the gastrointestinal tract, liver, and gallbladder)				
Histamine-2 Receptor Antagonists				
famotidine (Pepcid)	PO, INJ	PUD, GERD	HA, dizziness	Some strengths available OTC.
ranitidine (Zantac)	PO, INJ	PUD, GERD		
Proton Pump Inhibitors				
dexlansoprazole (Dexilant)	PO	PUD, GERD, esophagitis	HA, dizziness	
esomeprazole (Nexium)	PO, INJ	Erosive esophagitis, GERD, *Helicobacter pylori* infection		
lansoprazole (Prevacid)	PO, INJ	PUD, GERD, esophagitis, *H pylori* infection		
omeprazole (Prilosec)	PO	PUD, GERD, esophagitis		
pantoprazole (Protonix)	PO, INJ	Esophagitis, GERD		
rabeprazole (AcipHex)	PO	PUD, GERD, *H pylori* infection		
Monoclonal Antibodies (for immune-mediated GI and/or other disorders)				
adalimumab (Humira)	INJ	Crohn disease, rheumatoid arthritis, ulcerative colitis	*Most common:* rash, HA, SOB (infusion-related or injection site reactions) *Rare but serious:* rare infections, heart failure	Initial injection should be given by a health care professional.
infliximab (Remicade)	INJ	Crohn disease, ulcerative colitis, rheumatoid arthritis		Should be administered in a health care setting.
ENDOCRINOLOGIC AGENTS (for the pituitary, thyroid, and adrenal glands and the pancreas)				
Drugs for Diabetes (many also supplied as combination products)				
canagliflozin (Invokana)	PO	Diabetic nephropathy, reduction of cardiovascular mortality, type 2 diabetes	Candidiasis, diuresis, infection, vaginitis	
dapagliflozin (Farxiga)	PO	Type 2 diabetes, heart failure	Diuresis	

Table 1-3   (continued)

Generic Name (Brand Name)	Dosage Form	Common Uses	Common/Severe Adverse Effects	Comments
empagliflozin (Jardiance)	PO	Type 2 diabetes, reduction of cardiovascular mortality	Diuresis, hypoglycemia	
exenatide (Byetta, Bydureon)	SQ	Type 2 diabetes	*Most common:* N, V, D, feeling jittery, dizziness, HA, and dyspepsia *Rare but serious:* Not recommended in patients with severe GI disease, including gastroparesis, a complication of diabetes; pancreatic effects	Administered in the thigh, abdomen, or upper arm.
glimepiride (Amaryl)	PO	Type 2 diabetes	Low blood glucose, N, heartburn	
glipizide (Glucotrol)	PO	Type 2 diabetes		
glyburide (Diabeta)	PO	Type 2 diabetes		
insulin (example: Lantus, Novolog)	INJ	Type 1 and type 2 diabetes	Low blood glucose, injection-site reactions	Available in many different forms; some long acting, some short acting.
linagliptin (Tradjenta)	PO	Type 2 diabetes	Hypoglycemia, pharyngitis	
liraglutide (Victoza)	SQ	Type 2 diabetes	N, V *Rare but serious:* pancreatic effects	
metformin (Glucophage)	PO	Type 2 diabetes	*Most common:* D, N, V, flatulence (gas) *Rare but serious:* lactic acidosis	Avoid in patients with kidney disease or CHF.
pioglitazone (Actos)	PO	Type 2 diabetes	Edema (fluid retention)	Monitor liver function. Avoid in patients with moderate to severe CHF.
saxagliptin (Onglyza)	PO	Type 2 diabetes		
sitagliptin (Januvia)	PO	Type 2 diabetes		
Corticosteroids				
dexamethasone	PO, INJ	Anti-inflammatory agents; used in wide variety of conditions	*Most common:* insomnia, nervousness, increased appetite, indigestion *Rare but serious:* diabetes, cataracts, glaucoma, immunosuppression, PUD	Do not abruptly discontinue if taking high doses for prolonged period of time.
hydrocortisone	PO, INJ			
methylprednisolone	PO, INJ			
prednisone	PO			
triamcinolone	PO, INJ			

(table continues on next page)

Table 1-3 (continued)

GENERIC NAME (BRAND NAME)	DOSAGE FORM	COMMON USES	COMMON/SEVERE ADVERSE EFFECTS	COMMENTS
Estrogens and Progestins (sex hormones)				
conjugated estrogens (Premarin)	PO, INJ, vaginal	Menopausal symptoms	*Most common:* HA, dizziness, N, changes in vaginal bleeding patterns, fluid retention *Rare but serious:* blood clots (including heart attack and pulmonary embolism)	May increase risk for endometrial cancer in postmenopausal women.
estradiol (Estrace, Vivelle, Climara)	PO, INJ, TOP	Menopausal symptoms, atrophic vaginitis		
oral contraceptives (usually a combination of estrogen and progestin)	PO, TOP, vaginal	Birth control, emergency contraception (prevention of pregnancy after intercourse), menstrual problems		Smoking increases risk of cardiovascular side effects.
medroxyprogesterone (Provera)	PO	Menstrual and uterine problems	*Most common:* edema (swelling), breakthrough menstrual bleeding, changes in menstrual cycle (including no periods) *Rare but serious:* blood clots	
raloxifene (Evista)	PO	osteoporosis, breast cancer prevention	*Most common:* hot flashes, leg cramps *Rare but serious:* blood clots	
testosterone (example: AndroGel) (CS)	INJ, TOP	Delayed puberty, erectile dysfunction	Breast changes, libido changes, prostate abnormalities	
Other				
cinacalcet (Sensipar)	PO	High calcium levels, hyperparathyroidism	*Most common:* N, V, D, muscle pain, dizziness, increased blood pressure *Rare but serious:* seizures	
levothyroxine (example: Synthroid)	PO, INJ	Thyroid-replacement therapy	*Dose related (dose too high):* nervousness, fast heart rate, HA, insomnia, fever, weight loss, increased appetite, D	Do not change brands without prescriber's knowledge.

Table 1-3 (continued)

Generic Name (Brand Name)	Dosage Form	Common Uses	Common/Severe Adverse Effects	Comments
CARDIAC AGENTS (for the heart)				
Angiotensin-Converting Enzyme (ACE) Inhibitors				
benazepril (Lotensin)	PO	HTN	*Most common:* dizziness, cough	Avoid during second and third trimester of pregnancy. Monitor for hyperkalemia (high blood potassium levels).
enalapril (Vasotec)	PO, INJ	HTN, CHF		
fosinopril (Monopril)	PO	HTN, CHF, MI	*Rare but serious:* angioedema (severe allergic reaction causing throat swelling)	
		MI		
lisinopril (Zestril, Prinivil)	PO	HTN, CHF, acute		
quinapril (Accupril)	PO	HTN, CHF		
ramipril (Altace)	PO	HTN, CHF, prevention of cardiovascular disease in high-risk patients		
Angiotensin Receptor Blockers (ARBs)				
irbesartan (Avapro)	PO	HTN, kidney disease in diabetic patients	Cough (less common than with ACE inhibitors)	Avoid during second and third trimester of pregnancy. Monitor for hyperkalemia (high blood potassium levels).
losartan (Cozaar)	PO	HTN, kidney disease in diabetic patients, stroke prevention		
olmesartan (Benicar)	PO	HTN		
valsartan (Diovan)	PO	HTN, CHF		
Calcium Channel Blockers				
amlodipine (Norvasc)	PO	HTN, angina	*Most common:* peripheral edema (swelling of feet, ankles), low blood pressure, dizziness, C	
diltiazem (Cardizem)	PO, INJ	HTN, AF, angina, PSVT		
felodipine (Plendil)	PO	HTN	*Rare but serious:* heart problems (especially with verapamil)	
verapamil (Calan)	PO, INJ	Angina, HTN, PSVT, AF		
Other				
amiodarone (Cordarone, Pacerone)	PO, INJ	Arrhythmias (abnormal heart rhythms)	*Most common:* malaise, tremor, N, V, C, visual problems, slow heart rate, sensitivity to sun *Rare but serious:* lung problems, arrhythmias, liver problems, eye problems, thyroid problems	

(table continues on next page)

Table 1-3 (continued)

Generic Name (Brand Name)	Dosage Form	Common Uses	Common/Severe Adverse Effects	Comments
digoxin (Lanoxin)	PO, INJ	CHF, AF	*Dose related (dose too high):* anorexia, N, V, drowsiness, slow heart rate, confusion, visual changes	Drug concentrations in the blood should be monitored to avoid toxicity.
sacubitril; valsartan (Entresto)	PO	CHF, reduction of cardiovascular mortality and heart failure hospitalizations	Hyperkalemia, hypotension	
VASCULAR AGENTS (for the blood vessels)				
Beta-Blockers				
atenolol (Tenormin)	PO, INJ	HTN, angina, acute MI	Slow heart rate, dizziness, fatigue, wheezing	
metoprolol (example: Lopressor, Toprol)	PO, INJ	HTN, angina, MI, CHF		
nebivolol (Bystolic)	PO	HTN		
propranolol (Inderal)	PO, INJ	HTN, angina, migraine HA		
Other Antiadrenergic Agents				
carvedilol (Coreg)	PO	HTN, CHF	*Most common:* OH, D, dizziness, slow heart rate *Rare but serious:* liver problems	
labetalol (Trandate, Normodyne)	PO, INJ	HTN	*Most common:* dizziness, N, OH *Rare but serious:* liver problems	
Vasodilators				
isosorbide mononitrate (example: Imdur, Monoket)	PO	Angina	HA, dizziness, OH	
nitroglycerin (Nitrostat, Nitro-Dur, Transderm Nitro)	PO, INJ, TOP	Angina	OH, HA, flushing, dizziness, weakness	Sublingual tablets are placed under the tongue.
Antihyperlipidemic Agents (to lower cholesterol)				
atorvastatin (Lipitor)	PO	Hyperlipidemias, heart attack prevention	*Most common:* flatulence (gas) *Mild:* dyspepsia *Rare but serious:* muscle problems, liver problems	Contraindicated during pregnancy. Patient should avoid drinking grapefruit juice. Promptly report any muscle pain/weakness.
gemfibrozil (Lopid)	PO	Hypertriglyceridemia		
lovastatin (Mevacor)	PO	Hyperlipidemias, heart attack prevention		

Table 1-3   (continued)

Generic Name (Brand Name)	Dosage Form	Common Uses	Common/Severe Adverse Effects	Comments
pravastatin (Pravachol)	PO	Hyperlipidemias, heart attack prevention		
rosuvastatin (Crestor)	PO	Hyperlipidemias, heart attack and stroke prevention		
simvastatin (Zocor)	PO	Hyperlipidemias, heart attack and stroke prevention		
ezetimibe (Zetia)	PO	Hyperlipidemias	*Rare:* D	
fenofibrate (TriCor, others)	PO	Hyperlipidemias	*Most common:* N, C *Rare but serious:* liver problems, gallbladder problems (gallstones)	
niacin (Niaspan)	PO	Hyperlipidemias, heart attack prevention	Flushing, N, V, abdominal pain, D, liver effects, increased blood glucose	
Anticoagulant and Antiplatelet Agents (prevent blood clots)				
abciximab (ReoPro)	INJ	Acute MI		Bleeding is the major risk with all anticoagulant and antiplatelet agents. It can occur from any body site and range from mild to severe. It is usually dose related. The effects of the drug in blood should be monitored for abciximab, eptifibatide, heparin, tirofiban, and warfarin.
apixaban (Eliquis)	PO	AF, stroke prevention		
aspirin	PO	Prevention of stroke, MI		
clopidogrel (Plavix)	PO	Recent MI or stroke		
dalteparin (Fragmin)	INJ	Acute MI, prevention of DVT		
dabigatran (Pradaxa)	PO	AF, stroke prevention		
enoxaparin (Lovenox)	INJ	DVT, PE, acute MI		
eptifibatide (Integrilin)	INJ	Acute MI		
heparin	INJ	DVT, PE		
rivaroxaban (Xarelto)	PO	AF, DVT, PE, stroke prevention		
tenecteplase (TNKase)	INJ	Acute MI ("clot buster")		
tinzaparin (Innohep)	INJ	DVT		
tirofiban (Aggrastat)	INJ	Acute MI		
warfarin (Coumadin)	PO	Prevention and treatment of DVT, PE; AF		Avoid warfarin during pregnancy. Interactions are very common; caution should be exercised.

(table continues on next page)

Table 1-3 (continued)

Generic Name (Brand Name)	Dosage Form	Common Uses	Common/Severe Adverse Effects	Comments
RENAL AGENTS (work in the kidneys)				
bumetanide (Bumex)	PO, INJ	Edema, heart failure, nephrotic syndrome	Azotemia, hyperuricemia, hypochloremia, hypokalemia, polyuria	
chlorthalidone (Thalitone)	PO	HTN, edema, CHF	*Most common:* electrolyte (sodium, potassium, chloride) imbalance, OH, sun sensitivity	Should be taken in the morning to prevent nighttime urination.
furosemide (Lasix)	PO, INJ	HTN, edema, CHF	*Most common:* electrolyte (sodium, potassium, chloride) imbalance, OH, sun sensitivity *Rare but serious:* hearing loss	
hydrochlorothiazide (multiple combination products)	PO	HTN, edema	OH, low blood potassium, sun sensitivity	Often abbreviated HCTZ.
torsemide (Demadex)	PO, INJ	CHF, HTN, edema	*Most common:* electrolyte (sodium, potassium, chloride) imbalance, OH, sun sensitivity *Rare but serious:* hearing loss	
triamterene/HCTZ (Maxzide, Dyazide)	PO	Edema, HTN, CHF	Electrolyte imbalances, sun sensitivity	
GENITOURINARY AGENTS				
dutasteride (Avodart)	PO	Benign prostatic hyperplasia	Decreased libido	Do not use in women or children. Pregnant women should not even handle the drug.
finasteride (Proscar)	PO	Benign prostatic hyperplasia, male pattern baldness		
darifenacin (Enablex)	PO	Urinary incontinence	AC, C, hypertension (mirabegron)	
mirabegron (Myrbetriq)	PO			
oxybutynin (Ditropan)	PO, TOP			Topical patch available OTC.
solifenacin (Vesicare)	PO			
tamsulosin (Flomax)	PO			
tolterodine (Detrol)	PO			
trospium (Sanctura)	PO			

Table 1-3 (continued)

GENERIC NAME (BRAND NAME)	DOSAGE FORM	COMMON USES	COMMON/SEVERE ADVERSE EFFECTS	COMMENTS
sildenafil (Viagra)	PO	Erectile dysfunction (tadalafil also used for benign prostatic hypertrophy)	*Most common:* HA, flushing, dyspepsia (upset stomach), visual changes *Rare but serious:* heart problems (including death) in men who already have cardiac disease	
tadalafil (Cialis)	PO			
vardenafil (Levitra)	PO			

BONE AND JOINT AGENTS (including pain drugs that act peripherally)

Nonsteroidal Anti-Inflammatory Drugs (NSAIDs)

diclofenac (example: Voltaren)	PO, transdermal, eye drop, INJ, topical gel	Pain, fever, inflammation (arthritis)	Dyspepsia, edema, N, anemia	Available OTC. These NSAID agents can raise blood pressure, so caution should be used if advising on an OTC product.
ibuprofen (example: Motrin)	PO			
indomethacin (Indocin)	PO, INJ			
meloxicam (Mobic)	PO			
naproxen (Naprosyn)	PO			Available OTC.

COX-2 Inhibitors

celecoxib (Celebrex)	PO	Pain, inflammation (arthritis)	*Most common:* abdominal pain, prolonged bleeding time *Rare but serious:* cardiovascular events, kidney problems	The COX-2 inhibitors are regarded as less damaging to the GI tract than the NSAIDs, but they have been associated with cardiovascular adverse events, including MI.

Other Analgesics

acetaminophen (Tylenol)	PO, SUPP, INJ	Pain, fever	*Rare but serious:* liver problems (especially in overdose)	

Musculoskeletal Agents (Muscle Relaxants)

baclofen (Lioresal)	PO, INJ	Muscle spasm, spasticity	N, dizziness, drowsiness, hypotonia	
carisoprodol (Soma) (CS)	PO		Drowsiness, xerostomia	
cyclobenzaprine (Flexeril)	PO		AC, drowsiness, dizziness	
metaxalone (Skelaxin)	PO			
methocarbamol (Robaxin)	PO			

(table continues on next page)

Table 1-3 (continued)

Generic Name (Brand Name)	Dosage Form	Common Uses	Common/Severe Adverse Effects	Comments
Monoclonal Antibodies for Immune-Mediated Arthritis (see also Gastroenterologic Agents)				
etanercept (Enbrel)	INJ	Rheumatoid arthritis	*Most common:* rash, HA, SOB (infusion-related or injection site reactions) *Rare but serious:* rare infections, liver effects, heart failure	
Drugs for Osteoporosis				
alendronate (Fosamax)	PO	Osteoporosis	Esophageal irritation (prevent by taking with full glass of water and not lying down after taking)	May be dosed weekly or monthly.
denosumab (Prolia)	INJ	Osteoporosis	Bone pain, shortness of breath, hypocalcemia, hypophosphatemia	
ibandronate (Boniva)	PO	Osteoporosis	Esophageal irritation (prevent by taking with full glass of water and not lying down after taking)	
risedronate (Actonel)	PO	Osteoporosis		
Drugs for Gout				
allopurinol (Zyloprim)	PO	Gout	*Most common:* rash (stop drug—can become severe) *Rare but serious:* liver problems, severe rash, kidney problems	
colchicine (Colcrys)	PO	Gout	*Most common:* N, V, D *Rare but serious:* blood problems	
febuxostat (Uloric)	PO	Gout, gouty arthritis, hyperuricemia	Worsening gout symptoms, N, joint pain	

Table 1-3 (continued)

Generic Name (Brand Name)	Dosage Form	Common Uses	Common/Severe Adverse Effects	Comments
ANTI-INFECTIVE AGENTS (for bacterial and fungal infections)				
Penicillins				
amoxicillin (Amoxil)	PO	Infections of ear, nose, throat, skin, lungs, urinary tract	Allergic reactions, D	**Applicable to all antibiotics:** Antibiotic choice is determined by the infecting microorganism—if unknown, then the most likely infecting organism(s) is targeted. Organisms can develop resistance to antibiotics, requiring the use of different antibiotics. Antibiotics are ineffective against viral infections.
amoxicillin/clavulanic acid (Augmentin)	PO			
piperacillin/ tazobactam (Zosyn)	INJ	Intra-abdominal infections, pneumonia		
ticarcillin/clavulanic acid (Timentin)	INJ	Intra-abdominal infections, pneumonia		
Cephalosporins				
cefaclor (Ceclor)	PO	Otitis media (ear infection), UTI, bronchitis	Allergic reactions, D (including a severe form called pseudomembranous colitis)	
cephalexin (Keflex)	PO	Otitis media, UTI		
cefazolin (Ancef)	INJ	Surgical prophylaxis, pneumonia, UTI		
cefprozil (Cefzil)	PO	Otitis media, sinusitis		
cefuroxime (Ceftin, Zinacef)	PO, INJ	Otitis media, UTI		
cefotetan (Cefotan)	INJ	Intra-abdominal infections		
cefpodoxime (Vantin)	PO	Pneumonia, gonorrhea		
cefixime (Suprax)	PO	UTI, otitis media		
cefoperazone (Cefobid)	INJ	Pneumonia, intra-abdominal infections		
cefotaxime (Claforan)	INJ	Pneumonia, intra-abdominal infections		
ceftazidime (Fortaz)	INJ	Pneumonia		
ceftriaxone (Rocephin)	INJ	Pneumonia, gonorrhea, meningitis		
cefepime (Maxipime)	INJ	Pneumonia		
loracarbef (Lorabid)	PO	Otitis media, pneumonia, UTI		

(table continues on next page)

Table 1-3   (continued)

GENERIC NAME (BRAND NAME)	DOSAGE FORM	COMMON USES	COMMON/SEVERE ADVERSE EFFECTS	COMMENTS
Macrolides and Ketolides				
azithromycin (Zithromax)	PO, INJ	Pneumonia, sinusitis	*Most common:* N, D, abdominal pain (worse with erythromycin) *Rare but serious:* liver problems, heart problems, pseudomembranous colitis	
clarithromycin (Biaxin)	PO	Pneumonia, sinusitis, *H pylori* infections		
erythromycin	PO, INJ	Upper respiratory tract infection, pneumonia		
telithromycin (Ketek)	PO	Sinusitis, pneumonia	*Most common:* N, D, visual problems *Rare but serious:* pseudomembranous colitis, heart problems, liver problems	
Quinolones				
ciprofloxacin (Cipro)	PO, INJ	Pneumonia, UTI	*Most common:* sun sensitivity *Rare but serious:* tendon rupture, heart problems, pseudomembranous colitis	Patient should watch for tendon weakness/rupture. Promptly report any tendon weakness to the pharmacist as soon as possible.
gemifloxacin (Factive)	PO, INJ	Pneumonia		
levofloxacin (Levaquin)	PO, INJ	Pneumonia, UTI		
moxifloxacin (Avelox)	PO, INJ	Pneumonia, sinusitis		
Other Antibiotics				
aztreonam (Azactam, Cayston)	PO, INJ	UTI, sepsis (blood infection)	Rash, N, D	
clindamycin (Cleocin)	PO, INJ	Intra-abdominal infections	D (can be severe; severe diarrhea should be reported to the pharmacist immediately)	
doxycycline	PO	Acne, various bacterial infections	Influenza, Jarisch-Herxheimer reaction	
gentamicin	INJ	Sepsis, UTI	*Rare but serious:* kidney problems, ear problems	Blood levels should be monitored.
imipenem/cilastatin (Primaxin)	INJ	Intra-abdominal infections, foot infections in diabetics	*Rare but serious:* seizures, pseudomembranous colitis	

Table 1-3 (continued)

Generic Name (Brand Name)	Dosage Form	Common Uses	Common/Severe Adverse Effects	Comments
metronidazole (Flagyl)	PO, INJ, TOP	Intra-abdominal infections, foot infections in diabetics	*Most common:* N, D, metallic taste *Rare but serious:* seizures	Avoid alcohol while taking and for 3 additional days after the last dose.
tigecycline (Tygacil)	INJ	Intra-abdominal infections, skin infections	*Most common:* N, V *Rare but serious:* permanent tooth discoloration in infants, children	Avoid in children <8 years old and during pregnancy.
tobramycin (Nebcin)	INJ	Sepsis, pneumonia	*Rare but serious:* kidney problems, ear problems	Blood levels should be monitored.
trimethoprim/ sulfamethoxazole (Bactrim, Septra)	PO, INJ	UTI	N, V, anorexia, allergic reactions	This has a sulfa component, so if a patient reports a sulfa allergy, this is one of the drugs they cannot take.
vancomycin (Vancocin)	PO, INJ	Infections due to methicillin-resistant *Staphylococcus aureus*	*Most common:* infusion-related reactions *Rare but serious:* kidney problems, ear problems, blood problems	Blood levels should be monitored. Oral form of drug is only for treatment of pseudomembranous colitis.
Antifungal Agents				
amphotericin B	INJ	Severe systemic fungal infections	*Most common:* infusion reactions (fever, chills, N, V, HA) *Rare but serious:* kidney problems (less risk with lipid formulations)	Pretreatment with antihistamines, acetaminophen, and corticosteroids helps lessen infusion reactions.
fluconazole (Diflucan)	PO, INJ	Candidiasis, severe fungal infections	*Most common:* HA, N *Rare but serious:* liver damage, severe rash	
itraconazole (Sporanox)	PO, INJ	Severe fungal infections, toenail infections	*Most common:* N *Rare but serious:* CHF, liver damage	Avoid in patients with CHF.
ketoconazole (Nizoral)	PO	Severe fungal infections	*Most common:* N, V *Rare but serious:* liver damage	This commonly causes medication interactions; caution should be taken.
terbinafine (Lamisil)	PO	Severe fungal toenail infections	*Most common:* rash, D *Rare but serious:* liver damage	

(table continues on next page)

Table 1-3 (continued)

Generic Name (Brand Name)	Dosage Form	Common Uses	Common/Severe Adverse Effects	Comments
		ANTIVIRAL AGENTS		
Antiretroviral Agents (for HIV infection)				
Protease Inhibitors				
atazanavir (Reyataz)	PO	HIV (in combination with the nucleoside and nonnucleoside reverse transcriptase inhibitors)	*Most common:* N, sun sensitivity *Rare but serious:* heart rhythm problems, liver problems	All protease inhibitors (PIs) can cause high blood glucose, including diabetes, and redistribution of body fat (buffalo hump), sometimes with cholesterol abnormalities. There are many drug interactions. Many PIs should be stored in the refrigerator.
indinavir (Crixivan)	PO		*Most common:* N *Rare but serious:* kidney stones, liver problems, blood problems	
nelfinavir (Viracept)	PO		D	
ritonavir (Norvir)	PO		*Most common:* N, V, D, anorexia, abdominal pain *Rare but serious:* pancreas and liver problems	
saquinavir (Fortovase)	PO		Indigestion	
telaprevir (Incivek)	PO		*Most common:* N, V, D, anorexia, abdominal pain *Rare but serious:* skin reactions, blood problems	
tenofovir (Viread)	PO		*Most common:* N, V, D, anorexia, muscle pain *Rare but serious:* liver effects	
Nucleoside and Nonnucleoside Reverse Transcriptase Inhibitors				
didanosine (Videx)	PO	HIV	*Most common:* D, abdominal pain *Rare but serious:* pancreatitis, liver problems, lactic acidosis (buildup of lactic acid), peripheral neuropathy (pain, weakness, numbness in hands and feet)	Abbreviated as ddI.

Table 1-3 (continued)

Generic Name (Brand Name)	Dosage Form	Common Uses	Common/Severe Adverse Effects	Comments
efavirenz (Sustiva)	PO		Impaired concentration, drowsiness, nightmares, insomnia, depression, anxiety, skin effects, liver effects, N, V, D, blood problems	
emtricitabine (Emtriva)	PO		*Most common:* skin effects, N, V, D, muscle pain, depression, dizziness, cough *Rare but serious:* liver or kidney problems	
lamivudine (Epivir)	PO		*Rare but serious:* liver problems, lactic acidosis	Abbreviated as 3TC.
stavudine (Zerit)	PO		*Most common:* peripheral neuropathy (dose related) *Rare but serious:* liver problems, lactic acidosis	Abbreviated as d4T.
tenofovir (Viread)	PO		N, V, depression, back pain, D, HA, insomnia	
zalcitabine (Hivid)	PO		*Most common:* peripheral neuropathy *Rare but serious:* liver problems, lactic acidosis, pancreatitis	Abbreviated as ddC.
zidovudine (Retrovir)	PO, INJ		*Most common:* N, V, fatigue *Rare but serious:* blood problems, liver problems, lactic acidosis	Abbreviated as AZT.
Integrase Inhibitors				
raltegravir (Isentress)	PO	HIV	*Most common:* D, N, stomach pain, insomnia, depression, heartburn, HA	
elvitegravir (Vitekta)	PO		D, N, HA	
dolutegravir (Tivicay)	PO		HA, insomnia	

(table continues on next page)

Table 1-3 (continued)

Generic Name (Brand Name)	Dosage Form	Common Uses	Common/Severe Adverse Effects	Comments
Other Antiviral Agents				
acyclovir (Zovirax)	PO, INJ	Herpes, chickenpox	*Most common:* N, D *Rare but serious:* kidney problems	
famciclovir (Famvir)	PO			
ganciclovir (Cytovene)	PO, INJ			
valacyclovir (Valtrex)	PO			
amantadine (Symmetrel)	PO	Influenza A, Parkinson disease	*Most common:* dizziness, insomnia, N, edema *Rare but serious:* suicide	Dangerous in overdose.
baloxavir marboxil (Xofluza)	PO	Influenza A, B	N, D, HA, respiratory symptoms	
oseltamivir (Tamiflu)	PO	Influenza A and B	N, V	
ribavirin (Rebetol, Copegus)	PO, aerosol	Hepatitis C (with interferon alfa), RSV in infants	*Most common:* anxiety, depression, fatigue *Rare but serious:* blood and heart problems, suicide	Contraindicated in pregnancy.
zanamivir (Relenza)	Inhalation	Influenza A and B	Breathing problems	
ONCOLYTIC AGENTS (for cancers, both solid tumors and blood cancers)				
Alkylating Agents and Platinum Compounds				
busulfan (Myleran)	PO, INJ	Leukemia	*Most common:* N, V, D, stomatitis, myelosuppression *Rare but serious:* seizures, lung problems, liver problems	Myelosuppression is a reduction in blood cell components (reduction in red blood cells is anemia; white blood cells is leukopenia/ neutropenia; platelets is thrombocytopenia). This renders the patient susceptible to infections and bleeding. The development of myelosuppression limits the dose that can be used for many chemotherapy agents. Correct dosing of chemotherapy is absolutely essential to avoid life-threatening toxicity and death.
carboplatin (Paraplatin)	INJ	Ovarian cancer	*Most common:* N, V, myelosuppression *Rare but serious:* severe allergic reactions	
chlorambucil (Leukeran)	PO	Leukemia, lymphomas	*Most common:* myelosuppression *Rare but serious:* seizures, cancer	
cisplatin (Platinol)	INJ	Testicular, ovarian, and bladder cancers	*Most common:* N, V, myelosuppression *Rare but serious:* kidney problems, hearing problems, severe allergic reactions, peripheral neuropathy	

Table 1-3 (continued)

Generic Name (Brand Name)	Dosage Form	Common Uses	Common/Severe Adverse Effects	Comments
cyclophosphamide (Cytoxan)	PO, INJ	Lymphomas, leukemia, breast and ovarian cancers	*Most common:* N, V, stomatitis, hair loss, hemorrhagic cystitis (bladder bleeding), leukopenia *Rare but serious:* heart damage, cancer	
ifosfamide (Ifex)	INJ	Testicular cancer	*Most common:* N, V, myelosuppression, hair loss, hemorrhagic cystitis *Rare but serious:* coma	Use with mesna to lessen hemorrhagic cystitis.
melphalan (Alkeran)	PO, INJ	Multiple myeloma, ovarian cancer	*Most common:* N, V, D, hair loss, myelosuppression *Rare but serious:* severe allergic reactions, cancer	
oxaliplatin (Eloxatin)	INJ	Colon and rectal cancers	*Most common:* N, V, D, neuropathy *Rare but serious:* severe allergic reactions, myelosuppression	
Antimetabolites				
capecitabine (Xeloda)	PO	Breast and colorectal cancers	*Most common:* D, N, V, stomatitis, myelosuppression *Rare but serious:* heart problems, painful swelling of hands and feet	
cytarabine (Cytosar-U)	INJ	Leukemia	*Most common:* N, V, D, myelosuppression, fever, muscle pain *Rare but serious:* liver problems	Abbreviated as ARA-C.
5-fluorouracil (Adrucil)	INJ	Colon, rectal, breast, stomach, and pancreatic cancers	*Most common:* N, V, stomatitis, myelosuppression *Rare but serious:* angina, visual problems	Abbreviated as 5-FU.
gemcitabine (Gemzar)	INJ	Pancreatic and lung cancers	Myelosuppression, fever, rash	

(table continues on next page)

Table 1-3 (continued)

Generic Name (Brand Name)	Dosage Form	Common Uses	Common/Severe Adverse Effects	Comments
hydroxyurea (Hydrea)	PO	Melanoma, leukemia	*Most common:* myelosuppression, stomatitis *Rare but serious:* kidney problems	
mercaptopurine (Purinethol)	PO	Leukemia	*Most common:* myelosuppression *Rare but serious:* liver problems	
methotrexate	PO, INJ	Breast and lung cancers, leukemia, rheumatoid arthritis, psoriasis	*Most common:* stomatitis, leukopenia, N, malaise *Rare but serious:* myelosuppression; liver, lung, and heart problems; severe skin reaction	
pemetrexed (Alimta)	INJ	Lung cancer, mesothelioma	*Most common:* N, V, D, weight loss, stomatitis, fatigue, rash, hypersensitivity *Rare but serious:* blood effects, skin reactions	
Antimitotic Agents				
docetaxel (Taxotere)	INJ	Breast and lung cancers	*Most common:* myelosuppression, rash, N, V, edema, hair loss *Rare but serious:* severe fluid retention	Use corticosteroids to lessen fluid retention.
paclitaxel (Taxol)	INJ	Ovarian, breast, and lung cancers	*Most common:* myelosuppression, peripheral neuropathy, N, V, D *Rare but serious:* severe allergic reactions, heart problems	
vinblastine (Velban)	INJ	Lymphoma	*Most common:* leukopenia, hair loss, N, V *Rare but serious:* breathing problems	Intrathecal administration (around the spine) is usually fatal.
vincristine (Oncovin)	INJ	Leukemia, lymphoma	*Most common:* hair loss, C, peripheral neuropathy *Rare but serious:* nerve damage, breathing problems	

Table 1-3 (continued)

Generic Name (Brand Name)	Dosage Form	Common Uses	Common/Severe Adverse Effects	Comments
vinorelbine (Navelbine)	INJ	Lung cancer	*Most common:* myelosuppression, fatigue, C, N *Rare but serious:* lung problems	

Topoisomerase Inhibitors

Generic Name (Brand Name)	Dosage Form	Common Uses	Common/Severe Adverse Effects	Comments
etoposide (VePesid)	PO, INJ	Testicular and lung cancers	*Most common:* myelosuppression, N, V *Rare but serious:* severe allergic reactions	Abbreviated as VP-16.
irinotecan (Camptosar)	INJ	Colon and rectal cancers	D (can be severe), N, V, myelosuppression, hair loss	
topotecan (Hycamtin)	INJ	Ovarian and lung cancers	Myelosuppression, hair loss, N, V, D, C	

Antibiotics (used as chemotherapy)

Generic Name (Brand Name)	Dosage Form	Common Uses	Common/Severe Adverse Effects	Comments
bleomycin (Blenoxane)	INJ	Lymphoma, head/neck and testicular cancers, pleural effusion (fluid in lungs)	*Most common:* hair loss, rash, itching, stomatitis, fever, chills, N, V *Rare but serious:* lung damage	
daunorubicin (Cerubidine)	INJ	Leukemia	*Most common:* myelosuppression, hair loss, N, V, red-colored urine *Rare but serious:* heart damage (related to total dose)	
doxorubicin (Adriamycin)	INJ	Leukemia; breast, ovarian, bladder, and thyroid cancers; lymphoma	*Most common:* myelosuppression, N, V, stomatitis, red-colored urine, hair loss *Rare but serious:* heart damage (related to total dose)	
epirubicin (Ellence)	INJ	Breast cancer	*Most common:* hair loss, myelosuppression, N, V, stomatitis, red-colored urine, cessation of menstrual cycles *Rare but serious:* heart damage (related to total dose), leukemia	

(table continues on next page)

Table 1-3 (continued)

Generic Name (Brand Name)	Dosage Form	Common Uses	Common/Severe Adverse Effects	Comments
idarubicin (Idamycin)	INJ	Leukemia	*Most common:* N, V, D, myelosuppression, hair loss, stomatitis *Rare but serious:* heart damage	
mitoxantrone (Novantrone)	INJ	Prostate cancer, leukemia, multiple sclerosis	*Most common:* myelosuppression, N, V, menstrual changes, hair loss, blue-green–colored urine *Rare but serious:* heart damage (related to total dose), leukemia	
Hormones (used as chemotherapy)				
anastrozole (Arimidex)	PO	Breast cancer	Weight gain, flushing	
bicalutamide (Casodex)	PO	Prostate cancer	*Most common:* hot flushes, breast enlargement/pain in men, C *Rare but serious:* liver problems	
exemestane (Aromasin)	PO	Breast cancer	Fatigue, hot flashes, N	
letrozole (Femara)	PO	Breast cancer	Bone pain, hot flashes, N, back pain	
leuprolide (Lupron)	INJ, implant	Prostate cancer, endometriosis	Hot flushes, cessation of menstruation	
megestrol (Megace)	PO	Breast and endometrial cancers	*Most common:* weight gain *Rare but serious:* blood clots	
tamoxifen (Nolvadex)	PO	Breast cancer	*Most common:* hot flushes *Rare but serious:* blood clots, uterine cancer, eye problems	
Monoclonal Antibodies				
alemtuzumab (Campath)	INJ	Leukemia	*Most common:* fever, chills, myelosuppression, N, V *Rare but serious:* severe infusion reactions	

Table 1-3 (continued)

GENERIC NAME (BRAND NAME)	DOSAGE FORM	COMMON USES	COMMON/SEVERE ADVERSE EFFECTS	COMMENTS
bevacizumab (Avastin)	INJ	Colon and rectal cancers	*Most common:* nose bleeds, abdominal pain, anorexia, high blood pressure, C, D *Rare but serious:* GI perforation, severe bleeding, CHF	
cetuximab (Erbitux)	INJ	Colorectal cancer	*Most common:* rash, sun sensitivity, N, D, C *Rare but serious:* severe infusion reactions, lung problems	
denosumab (Xgeva)	INJ	Bone metastases, osteoporosis, bone cancer	*Most common:* N, shortness of breath, dizziness, infection *Rare but serious:* jaw osteonecrosis, secondary cancers, pancreatitis	
gefitinib (Iressa)	PO	Lung cancer	*Most common:* D, rash, acne, N *Rare but serious:* lung problems	
gemtuzumab ozogamicin (Mylotarg)	INJ	Leukemia	*Most common:* myelosuppression, N, V, D, fever *Rare but serious:* severe allergic/infusion reactions, liver problems	
imatinib (Gleevec)	PO	Leukemia	*Most common:* edema (fluid retention), D, N, V, myelosuppression, muscle cramps, sun sensitivity *Rare but serious:* severe rash, liver problems	
pembrolizumab (Keytruda)	INJ	Certain types of lung cancer	Tiredness, edema, N, V, insomnia	
rituximab (Rituxan)	INJ	Lymphoma	*Most common:* N, night sweats, fever, chills, leukopenia *Rare but serious:* fatal infusion reactions, kidney problems, severe rash, heart problems	

(table continues on next page)

Table 1-3   (continued)

GENERIC NAME (BRAND NAME)	DOSAGE FORM	COMMON USES	COMMON/SEVERE ADVERSE EFFECTS	COMMENTS
trastuzumab (Herceptin)	INJ	Breast cancer	*Most common:* D, N, fever, chills *Rare but serious:* CHF, severe infusion reactions	
Kinase Inhibitors				
erlotinib (Tarceva)	PO	Lung and pancreatic cancers	*Most common:* N, V, D, anorexia, mouth ulcers, stomach pain, constipation *Rare but serious:* eye effects, lung toxicity, liver and kidney effects	Taking with food increases side effects.
sorafenib (Nexavar)	PO	Liver and kidney cancers	*Most common:* hand-foot syndrome, rash, increased blood pressure, hair loss *Rare but serious:* CHF, heart and blood effects	
sunitinib (Sutent)	PO	GI, kidney, and pancreatic cancers	*Most common:* N, V, D, abdominal pain, constipation, mouth ulcers *Rare but serious:* arrhythmias, heart events, bleeding or clotting, liver effects	Must be ordered through a specialty pharmacy.
Hematopoietic Agents (to treat myelosuppression caused by chemotherapy)				
darbepoetin alfa (Aranesp)	INJ	Anemia	*Most common:* elevated blood pressure *Rare but serious:* death, heart attack, blood clots, stroke	Must be dispensed through the ESA APPRISE Oncology Program.
epoetin alfa (Epogen)	INJ	Anemia		
filgrastim (Neupogen)	INJ	Neutropenia	*Rare but serious:* severe allergic reactions	Abbreviated as G-CSF.
pegfilgrastim (Neulasta)	INJ			
DERMATOLOGIC AGENTS (for the skin)				
Anti-Infective Agents (antibiotic, antifungal, and antiviral drugs)				
acyclovir (Zovirax)	TOP	Herpes genitalis, cold sores	Burning, stinging	
clotrimazole (Lotrimin)	TOP	Athlete's foot, jock itch, other mild fungal infections	Redness, stinging	Some forms available OTC.

Table 1-3   (continued)

GENERIC NAME (BRAND NAME)	DOSAGE FORM	COMMON USES	COMMON/SEVERE ADVERSE EFFECTS	COMMENTS
mupirocin (Bactroban)	TOP	Impetigo, bacterial infections	Burning, stinging	
polymyxin B/neomycin/ bacitracin (Neosporin)	TOP	To prevent bacterial infection after minor injury	Allergic reaction	Available OTC.
terbinafine (Lamisil)	TOP	Athlete's foot, jock itch, other fungal infections	Irritation, burning	Some forms available OTC.
tolnaftate (Tinactin)	TOP	Athlete's foot, jock itch, other mild fungal infections	Irritation	Available OTC.
Topical Corticosteroids				
betamethasone (Diprolene, Valisone)	TOP	Inflammation and itching	Burning, irritation	
hydrocortisone (Hytone)	TOP			Some forms available OTC.
triamcinolone (Kenalog)	TOP			
Other Dermatologic Agents				
capsaicin (Zostrix)	TOP	Pain (for conditions such as arthritis and shingles)	Significant burning	Available OTC.
isotretinoin (Accutane)	PO	Severe acne	*Most common:* dry skin, dry eyes *Rare but serious:* depression, visual problems	Contraindicated in pregnancy; dispensing restrictions.
minoxidil (Rogaine)	TOP	Hair growth in men	*Most common:* local irritation *Rare but serious:* fast heart rate, dizziness, blood pressure changes	Available OTC.
pimecrolimus (Elidel)	TOP	Dermatitis	burning	
NUTRITIONAL AGENTS (vitamins, nutritional aids, and supplements)				
calcium	PO, INJ	Hypocalcemia (osteoporosis)	*Most common:* C *Rare but serious:* hypercalcemia, heart problems (IV administration)	
iron	PO, INJ	Iron-deficiency anemia	*Most common:* N *Rare but serious:* iron overload, severe allergic reactions (IV or IM administration)	Overdose dangerous for young children.

(table continues on next page)

Table 1-3 (continued)

Generic Name (Brand Name)	Dosage Form	Common Uses	Common/Severe Adverse Effects	Comments
potassium supplements (K-Dur, others)	PO, INJ	Hypokalemia (potassium deficiency)	*Most common:* D, N *Rare but serious:* hyperkalemia	IV administration can be dangerous and requires heart monitoring.
vitamin D	PO	Nutritional supplementation, rickets, vitamin D deficiency		Also called cholecalciferol.

Abbreviations Used:

AC = anticholinergic side effects (dry mouth, blurred vision, and urinary retention)

AF = atrial fibrillation

C = constipation

CS = controlled substance

CHF = congestive heart failure

COPD = chronic obstructive pulmonary disease

DVT = deep venous thrombosis (blood clot in leg)

D = diarrhea

EPS = extrapyramidal symptoms (dyskinesia [abnormal involuntary movements, also called tardive dyskinesia], dystonias [muscle spasms], akathisia [feeling of a need to move around], akinesia [decreased motor activity], and pseudoparkinsonism [drug-induced effects that resemble Parkinson disease, including decreased motor activity, tremor and pill-rolling motion, cogwheel rigidity in which patients' limbs jerk when moved, and postural problems])

GERD = gastroesophageal reflux disease

GI = gastrointestinal

HA = headache

HIV = human immunodeficiency virus

HTN = hypertension (high blood pressure)

IM = intramuscular

INJ = injection (could be intravenous, intramuscular, subcutaneous)

IV = intravenous

MI = myocardial infarction (heart attack)

N = nausea

OCD = obsessive-compulsive disorder

ODT = orally disintegrating tablet

OH = orthostatic hypotension (low blood pressure upon standing up, especially from a lying position, causing the person to feel dizzy or fall)

OTC = over the counter (nonprescription)

PE = pulmonary embolism (blood clot in lung)

PO = oral

PSVT = paroxysmal supraventricular tachycardia

PUD = peptic ulcer disease (can be in the stomach [gastric] or first part of the small intestine [duodenal])

RSV = respiratory syncytial virus

SL = sublingual

SOB = shortness of breath

SQ = subcutaneous

SUPP = suppository

TOP = topical (example: cream, ointment, patch)

UTI = urinary tract infection

V = vomiting

that many patients will encounter, and pharmacists typically warn patients about these problems and what to do if they occur. Serious adverse effects, which usually occur rarely, are the problems that prescribers and pharmacists watch for during medication therapy.

Contraindications/Precautions
Because of their effects on multiple organs or organ systems in the body, certain drugs either cannot be used or must be used with caution in patients with more than 1 disease. For instance, some of the drugs found in nonprescription cough and cold products—decongestants—can raise blood pressure and affect blood glucose levels. Therefore, the contraindications for decongestants include patients with diseases of blood pressure or blood glucose, and they should not be used by patients with hypertension or diabetes before discussion with their doctor.

Another common contraindication is patient **allergy** to a drug. When patients allergic to one drug tend to react to other similar drugs (such as the penicillins), the drugs are said to exhibit **cross sensitivities**. Sometimes drugs can be used in patients with certain diseases, but only with caution. These warnings are listed as **precautions** to use of a drug. A common type of precaution is the use of the drug in special patient populations, including women who are or may become pregnant, newborn babies (neonates), children, the elderly, and those with diseases of the liver (affecting metabolism) or kidneys (affecting excretion).

Storage Considerations

All drugs will degrade or be changed into other substances when exposed to oxygen and/or water, even the amounts present in the air. The rate at which drugs degrade is a function of their chemical structure and the conditions under which they are stored. Because colder temperatures slow these degradation processes, some drugs must be frozen (below 0°C or 32°F) or stored in the refrigerator (2°C-8°C, or 36°F-46°F). Other agents can be stored at room temperature (15°C-30°C, or 59°F-86°F) but must be protected from extreme temperatures (high and freezing temperatures). It can be very important that patients store drugs properly so as to prevent degradation and to ensure that the drug is fully potent when taken. Technicians can play a valuable role in patient care by noting storage requirements and promoting safe medication use. For example, if a patient mentions that a drug appears to have changed shades of color, it could be a sign that the medication was kept in a hot car for too long or another inappropriate place. Being aware of the importance of storage conditions can make a big difference in a patient's therapy.

Drug Interactions

Medications sometimes "interact" with each other, and as a result, the anticipated effect of the drug does not occur or adverse reactions are produced. There are many causes of drug interactions, and some drugs are more likely to cause interactions than other drugs. An interaction can occur when one drug prevents the absorption of another. For example, many antacids should not be taken with quinolone antibiotics because the elements in the antacids can bind the quinolone and prevent its absorption, resulting in lack of antibiotic effect.

Most drug interactions involve interference with or changes in drug metabolism in the liver. Recall that the liver metabolizes many drugs by the CYP 450 enzymes, including CYP 3A4 and CYP 2C9. These isoenzymes can be affected by certain drugs to speed up (induce) or slow down (inhibit) the actions of other drugs. For example, erythromycin is a known inhibitor of CYP 3A4. Carbamazepine, an antiseizure or antiepileptic medication, is metabolized by this pathway. If these drugs are taken together, erythromycin can be expected to slow the metabolism of carbamazepine and thereby increase the blood levels of carbamazepine and possibly cause symptoms of toxicity.

Food and herbal remedies can also interact with drugs. It is the duty of the pharmacist, with the aid of the technician, to screen for and minimize drug interactions.

While computer systems used in pharmacies today help to catch drug interactions, professional judgment often comes into play. For example, if the interaction is not anticipated to cause a clinically significant problem and the prescribed drug is really needed for the patient, the pharmacist may decide to proceed with dispensing.

Conclusion

An understanding of diseases and the medications that are used to treat them is an essential component of pharmacy practice. Continue to refer to the information in this chapter as you learn and grow on your path to becoming a successful pharmacy technician.

REFERENCES

1. Seeley RR, Stephens TD, Tate P. *Essentials of Anatomy and Physiology*. 3rd ed. St. Louis, MO: Mosby-Year Book, Inc; 1999:Table 2-1.
2. Tortora GJ, Derrickson B. *Principles of Anatomy & Physiology*. 13th ed. New York, NY: John Wiley & Sons; 2011.

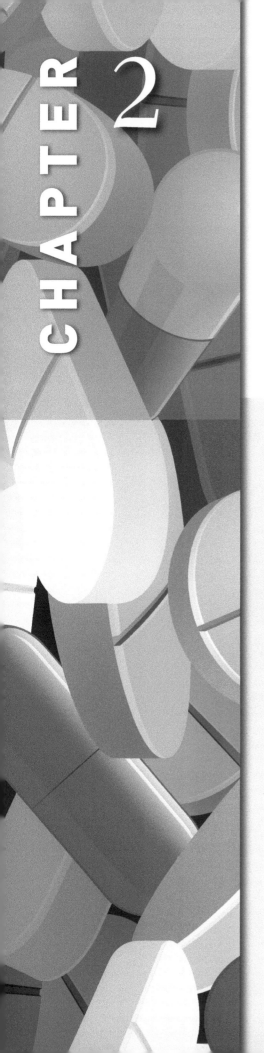

Pharmacy Calculations, Abbreviations, and Terminology

Chapter 2 presents information in 3 key areas of
knowledge. First, it presents calculations as a mixture
of straightforward explanations and practical problems.
Next, it presents abbreviations, primarily in a table, with
a brief explanation of their Latin origins. Then it presents
commonly used medical terminology in a list form, again
with a brief description of word origins and roots.

Pharmacy Calculations

Calculations are an integral part of pharmacy practice. From calculating prices to determining a patient-specific dose, pharmacists and technicians use arithmetic and simple algebra many times every day.

You can solve virtually every common problem in pharmacy by using the mathematical technique known as ratio and proportion. By thinking through what you know and what you are trying to figure out, ratio and proportion will enable you to determine the answer by simply cross multiplying and then dividing. Let's look at this technique and then consider some practical applications.

Ratio and Proportion

When using the ratio and proportion method, start by setting up 2 common fractions, one showing what you know and the other containing the value that you are trying to calculate. Be sure to keep the units of measurement (eg, milligram [mg]) that are above and below each line consistent. For instance, suppose you want to know how many milligrams are in 0.5 g. As shown in Table 2-1, you can see that 1 g is equivalent to 1000 mg. Using this information, the following ratios can be set up:

$$\frac{1000 \text{ mg}}{1 \text{ g}} = \frac{?}{0.5 \text{ g}}$$

This can be read as, "1000 mg is to 1 g as the unknown quantity is to 0.5 g."

By cross-multiplying the top of each fraction (the numerators) by the bottom of the other fraction (the denominators), you get the following equation:

$$\frac{1000 \text{ mg}}{1 \text{ g}} \diagdown\!\!\!= \frac{?}{0.5 \text{ g}}$$
$$? \times 1 \text{ g} = 1000 \text{ mg} \times 0.5 \text{ g}$$

Now move all the numbers to the right side of the equation and leave only the ? on the left. You can do this by dividing both sides by 1 g and canceling common units. The calculations on the right then provide your answer:

$$? = \frac{1000 \text{ mg} \times 0.5 \text{ g}}{1 \text{ g}}$$
$$? = 1000 \text{ mg} \times 0.5$$
$$? = 500 \text{ mg}$$

Table 2-1	Metric Measures: Prefixes and Units of Weight, Length, and Volume

PREFIXES

kilo = 1000 times (abbreviated k)

deci = $\dfrac{1 \text{ times}}{10}$ (0.1; abbreviated d)

centi = $\dfrac{1 \text{ times}}{100}$ (0.01; abbreviated c)

milli = $\dfrac{1 \text{ times}}{1000}$ (0.001; abbreviated m)

micro = $\dfrac{1 \text{ times}}{1,000,000}$ (0.000001; abbreviated mc or μ)

WEIGHT (ALSO REFERRED TO AS MASS)

Basic unit: gram (g)
Units commonly encountered:
    milligrams (mg), as in 1 g = 1000 mg
    micrograms (mcg or μg), as in 1 mcg = 0.001 mg
    kilogram (kg), as in 1 kg = 1000 g

LENGTH

Basic unit: meter (m)
Units commonly encountered:
    centimeters (cm), as in 100 cm = 1 m
    millimeters (mm), as in 1 cm = 10 mm = 0.01 m

VOLUME

Basic unit: liter (L)
Units commonly encountered:
    milliliter (mL), as in 1 L = 1000 mL
    deciliter (dL), as in 100 mL = 1 dL = 0.1 L

You can quickly solve problems by converting most calculations into this format. Just remember—always set up 2 proportions, one showing the information you're given or what you know and the other putting the question mark in the appropriate place, depending on the information you're looking for.

Units of Measure and Common Equivalents

A common type of calculation in pharmacy is converting between metric measurements (see Table 2-1) and common equivalents that you typically encounter in the United States, such as pounds, inches, or quarts. The common system is also called the avoirdupois (pronounced AV-WA-DU-PWA) system, and it uses the units shown in Table 2-2.

Pharmacy uses a third set of measurements referred to as the apothecary system, which you may see occasionally in practice (Table 2-3). In the apothecary system, remember that the grains are the same as grains in the avoirdupois system, but the ounces and pounds are different. The 3 drugs for which the apothecary system continues to be used most often are aspirin (a 325-mg aspirin tablet contains 5 grains of this drug), thyroid products, and phenobarbital. Table 2-4 shows the mathematical relationships among the metric, apothecary, and avoirdupois systems.

These various units and systems give us a good chance to try using ratio and proportion to solve simple problems. Here are examples of questions you may encounter and problems you can use to test yourself. The answers to those problems not solved for you are shown at the end of this chapter.

1. **How many inches are in 4 feet?**

$$\frac{12 \text{ in}}{1 \text{ ft}} = \frac{?}{4 \text{ ft}}$$

$? \times 1 \text{ ft} = 12 \text{ in} \times 4 \text{ ft}$

$? = \dfrac{12 \text{ in} \times 4 \text{ ft}}{1 \text{ ft}}$

$? = 12 \text{ in} \times 4$

$? = 48 \text{ in}$

> You can quickly solve problems by converting most calculations into the ratio and proportion format.

2. **How many milligrams are in 4 grams?**

$$\frac{1000 \text{ mg}}{1 \text{ g}} = \frac{?}{4 \text{ g}}$$

$? \times 1 \text{ g} = 1000 \text{ mg} \times 4 \text{ g}$

$? = \dfrac{1000 \text{ mg} \times 4 \text{ g}}{1 \text{ g}}$

$? = 1000 \text{ mg} \times 4$

$? = 4000 \text{ mg}$

3. **How many milligrams are in 5 grains?**

$$\frac{65 \text{ mg}}{1 \text{ gr}} = \frac{?}{5 \text{ gr}}$$

$? \times 1 \text{ gr} = 65 \text{ mg} \times 5 \text{ gr}$

$? = \dfrac{65 \text{ mg} \times 5 \text{ gr}}{1 \text{ gr}}$

$? = 65 \text{ mg} \times 5$

$? = 325 \text{ mg}$

Note: As mentioned earlier in this chapter, a 5-grain aspirin tablet contains 325 mg. This is also the weight of a regular-dose acetaminophen (Tylenol) tablet or capsule.

Table 2-2	Avoirdupois Units of Weight, Length, and Volume

WEIGHT	LENGTH	VOLUME
Basic unit: ounce (oz)	Basic unit: inch (in)	Basic unit: ounce
Units commonly encountered:	*Units commonly encountered:*	*Units commonly encountered:*
1 oz = 437.5 grains (gr)	12 in = 1 foot (ft)	8 oz = 1 cup
1 pound (lb) = 16 oz = 7000 gr	3 ft = 1 yard (yd)	2 cups = 1 pint (pt)
		2 pt = 1 quart (qt)
		4 qt = 1 gallon (gal)

Table 2-3   Apothecary Units of Weight and Volume[a]

WEIGHT

Basic unit: grain (gr)
Units commonly encountered:

     20 gr = 1 scruple (∋)
     3 scruples = 1 dram (ʒ)
     8 drams = 1 oz (℥)
     12 oz = 1 pound (lb)

VOLUME

Basic unit: minim (♏)
Units commonly encountered:

     60 minims = 1 fluid dram
     8 fluid drams = 1 fluid oz
     16 fluid oz = 1 pt
     2 pt = 1 qt
     4 qt = 1 gal

[a]The Pharmacy Technician Certification Board examination does not test on knowledge of this system.

4. **How many kilograms does a 154-pound person weigh?**

$$\frac{1 \text{ kg}}{2.2 \text{ lb}} = \frac{?}{154 \text{ lb}}$$

$$? \times 2.2 \text{ lb} = 1 \text{ kg} \times 154 \text{ lb}$$

$$? = \frac{1 \text{ kg} \times 154 \text{ lb}}{2.2 \text{ lb}}$$

$$? = \frac{154 \text{ kg}}{2.2}$$

$$? = 70 \text{ kg}$$

Did you know? Most pharmacokinetic calculations—those used by pharmacists to calculate drug dosages—are based on a 70-kg person. The equations are adjusted for the patient's actual body mass as part of the calculation.

Table 2-4   Metric, Apothecary,[a] and Avoirdupois Conversions

LENGTH

1 m = 39.4 in
1 in = 2.54 cm

VOLUME

1 fluid oz (f℥) = 30 mL
1 pt = 473 mL
1 gal = 3785 mL

WEIGHT

1 kg = 2.2 lb avoirdupois
1 lb avoirdupois = 454 g
1 oz avoirdupois (℥) = 28.4 g
1 oz apothecary = 31 g
1 g = 15.4 grains (gr)
1 gr = 65 mg

[a]The Pharmacy Technician Certification Board examination does not test on knowledge of the apothecary system or conversions to and from it.

5. **How many milliliters are in 1 quart?**

Tip: First convert the quart unit to ounces; then solve for milliliters!

1 qt = 2 pt = 32 oz

$$\frac{30 \text{ mL}}{1 \text{ oz}} = \frac{?}{32 \text{ oz}}$$

$$? \times 1 \text{ oz} = 30 \text{ mL} \times 32 \text{ oz}$$

$$? = \frac{30 \text{ mL} \times 32 \text{ oz}}{1 \text{ oz}}$$

$$? = 30 \text{ mL} \times 32$$

$$? = 960 \text{ mL}$$

Now you complete some problems!

6. **How many grams are in 3 kilograms?**

$$\frac{1000 \text{ g}}{1 \text{ kg}} = \frac{?}{3 \text{ kg}}$$

7. **How many milliliters are in 5 deciliters?**

$$\frac{100 \text{ mL}}{1 \text{ dL}} = \frac{?}{5 \text{ dL}}$$

8. **How many inches are in 5 meters?**

$$\frac{39.4 \text{ in}}{1 \text{ m}} = \frac{?}{5 \text{ m}}$$

9. **If a patient weighs 22.4 kilograms, how many pounds is that?**

$$\frac{1 \text{ kg}}{2.2 \text{ lb}} = \frac{22.4 \text{ kg}}{?}$$

A new way to diet: Just give your weight in kilograms!

10. **How many avoirdupois ounces are in 1 kilogram?**

Tip: Use the 1 oz (avoirdupois) = 28.4 g conversion, but convert grams to kilograms by dividing by 1000.

For example: $\left(\dfrac{28.4}{1000} = 0.0284 \text{ kg} \right)$

$$\frac{1 \text{ oz}}{0.0284 \text{ kg}} = \frac{?}{1 \text{ kg}}$$

$$? \times 0.0284 \text{ kg} = 1 \text{ oz} \times 1 \text{ kg}$$

$$? = \frac{1 \text{ oz} \times 1 \text{ kg}}{0.0284 \text{ kg}}$$

$$? = \frac{1}{0.0284 \text{ oz}}$$

11. How many centimeters are in 6 inches?

12. How many milliliters are in 15 liters?

13. If an extra-strength tablet of Tylenol contains 500 mg of acetaminophen, how many grams are in 100 tablets? How many grams are in 1 tablet?

    Hint: For the first part of this problem, the proportion would be $\dfrac{500\ mg}{1\ tablet} = \dfrac{?}{100\ tablets}$.

    After you get an answer in milligrams, convert it to grams.

14. If a solution has 10 mg of drug per milliliter, how much drug is in 10 mL?

    $Hint: \dfrac{10\ mg}{1\ mL} = \dfrac{?}{10\ mL}$

Percentage Calculations

While most medications are commercially available in ready-to-dispense form, pharmacists and pharmacy technicians sometimes make prescriptions from other ingredients through a process called compounding. This process will be described in more detail in Chapters 9 and 10.

Percentage calculations come into play during compounding when one substance (usually the drug) is dissolved or incorporated into a larger amount of a second substance. This is most often a solution in which a drug powder is dissolved in water or some other vehicle. The percentage then refers to the amount of drug (the solute) that is dispersed in the vehicle (the solvent). An example would be a solution of salt, or sodium chloride, dissolved in water.

Many of these products are prepared for injection into the veins and may contain very powerful drugs. Because there is little room for error in these or any other pharmaceutical calculation, you need to be completely certain of the accuracy of your work. Always double- or triple-check your calculations or ask someone else to confirm them.

Fortunately, percentage calculations can be solved using the same ratio and proportion technique

presented in the previous section, Units of Measure and Common Equivalents. All you have to remember is what "percentage" means: the amount of solute in milliliters or grams contained in 100 mL or 100 g of the final solution.

Weight-in-Volume Solutions (w/v)

If 5 g of dextrose (the chemical name for table sugar) is dissolved in water such that 100 mL of total solution is prepared (5 g per 100 mL), the result is a 5% solution of dextrose in water. Because this type of solution involves a certain weight of drug in a total volume of solution, it is sometimes called a weight-in-volume solution, and you will sometimes see the concentration expressed as 5% w/v to denote this relationship. Because this is the most common kind of solution, it is often understood that the percentage is w/v if nothing indicates otherwise.

Volume-in-Volume Solutions (v/v)

An example involving 2 liquids would be alcohol dissolved in water. A 70% ethanol solution in water is made up of 70 mL of ethanol mixed with enough water to make 100 mL of solution (70 mL per 100 mL). These types of solutions are sometimes called volume-in-volume solutions, and the percentage is written as 70% v/v.

Weight-in-Weight Percentages (w/w)

When a drug is incorporated into another solid or semisolid product, such as a cream or ointment, the product is expressed as a weight-in-weight percentage. For example, 2 g of lidocaine mixed with enough of a compounding base to make 100 g of ointment (2 g per 100 g) would be a 2% w/w lidocaine ointment.

> Because there is little room for error in pharmaceutical calculations, you need to be completely certain of the accuracy of your work. Double- or triple-check your calculations or ask someone else to confirm them.

Let's try a few problems using percentage calculations.

15. **How many grams of dextrose are in 50 mL of a 5% w/v solution?**

    First, set up 2 common fractions that express the proportional relationships:

    $$\frac{5\text{ g}}{100\text{ mL}} = \frac{?}{50\text{ mL}}$$

    $$? \times 100\text{ mL} = 5\text{ g} \times 50\text{ mL}$$

    $$? = \frac{5\text{ g} \times 50\text{ mL}}{100\text{ mL}}$$

    $$? = \frac{5\text{ g} \times 50}{100}$$

    $$? = 2.5\text{ g}$$

16. **How many liters of a 5% dextrose solution contain 100 g of dextrose?**

    $$\frac{5\text{ g}}{100\text{ mL}} = \frac{100\text{ g}}{?}$$

    $$? \times 5\text{ g} = 100\text{ mL} \times 100\text{ g}$$

    $$? = \frac{100\text{ mL} \times 100\text{ g}}{5\text{ g}}$$

    $$? = \frac{100\text{ mL} \times 100}{5}$$

    $$? = 2000\text{ mL}$$

    Now, convert 2000 mL to liters:

    $$\frac{1000\text{ mL}}{1\text{ L}} = \frac{2000\text{ mL}}{?}$$

    $$? \times 1000\text{ mL} = 1\text{ L} \times 2000\text{ mL}$$

    $$? = \frac{1\text{ L} \times 2000\text{ mL}}{1000\text{ mL}}$$

    $$? = \frac{1\text{ L} \times 2000}{1000}$$

    $$? = 2\text{ L}$$

17. **How many grams of lidocaine are in 75 g of a 2% w/w ointment?**

    $$\frac{2\text{ g of lidocaine}}{100\text{ g of ointment}} = \frac{?}{75\text{ g of ointment}}$$

    $$? \times 100\text{ g of ointment} = 2\text{ g of lidocaine} \times 75\text{ g of ointment}$$

    $$? = 2\text{ g of lidocaine} \times \frac{75\text{ g of ointment}}{100\text{ g of ointment}}$$

    $$? = 2\text{ g} \times \frac{75}{100}$$

    $$? = 1.5\text{ g of lidocaine}$$

18. **How many milliliters of ethanol are in 35 mL of a 70% v/v ethanol solution?**

    $$\frac{70\text{ mL of ethanol}}{100\text{ mL of solution}} = \frac{?}{35\text{ mL of solution}}$$

    $$? \times 100\text{ mL of solution} = 70\text{ mL of ethanol} \times 35\text{ mL of solution}$$

    $$? = 70\text{ mL of ethanol} \times \frac{35\text{ mL of solution}}{100\text{ mL of solution}}$$

    $$? = \frac{70\text{ mL of ethanol} \times 35}{100}$$

    $$? = 24.5\text{ mL of ethanol}$$

19. **How many grams of a 1% hydrocortisone cream contain 0.5 g of hydrocortisone?**

    $$\frac{1\text{ g of hydrocortisone}}{100\text{ g of cream}} = \frac{0.5\text{ g of hydrocortisone}}{?}$$

    $$? \times 1\text{ g of hydrocortisone} = 100\text{ g of cream} \times 0.5\text{ g of hydrocortisone}$$

    $$? = 100\text{ g of cream} \times \frac{0.5\text{ g of hydrocortisone}}{1\text{ g of hydrocortisone}}$$

    $$? = 100\text{ g of cream} \times \frac{0.5}{1}$$

    $$? = 50\text{ g of cream}$$

20. **How much sodium chloride is in 200 mL of a 0.9% solution?**

    $$\frac{0.9\text{ g}}{100\text{ mL}} = \frac{?}{200\text{ mL}}$$

    $$? \times 100\text{ mL} = 0.9\text{ g} \times 200\text{ mL}$$

    $$? = 0.9\text{ g} \times \frac{200\text{ mL}}{100\text{ mL}}$$

    $$? = 0.9\text{ g} \times \frac{200}{100}$$

    $$? = 1.8\text{ g}$$

21. **How much of a 70% v/v ethanol solution would contain 140 mL of ethanol?**

    $$\frac{70\text{ mL ethanol}}{100\text{ mL solution}} = \frac{140\text{ mL ethanol}}{?}$$

    $$? \times 70\text{ mL ethanol} = 100\text{ mL solution} \times 140\text{ mL ethanol}$$

    $$? = 100\text{ mL solution} \times \frac{140\text{ mL ethanol}}{70\text{ mL ethanol}}$$

    $$? = 100\text{ mL solution} \times \frac{140}{70}$$

    $$? = 200\text{ mL solution}$$

Now try some on your own.

22. How many grams of dextrose would be needed to make 300 mL of a 5% dextrose solution?

$$\frac{5 \text{ g}}{100 \text{ mL}} = \frac{?}{300 \text{ mL}}$$

23. How many milliliters of ethanol are in 50 mL of a 50% v/v solution?

24. To prepare 150 g of a 2% w/w lidocaine ointment, how many grams of lidocaine would you need?

Ratio Strengths

Ratio strengths are another type of pharmaceutical calculation, and they are quite similar to percentage concentration problems. The amount of drug in a preparation is expressed as a ratio strength (for example, a 1:10 strength).

Similar to percentage calculations, ratio strength problems can be weight in volume, volume in volume, or weight in weight, depending on whether the preparation involves liquids or solids. This calculation most often involves a solution in which a drug powder is dissolved in water or some other vehicle. But it could also be a liquid dissolved in a liquid, as with alcohol in water, or a mixture of 2 solids, as with a drug in a cream or ointment. The percentage refers to the amount of drug (the solute) that is dispersed in the vehicle (the solvent).

With ratio strengths, you always assume that the solute is 1 part. Then you calculate how many parts of the final preparation contain that 1 part. For instance, in a 1:10 solution of sodium chloride, there is 1 part of sodium chloride in 10 parts of solution. This is basically the opposite of a percentage calculation where you are calculating the amount of solute present in 100 g or 100 mL of final product.

Here are some examples of ratio strength problems.

25. What is the ratio strength (w/v) of a solution with 2 g of drug in 50 mL of solution?

First, set up 2 common fractions that express the proportional relationships:

$$\frac{1 \text{ g}}{?} = \frac{2 \text{ g}}{50 \text{ mL}}$$
$$? \times 2 \text{ g} = 1 \text{ g} \times 50 \text{ mL}$$
$$? = 1 \text{ g} \times \frac{50 \text{ mL}}{2 \text{ g}}$$
$$? = \frac{50 \text{ mL}}{2}$$
$$? = 25 \text{ mL}$$

Therefore, the ratio strength is expressed as 1:25.

26. How many liters of a 1:20 dextrose solution contain 100 g of dextrose?

$$\frac{100 \text{ g}}{?} = \frac{1 \text{ g}}{20 \text{ mL}}$$
$$? \times 1 \text{ g} = 100 \text{ g} \times 20 \text{ mL}$$
$$? = 100 \text{ g} \times \frac{20 \text{ mL}}{1 \text{ g}}$$
$$? = 100 \times \frac{20 \text{ mL}}{1}$$
$$? = 2000 \text{ mL}$$
$$\frac{1000 \text{ mL}}{1 \text{ L}} = \frac{2000 \text{ mL}}{?}$$
$$? \times 1000 \text{ mL} = 1 \text{ L} \times 2000 \text{ mL}$$
$$? = 1 \text{ L} \times \frac{2000 \text{ mL}}{1000 \text{ mL}}$$
$$? = 1 \text{ L} \times \frac{2000}{1000}$$
$$? = 2 \text{ L}$$

27. How many grams of lidocaine are in 75 g of a 1:50 w/w ointment?

$$\frac{1 \text{ g of lidocaine}}{50 \text{ g of ointment}} = \frac{?}{75 \text{ g of ointment}}$$
$$? \times 50 \text{ g of ointment} = 1 \text{ g of lidocaine} \times 75 \text{ g of ointment}$$
$$? = 1 \text{ g of lidocaine} \times \frac{75 \text{ g of ointment}}{50 \text{ g of ointment}}$$
$$? = 1 \text{ g of lidocaine} \times \frac{75}{50}$$
$$? = 1.5 \text{ g of lidocaine}$$

Similar to percentage calculations, ratio strength problems can be weight in volume, volume in volume, or weight in weight depending on whether the preparation involves liquids or solids.

28. **How many milliliters of ethanol are in 35 mL of a 1:2 v/v ethanol solution?**

$$\frac{1 \text{ mL of ethanol}}{2 \text{ mL of solution}} = \frac{?}{35 \text{ mL of solution}}$$

$? \times 2 \text{ mL of solution} = 1 \text{ mL of ethanol}$
$\qquad\qquad\qquad \times 35 \text{ mL of solution}$

$? = 1 \text{ mL of ethanol} \times \dfrac{35 \text{ mL of solution}}{2 \text{ mL of solution}}$

$? = 1 \text{ mL of ethanol} \times \dfrac{35}{2}$

$? = 17.5 \text{ mL of ethanol}$

29. **How many grams of a 1:100 hydrocortisone cream contain 0.5 g of hydrocortisone?**

$$\frac{1 \text{ g of hydrocortisone}}{100 \text{ g of cream}} = \frac{0.5 \text{ g of hydrocortisone}}{?}$$

$? \times 1 \text{ g of hydrocortisone} = 100 \text{ g of cream}$
$\qquad\qquad\qquad \times 0.5 \text{ g of hydrocortisone}$

$? = 100 \text{ g of cream} \times \dfrac{0.5 \text{ g of hydrocortisone}}{1 \text{ g of hydrocortisone}}$

$? = 100 \text{ g of cream} \times \dfrac{0.5}{1}$

$? = 50 \text{ g of cream}$

30. **How much sodium chloride is in 200 mL of a 1:111 solution?**

$$\frac{1 \text{ g}}{111 \text{ mL}} = \frac{?}{200 \text{ mL}}$$

$? \times 111 \text{ mL} = 1 \text{ g} \times 200 \text{ mL}$

$? = 1 \text{ g} \times \dfrac{200 \text{ mL}}{111 \text{ mL}}$

$? = 1 \text{ g} \times \dfrac{200}{111}$

$? = 1.8 \text{ g}$

31. **How much of a 1:1.43 v/v ethanol solution would contain 140 mL of ethanol?**

$$\frac{1 \text{ mL ethanol}}{1.43 \text{ mL solution}} = \frac{140 \text{ mL ethanol}}{?}$$

$? \times 1 \text{ mL ethanol} = 1.43 \text{ mL solution}$
$\qquad\qquad\qquad \times 140 \text{ mL ethanol}$

$? = 1.43 \text{ mL solution} \times \dfrac{140 \text{ mL ethanol}}{1 \text{ mL ethanol}}$

$? = 1.43 \text{ mL solution} \times \dfrac{140}{1}$

$? = 200 \text{ mL solution}$

Here are some problems for you to try.

32. **How many grams of dexamethasone are in 75 g of a 1:100 cream?**

33. **How many liters of a 1:2 alcohol solution contain 4 L of alcohol?**

34. **How many grams of dextrose are in 300 mL of a 1:20 solution?**

Temperature Conversion

Although Americans are more familiar with Fahrenheit temperatures, most medical temperature measurements are taken using the centigrade or Celsius system. The Celsius scale is based on the freezing and boiling points of water, which are denoted as 0°C and 100°C. These 2 points are equivalent to 32°F and 212°F, respectively. To convert between the 2 systems, use the following equation:

$$9(°C) = 5(°F) - 160$$

Use this equation to solve some problems.

35. **Convert 39°F to °C.**

$9(°C) = 5(°F) - 160$
$9(°C) = 5(39) - 160$
$9(°C) = 195 - 160$
$9(°C) = 35$
$9°C = \dfrac{35}{9}$
$°C = 3.9$

36. **Convert 80°C to °F.**

$9(°C) = 5(°F) - 160$
$9(80) = 5(°F) - 160$
$5(°F) = 720 + 160$
$5(°F) = 880$
$°F = \dfrac{880}{5}$
$°F = 176$

Now try some problems on your own.

37. **Convert 98.6°F (normal body temperature) to °C.**

38. **Convert 20°C to °F.**

Household Equivalents

In the community and ambulatory pharmacy settings, patients need to use common household measures to administer liquid medications. Table 2-5 provides conversions between metric quantities and household measurements. Use these conversions to calculate drug dosages.

39. How much drug is in 2 tsp of a $\frac{10 \text{ mg}}{5 \text{ mL}}$ solution?

    First, convert the common household measure to the metric system using ratio and proportion.

    $$\frac{1 \text{ tsp}}{5 \text{ mL}} = \frac{2 \text{ tsp}}{?}$$

    $$? \times 1 \text{ tsp} = 5 \text{ mL} \times 2 \text{ tsp}$$

    $$? = 5 \text{ mL} \times \frac{2 \text{ tsp}}{1 \text{ tsp}}$$

    $$? = 5 \text{ mL} \times \frac{2}{1}$$

    $$? = 10 \text{ mL}$$

    Then, calculate the amount of drug in 10 mL using ratio and proportion.

    $$\frac{10 \text{ mg}}{5 \text{ mL}} = \frac{?}{10 \text{ mL}}$$

    $$? \times 5 \text{ mL} = 10 \text{ mg} \times 10 \text{ mL}$$

    $$? = 10 \text{ mg} \times \frac{10 \text{ mL}}{5 \text{ mL}}$$

    $$? = 10 \text{ mg} \times \frac{10}{5}$$

    $$? = 20 \text{ mg}$$

40. How many teaspoonfuls are in a 1-pt bottle of medication?

    Since 1 pt contains 473 mL and 1 tsp contains 5 mL, the following ratio and proportion can be set up:

    $$\frac{1 \text{ tsp}}{5 \text{ mL}} = \frac{?}{473 \text{ mL}}$$

    $$? \times 5 \text{ mL} = 1 \text{ tsp} \times 473 \text{ mL}$$

    $$? = 1 \text{ tsp} \times \frac{473 \text{ mL}}{5 \text{ mL}}$$

    $$? = 1 \text{ tsp} \times \frac{473}{5}$$

    $$? = 94.6 \text{ tsp} \left(\text{meaning that 94 full teaspoonfuls can be obtained from a 1 pt bottle}\right)$$

Table 2-5	Common Household Equivalents of Metric Liquid Measures
METRIC MEASURE (mL)	**HOUSEHOLD EQUIVALENT**
5	1 teaspoonful (tsp)
15	1 tablespoonful (Tbs) or 3 tsp
30 (equal to 1 fluid oz)	2 Tbs

Now try some calculations on your own.

41. How many 1-Tbs (tablespoonful) doses can be obtained from a 90-mL bottle of medicine?

42. If an antibiotic suspension has 150 mg per 5 mL, how much drug is in 1 Tbs?

Pharmaceutical Abbreviations

When writing prescriptions or entering prescription information into the electronic health record, prescribers often use abbreviations for Latin terms to indicate how patients should take medications. For instance, instead of writing "two times a day," they just write "bid," which is an abbreviation for 2 times a day in Latin.

Table 2-6 lists the most commonly used abbreviations that you will need to memorize. To help you learn these abbreviations, notice certain commonalities:

- *a* can be an abbreviation for *ante*, meaning before, or *aura*, meaning ear.
- *d* can mean *die*, for day, or *dextro*, meaning right.

> When writing prescriptions or entering prescription information into the electronic health record, prescribers often use abbreviations for Latin terms to indicate how patients should take medications.

LATIN-BASED ABBREVIATIONS

a	before
ac	before meals
ad	right ear
as	left ear
au	both ears or each ear
bid	2 times a day
c	with
dtd	dispense such doses
gtt, gtts	drop or drops
h, hr	hour
hs	at bedtime (at the hour of sleep)
non rep	do not repeat, no refills
p	after
po	by mouth
prn	as needed
q	every
qd	every day
q am	every morning
q pm	every evening
q hs	every bedtime
qod	every other day (every second day)

q 4 h	every 4 hours (or 3, 6, 8, 12, 24 hours, or other intervals)
qid	4 times a day
tid	3 times a day
os	left eye
od	right eye
ou	both eyes or each eye
ut dict, ud	as directed
stat	at once, now

OTHER COMMON ABBREVIATIONS

APAP	acetaminophen
ASA	aspirin
DAW	dispense as written
IM	intramuscular
IV	intravenous
MOM	milk of magnesia
NSAID	nonsteroidal anti-inflammatory drug
OTC	over-the-counter (as in nonprescription)
PCN	penicillin
SC	subcutaneous
TCN	tetracycline

- *h* stands for *hora* or hour.
- *b*, *t*, and *q* usually refer to how many times a day to give a medicine, standing for 2 times, 3 times, and 4 times daily, respectively.
- *q* stands for *quaque*, meaning every.
- *o* stands for *oculo*, for eye.

Examples:

ac	=	before meals
ad	=	right ear
as	=	left ear
qd	=	every day
q 4 h	=	every 4 hours
q 8 h	=	every 8 hours
bid	=	2 times a day
tid	=	3 times a day
qid	=	4 times a day
od	=	right eye
os	=	left eye

Medical Terminology

While the words used to describe parts of the body, medical procedures, and diseases can certainly be formidable, many of them can be broken down to common prefixes, roots, and suffixes that help you deduce their meaning. According to *Stedman's Medical Dictionary*, about 400 such word parts make up 90%-95% of all medical terminology. By learning these word parts, you can decipher most medical terms, even if you have never encountered them before.

The most common of these 400 word parts are shown in Table 2-7 with explanatory examples. The entries under "prefixes and combining forms" are used at the beginning of words, in the middle of terms, or with root words, as follows:

- an- (without) + hedonia (pleasure) = anhedonia (without pleasure)
- poly- (many) + dactyl (fingers or toes) = polydactyly (having more than 5 fingers or toes)

Similarly, suffixes can be added to prefixes, combining forms, or root words to form medical terms, as follows:

- splen- (referring to the spleen) + -ectomy (removal) = splenectomy (removal of the spleen)
- laryng- (referring to the larynx) + -itis (inflammation) = laryngitis (loss of voice caused by inflammation of the larynx, or voice box)

Now, using the information in Table 2-7, try to decipher the meaning of the following medical terms:

- photophobic
- stomatitis
- nephrectomy
- thoracotomy
- gastroscopy

Table 2-7 Common Medical Prefixes and Suffixes, Their Meanings, and Examples

Element	Meaning	Example
Prefixes and Combining Forms		
a-, an-	without	aplastic, anhedonia
arteri-, arterio-	artery	arteriosclerosis
arthro-	bone joint	arthroscope
auto-	self	autoimmune
bacteri-, bacterio-	bacteria	bacteriostatic
bi-	twice, double	bisexual, binocular
bronch-, bronchi-	bronchus	bronchitis
carcin-, carcino-	cancer	carcinogenic
cardi-, cardio-	heart	cardiology
chlor-, chloro-	chlorine	hydrochloric acid
chol-	bile	cholestasis
chondro-	cartilage	chondrocyte
cis-	on the same side as (chemistry)	cis-retinoic acid (see trans-)
co-, col-, com-, con-, cor-	together with	cofactor
crani-, cranio-	cranium (head, skull)	craniotomy
cry-	cold	cryogenic
cyst-	bladder	cystitis
cyt-	cell	cytology
dactyl-	fingers, toes	dactyledema
de-	away, cessation	decompose
derm-	skin	dermatology
dextr-	toward the right	dextroamphetamine
duodeno-	duodenum (small intestine)	duodenal ulcer
dys-	bad, difficult	dysfunctional
ect-	outer, outside	ectoderm
encephalo-	brain	encephalogram
end-, endo-	within, inner	endoderm

Element	Meaning	Example
enter-, entero-	intestines	gastroenterology
erythro-	red	erythrocyte (red blood cell)
eu-	good, well	eugenics, eutectic
ex-	out, away from	exhalation
extra-	without, outside of	extrachromosomal
ferri-, ferro-	iron	ferric sulfate, ferrous citrate
gastro-	stomach	gastroscopy
gloss-	tongue	glossitis
gyn-, gyne-, gyneco-, gyno-	woman	gynecology
hem-, hema-, hemat-, hemato-	blood	hematology, hemoglobin
hist-, histio-	tissue	histology
hydr-, hydro-	water, hydrogen	hydrolysis
hyper-	excessive, above normal	hyperactive
hypo-	beneath, less than normal	hypotonic
hyster-	uterus	hysterectomy
ileo-	ileum (small intestine)	ileotomy
infra-	below	infrared
inter-	among, between	intervascular (between blood and lymph vessels)
intra-	within	intravenous (within veins)
irid-	iris (of the eye)	iridology, iritis
kerat-, kerato-	cornea (of the eye)	keratectomy

(table continues on next page)

Table 2-7 (continued)

Element	Meaning	Example	Element	Meaning	Example
kinesi-, kinesio-	movement	kinesiology	oxa-, oxo-	addition of oxygen	oxalic acid, oxalate
lact-, lacto-	milk	lactose, lactase	pan-, pant-, panto-	all, entire	pandemic (worldwide epidemic)
laryng-	larynx (in the throat)	laryngitis			
latero-	to one side	lateral, lateroflexion	path-, patho-	disease	pathology
lepto-	frail, slender, thin	leptin	ped-, pedi-, pedo-	child or foot	pediatrics, pedograph
leuko-	white	leukocyte (white blood cell)	peri-	around	pericardium
lip-, lipo-	fat, lipid	liposome	pharmaco-	drugs, medicine	pharmacotherapy
lymph-	lymph system, glands	lymphatic	pharyng-, pharyngo-	pharynx (of the throat)	pharyngotomy
lys-	breaking up, dissolution	lysis	phleb-, phlebo-	vein	phlebotomy
			phos-, phot-, photo-	light	photophobic
macro-	large	macrocyte			
mast-, masto-	breast	mastectomy	phren-, phreni-	diaphragm	phrenoplegia
meg-, mega-, megalo-	large	megalocytes	physi-, physio-	physical, natural	physiology
			plasma-, plasmat-, plasmato-	plasma	plasmapheresis
melan-, melano-	black	melanoma			
mening-, meningo-	meninges	meningitis	pleur-, pleura-, pleuro-	rib, side, pleura	pleural, pleurisy
morph-, morpho-	form, shape, structure	morphology	pneum-, pneuma-, pneumata-, pneumato-	air, gas, lungs, breathing	pneumonitis
myx-, myxo-	mucus	myxedema, myxoid			
necr-, necro-	death	necrosis	poly-	multiple	polydactyly, polyuria
nephr-, nephro-	kidney	nephritis, nephrology	post-	after, behind	postpartum (after childbirth)
neur-, neuri-, neuro-	nerve, nervous system	neurology	pre-	before	preprandial (before eating)
oculo-	eye	oculoscope			
olig-, oligo-	few, little	oligospermia	pro-	before, precursor of	prodrug
onco-	tumor	oncology			
onych-, onycho-	fingernail, toenail	onychectomy	proct-, procto-	anus, rectum	proctologist
oo-, oophor-, oophoro-	ovary, ovum	oophorectomy	psych-, psyche-, psycho-	mind	psychopathology
			pyel-, pyelo-	renal pelvis	pyelonephritis
ophthalm-, ophthalmo-	eyes	ophthalmology	pyreto-, pyro-	heat, fever	pyretics (drugs that relieve fever)
orchi-, orchido-, orchio-	testis	orchidectomy	radio-	radiation, X-rays	radiology
ossi-, osseo-, ost-, oste-, osteo-	bone	osteoporosis	re-, retro-	again, backward	reconstructive, retrograde
ovari-, ovario-	ovary	ovariectomy	rhin-, rhino-	nose	rhinitis
ovi-, ovo-	egg	oviduct	schiz-, schizo-	split, cleft, division	schizophrenia

Table 2-7 (continued)

Element	Meaning	Example
scler-, sclero-	hardness, the sclera	scleroderma
semi-	one-half, partly	semicomatose
sigmoid-, sigmoido-	sigmoid colon (large intestine)	sigmoidoscopy
somat-, somato-, somatico-	the body	somatotropic
spermato-, spermo-, sperma-	semen, sperm	spermatozoa
splen-, spleno-	spleen	splenectomy
staphyl-, staphylo-	staphylococci	staphylococcal
steno-	narrowness, constriction	stenosis
stom-, stoma-, stomat-, stomato-	mouth	stomatitis
sub-	beneath, less than normal	subdural
super-	in excess, above, superior	supersaturate, superovulation
therm-, thermo-	heat	thermometer
thorac-, thoracico-	chest, thorax	thoracotomy
thromb-, thrombo-	blood clot	thrombosis
thyr-, thyro-	thyroid gland	thyrotoxicosis
toco-	childbirth	tocolytic
tox-, toxico-, toxo-	toxin, poison	toxicology
trache-, tracheo-	trachea	tracheotomy
trans-	across (chemical designation)	trans-retinoic acid (see cis-)
trich-, trichi-, trichia-, tricho-	hair, hairlike structure	trichitis
tropho-	food, nutrition	trophoblast, trophoderm
uri-, uric-, urico-	uric acid	uricosuric
vas-	duct, blood vessel	vas deferens
vasculo-, vaso-	blood vessel	vasculogenesis
vesic-, vesico-	vesica, vesicle	vesiculitis
zo-, zoo-	animal, animal life	zoonoses
zy-	fertilization	zygote, zygospore
zym-, zymo-	enzymes	zymology, zymogen

Element	Meaning	Example
Suffixes		
-ase	an enzyme	sucrase
-ate	a salt or ester of an acid	sulfate
-cidal, -cide	killing, destroying	bactericidal
-cyte	cell	macrocyte
-ectomy	excision, removal	splenectomy
-gram	recording	electrocardiogram
-graph	recording instrument	polygraph
-ia, -iasis	condition	trichomoniasis
-ic	pertaining to	physiologic
-ism	condition, disease	trophism
-itis	inflammation	nephritis
-lepsis, -lepsy	seizure	epilepsy
-megaly	large	acromegaly
-oid	resemblance to	lymphoid
-ology	study of	biology, nephrology
-oma, -omata	tumor, neoplasm	keratoma
-one	chemical ketone group	acetone
-otomy	incision, cutting into	lobotomy
-pathy	disease	cardiopathy
-penia	deficiency	leukopenia
-phage, -phagia	eating	polyphagia
-phobe, -phobic	afraid of	claustrophobic
-plegia	paralysis	paraplegia
-poiesis	production	hematopoiesis
-rrhagia, -rrhage	discharge	hemorrhage
-rrhea	flowing	rhinorrhea, diarrhea
-scope	instrument for viewing	microscope
-scopy	use of instrument for viewing	microscopy
-stat	agent to prevent change	bacteriostat
-trophic	food, nutrition	lymphotrophic
-uria	urine	glycosuria

Conclusion

While much of the information in this chapter requires memorization, it will serve you well as you begin to process prescriptions in the pharmacy. Through a minimal amount of memorization and a large measure of understanding the way calculations are performed, conversions are made, and medical terms are formed, you will feel quite confident in your everyday duties and your interactions with pharmacists and other health care professionals.

Answers to Unsolved Problems in This Chapter

6. 3000
7. 500
8. 197
9. 49.28
10. 35.21
11. 15.24
12. 15,000
13. 50 (100 tablets); 0.5 (1 tablet)
14. 100
22. 15
23. 25
24. 3
32. 0.75
33. 8
34. 15
37. 37
38. 68
41. 6
42. 450

Answers to Medical Terms

Photophobic = photo- (light) + -phobic (afraid of) = photophobic (fear or avoidance of light)

Stomatitis = stomat- (mouth) + -itis (inflammation) = stomatitis (inflammation in the mouth)

Nephrectomy = nephr- (referring to the kidney) + -ectomy (removal) = nephrectomy (removal of the kidney)

Thoracotomy = thorac- (chest, thorax) + -otomy (incision, cutting into) = thoracotomy (an incision into the chest such as for surgery)

Gastroscopy = gastro- (stomach) + -scopy (use of instrument for viewing) = gastroscopy (visual examination of the stomach, usually with a special scoping instrument)

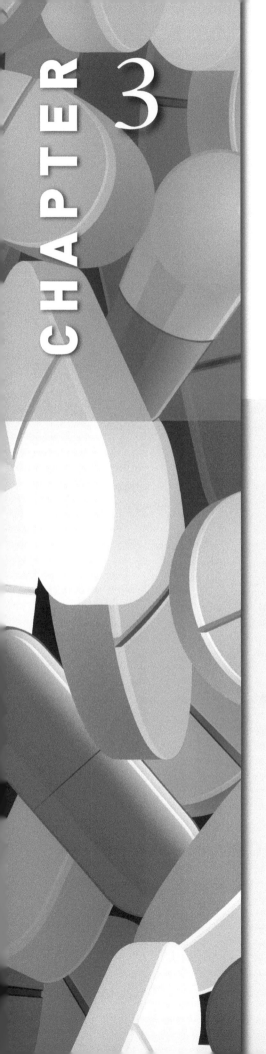

CHAPTER 3

Pharmacy Law and Regulation

This chapter focuses on the Food and Drug Administration (FDA), the Centers for Medicare and Medicaid Services (CMS), the Drug Enforcement Administration (DEA), the United States Pharmacopeia (USP), and state boards of pharmacy. It describes the drug approval process and introduces FDA regulatory actions such as drug recalls and Risk Evaluation and Mitigation Strategies. Then it covers DEA regulation of controlled substances in detail and patient privacy requirements under the Health Insurance Portability and Accountability Act. Although state-specific board of pharmacy regulations cannot be covered, this chapter emphasizes the important roles that these agencies play in the daily operation and regulation of pharmacies.

Introduction

Because medications have such powerful effects on the human body and are such specialized entities, they are subject to regulation at both the federal and state levels. Some types of pharmacies are subject to additional government regulations based on the ways these facilities are paid for pharmaceuticals and patient care services with federal monies. In addition, the pharmacy profession regulates itself through voluntary programs involving accreditation of training programs and certification of individuals. In this chapter, these government and voluntary programs are described as they apply to you, the pharmacy technician.

Food and Drug Administration

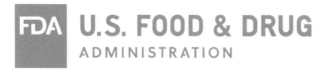

FDA's decisions have profound effects on medical care. The FDA is the part of the federal government that controls which medications can be legally sold in the United States. FDA also oversees medical devices (including pumps used to infuse drugs), dietary supplements (herbal and alternative medicines), cosmetics and other beauty aids, and foods.

History

FDA was created through the passage of the Federal Food and Drugs Act of 1906. In addition to oversight of food, the FDA initially had authority to pursue manufacturers of pharmaceutical products that were **adulterated** or **misbranded**. A product that is adulterated is altered, dirty, or unclean; prepared, packaged, or stored under unsanitary conditions; or prepared in unsafe containers. Misbranding refers to package labeling that contains false or misleading information about the identity of the substance in the container or that fails to carry required warnings or instructions on product labeling.

In 1937, a tragedy struck the United States when a toxic preparation of Elixir Sulfanilamide caused 73 deaths. This tragedy led to the passage of the Food, Drug, and Cosmetic Act of 1938, which expanded the FDA's oversight to include approval of new drug products, medical devices, and cosmetics based on their safety for use in humans.

Two important amendments have been made to the Food, Drug, and Cosmetic Act of 1938. In 1952, Congress passed the Durham-Humphrey Amendment, which directed the FDA to divide drug products into 2 categories: those that require a prescription and those that may be sold without a prescription. Prescription medications are referred to as legend drugs because the FDA requires a symbol or statement on the product's packaging. Drugs that do not require prescriptions are called nonprescription, nonlegend, or over-the-counter (OTC) drugs.

In response to birth defects reported in Europe caused by the drug thalidomide, Congress later gave the FDA more authority by passing the Kefauver-Harris Drug Amendments of 1962. These amendments allowed the FDA to control research into new drugs; require that new drugs be safe and effective for the conditions listed in product labeling; facilitate easier removal of drugs from the market whenever necessary; and more easily regulate prescription drug advertisements.

Drug Approval Process

FDA has extensive authority to determine which drug products can be marketed in the United States. A pharmaceutical company that wants to market a product must prove that the drug is both safe to use in humans and effective for its claimed uses. FDA requires evidence from research studies called controlled clinical trials. In these trials, the pharmaceutical company must compare the new drug with either a placebo (dosage forms that appear similar to the real product but contain no active ingredient) or a known, effective alternative agent.

Medications going through this FDA premarketing process are called investigational drugs. In 2019,

> A pharmaceutical company that wants to market a product must prove to the FDA that the drug is both safe to use in people and effective for the claimed uses.

pharmaceutical companies spent $186 billion globally searching for compounds to test and conduct investigational drug studies. Through chemical and animal studies, company researchers identify a compound they believe will be useful in humans. Then, the company files an Investigational New Drug (IND) application with the FDA.

Figure 3-1 shows why this is such an expensive process. For each drug that is eventually approved by the FDA, companies screen 5000-10,000 compounds. The Tufts Center of Drug Development estimates that pharmaceutical companies spend $2.6 billion to successfully bring a drug to market. Only 12% of compounds that start the research and development process actually gain FDA approval.

If the FDA approves the initial IND application, the company begins testing in humans. As shown in Figure 3-1, these tests progress through 3 phases:

- **Phase I:** The investigational drug is tested in a small number (20-80) of healthy volunteers, who do not have any active disease, to ensure its safety and determine appropriate dosage in humans.
- **Phase II:** A slightly larger number (100-300) of patient volunteers who have the target disease use the drug to see if it continues to prove safe and determine its effectiveness.
- **Phase III:** If the FDA allows the company to proceed into phase III, the company recruits 1000-5000 patient volunteers to participate in a controlled clinical trial. These trials are used to test for efficacy as well as to identify adverse effects (harmful and unintended side effects) of the drug during short- and long-term use.

After phase III trials are complete, the pharmaceutical company reviews the data. If the numbers indicate safety and efficacy of the drug, the company files a New Drug Application (NDA) with the FDA. The FDA can take several months, or even years, to review the NDA before either approving or denying the application. Even when the NDA is approved, the FDA usually requires further postmarket testing, sometimes called phase IV, to check for adverse effects that occur in very small percentages of patients taking the drug.

Despite the complexity of this process, around 40 drugs are approved by the FDA each year. According to Pharmaceutical Research and Manufacturers of America (PhRMA), more than 8000 medications were in development in 2019. Now, with the new knowledge we have about the human genome (the 46 human chromosomes) and the need to meet needs of the coronavirus disease (COVID-19) pandemic, companies are increasing both the number and the types of new drugs they are researching. As a pharmacy technician, you may encounter patients who are receiving new, investigational drugs. Especially in large teaching hospitals, your pharmacy may be assisting with numerous drug protocols. Special procedures and record keeping must be followed when handling these agents.

For instance, these studies are usually placebo controlled. This means that up to one-half of the patients in the study are receiving tablets or capsules that are identical in appearance but have no active drug. By using these placebos, the researchers can measure the improvements in patients' conditions that are attributable to the new drug.

The studies are usually double blinded, which means that neither the researchers nor the patients know who is receiving the active drug or who is receiving a placebo. For this purpose, the pharmacy often prepares identical dosage forms (tablets or capsules), some with active drug and some with placebo. It is important to properly label these products to ensure the study is conducted correctly.

In unprecedented or extreme circumstances, as were seen with the start of the COVID-19 pandemic, the FDA may enact or rely on specific programs to meet the needs of the public. In 2020, the FDA launched the Coronavirus Treatment Acceleration Program (CTAP) to move new COVID-19 treatments

> As a pharmacy technician, you may encounter patients who are receiving investigational new drugs. Special procedures and record keeping must be followed when handling these agents.

Figure 3-1 Drug Development: How Compounds Move From the Laboratory to Clinical Use. For full resolution images, please see the complementary supplemental files posted on PharmacyLibrary.com/updates

FDA U.S. Food and Drug Administration
Drug Approval Process

What is a drug as defined by the FDA?

A drug is any product that is intended for use in the diagnosis, cure, mitigation, treatment, or prevention of disease and that is intended to affect the structure or any function of the body.

PRE-CLINICAL

Drug Sponsor's Discovery and Screening Phase

Drug Developed

Drug sponsor develops a new drug compound and seeks to have it approved by FDA for sale in the United States.

Animals Tested

Sponsor must test new drug on animals for toxicity. Multiple species are used to gather basic information on the safety and efficacy of the compound being investigated/researched.

IND Application

The sponsor submits an Investigational New Drug (IND) application to FDA based on the results from intial testing that include, the drug's composition and manufacturing, and develops a plan for testing the drug on humans.

IND REVIEW

FDA reviews the IND to assure that the proposed studies, generally referred to as clinical trials, do not place human subjects at unreasonable risk of harm. FDA also verifies that there are adequate informed consent and human subject protection.

FDA's Center for Drug Evaluation and Research (CDER) evaluates new drugs before they can be sold.

The centers evaluation not only prevent, quackery, but also provide doctors and patients the information they need to use medicines wisely. CDER ensures that drugs, both brand-name and generic, are effective and their health benefits outweigh their known risks.

CLINICAL

Drug Sponsor's Clinical Studies/Trials

PHASE 1

20-80

The typical number of healthy volunteers used in Phase 1; this phase emphasizes safety. The goal here in this phase is to determine what the drug's most frequent side effects are and, often, how the drug is metabolized and excreted.

PHASE 2

100's

The typical number of patients used in Phase 2; this phase emphasizes effectiveness. This goal is to obtain preliminary data on whether the drug works in people who have a certain disease or condition. For controlled trials, patients receiving the drug are compared with similar patients receiving a different treatment—usually a placebo, or a different drug. Safety continues to be evaluated, and short-term side effects are studied.

At the end of Phase 2, FDA and sponsors discuss how large-scale studies in Phase 3 will be done.

DRUG SPONSOR
FDA

PHASE 3

1000's

The typical number of patients used in Phase 3. These studies gather more information about safety and effectiveness, study different populations and different dosages, and uses the drug in combination with other drugs.

Figure 3-1 (continued)

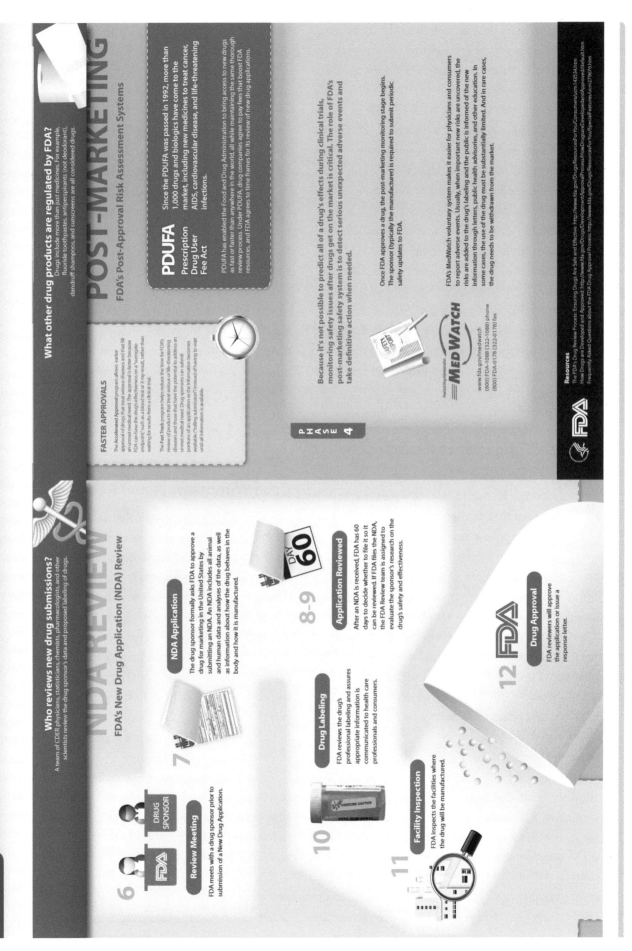

Who reviews new drug submissions?

A team of CDER physicians, statisticians, chemists, pharmacologists, and other scientists review the drug sponsor's data and proposed labeling of drugs.

NDA REVIEW

FDA's New Drug Application (NDA) Review

6

Review Meeting

FDA meets with a drug sponsor prior to submission of a New Drug Application.

7

NDA Application

The drug sponsor formally asks FDA to approve a drug for marketing in the United States by submitting an NDA. An NDA includes all animal and human data and analyses of the data, as well as information about how the drug behaves in the body and how it is manufactured.

DAY 60

8-9

Application Reviewed

After an NDA is received, FDA has 60 days to decide whether to file it so it can be reviewed. If FDA files the NDA, the FDA Review team is assigned to evaluate the sponsor's research on the drug's safety and effectiveness.

10

Drug Labeling

FDA reviews the drug's professional labeling and assures appropriate information is communicated to health care professionals and consumers.

11

Facility Inspection

FDA inspects the facilities where the drug will be manufactured.

12

Drug Approval

FDA reviewers will approve the application or issue a response letter.

What other drug products are regulated by FDA?

Drugs include more than just medicines. For example, fluoride toothpastes, antiperspirants (not deodorant), dandruff shampoos, and sunscreens are all considered drugs.

POST-MARKETING

FDA's Post-Approval Risk Assessment Systems

FASTER APPROVALS

The Accelerated Approval program allows earlier approval of drugs that treat serious diseases and that fill an unmet medical need. The approval is faster because FDA can base the drug's effectiveness on a "surrogate endpoint," such as a blood test or X-ray result, rather than waiting for results from a clinical trial.

The Fast Track program helps reduce the time for FDA's review of products that treat serious or life-threatening disease and those that have the potential to address an unmet medical need. Drug sponsors can submit portions of an application as the information becomes available ("rolling submission") instead of having to wait until all information is available.

PDUFA

Prescription Drug User Fee Act

Since the PDUFA was passed in 1992, more than 1,000 drugs and biologics have come to the market, including new medicines to treat cancer, AIDS, cardiovascular disease, and life-threatening infections.

PDUFA has enabled the Food and Drug Administration to bring access to new drugs as fast or faster than anywhere in the world, all while maintaining the same thorough review process. Under PDUFA, drug companies agree to pay fees that boost FDA resources, and FDA agrees to time frames for its review of new drug applications.

PHASE 4

Because it's not possible to predict all of a drug's effects during clinical trials, monitoring safety issues after drugs get on the market is critical. The role of FDA's post-marketing safety system is to detect serious unexpected adverse events and take definitive action when needed.

Once FDA approves a drug, the post-marketing monitoring stage begins. The sponsor (typically the manufacturer) is required to submit periodic safety updates to FDA.

MEDWATCH

www.fda.gov/medwatch
(800) FDA-1088 (322-1088) phone
(800) FDA-0178 (322-0178) fax

FDA's MedWatch voluntary system makes it easier for physicians and consumers to report adverse events. Usually, when important new risks are uncovered, the risks are added to the drug's labeling and the public is informed of the new information through letters, public health advisories, and other education. In some cases, the use of the drug must be substantially limited. And in rare cases, the drug needs to be withdrawn from the market.

Resources
The FDA's Drug Review Process: Ensuring Drugs Are Safe and Effective: http://www.fda.gov/Drugs/ResourcesForYou/Consumers/ucm143534.htm
How Drugs are Developed and Approved: http://www.fda.gov/Drugs/DevelopmentApprovalProcess/HowDrugsareDevelopedandApproved/default.htm
Frequently Asked Questions about the FDA Drug Approval Process: http://www.fda.gov/Drugs/ResourcesForYou/SpecialFeatures/ucm279676htm

Source: US Food and Drug Administration.

to patients as soon as possible while at the same time finding out whether they are helpful or harmful. As of November 2020, more than 560 drug products were in the development stage and over 370 trials had been reviewed by the FDA for COVID-19 treatments. The FDA has also granted selected COVID-19 treatments **Emergency Use Authorization**, which allows unapproved medical products or unapproved uses of approved medical products to be used in emergency situations to diagnose, treat, or prevent serious or life-threatening diseases or conditions in selected situations when there are no adequate, approved, and available alternatives. As of November 2020, there are a total of 5 COVID-19 treatments authorized for emergency use by the FDA.

If your responsibilities include investigational or emergency use agents, be sure that you understand the relevant policies and procedures established in your facility.

Therapeutic Equivalence Ratings

Once a drug product's patent expires, any pharmaceutical manufacturer can pursue approval and marketing of a generic form of that medication through an Abbreviated New Drug Application (ANDA) process. After an ANDA is approved by the FDA, the manufacturer can produce and market the generic medication.

The FDA oversees the process for determining whether generic and brand medications can be substituted for one another. In other words, when a patient presents a prescription for a brand-name product in the pharmacy, the pharmacist and pharmacy technician are obligated to fill the prescription with that specific product or a generic alternative that is considered to be equivalent by the FDA.

Drug products are classified as **therapeutically equivalent** by the FDA if they can be substituted for one another with the full expectation that the substituted agent will have the same efficacy and safety profile as the prescribed brand-name drug product. The FDA considers medications to be therapeutically equivalent if they are pharmaceutical equivalents (same ingredient, dosage form, route of administration, and strength) and meet criteria for bioequivalence

(substituted product performs the same in the body as the prescribed drug).

The **Orange Book** is an FDA reference first published in 1980 that includes the therapeutic equivalence ratings, or "codes," for generic and branded drugs. It is available online (https://www.fda.gov/drugs/information-healthcare-professionals-drugs/electronic-orange-book) and is updated regularly.

The most commonly used equivalence code is an "AB" rating for oral medications. You may hear in the pharmacy that 2 drug products that are pharmaceutically equivalent (same ingredient, dose, route, and strength) are "AB rated," signifying that they are substitutable according to the FDA. Keep in mind, though, that rules for applying therapeutic equivalence ratings are set by state boards of pharmacy and differ in each state. Ask your pharmacist if you are unsure if 2 drug products are therapeutically equivalent and, therefore, substitutable in the pharmacy.

Chapter 10 contains additional information on brands and generics in the dispensing process.

Drug Withdrawals and Recalls

Despite efforts to ensure the safety and efficacy of drugs before they come onto the market, serious or fatal adverse effects sometimes occur after a medication is used widely. Even when a drug is tested in a few thousand people, rare but serious side effects may not occur until millions of people are exposed to the drug. When these situations develop, the drug is withdrawn from the market, either temporarily or permanently. Although the withdrawals are often termed voluntary, the companies usually act after they and FDA officials conclude that the risk of continued use of the drug outweighs the possible benefits of keeping the drug on the market.

The FDA may also ask companies to recall specific batches, or lots/lot numbers, of their products. Reasons for recalls vary from serious, high-risk situations to lower-risk situations. For example, in a serious situation, a product may contain the wrong drug or a much higher dose of the correct drug than is listed on the product's label. An instance of a lower-risk situation could involve manufacturing processes being called into question despite there being nothing necessarily wrong with the drug product itself.

To place recalls into perspective, the FDA divides them into 3 types, as follows:

- **Class I:** Continued use of the product is very likely to cause serious adverse effects or death in people.
- **Class II:** Use of the product could cause temporary but reversible effects, or there is little chance that serious adverse effects would result from use of the product.
- **Class III:** Use of the recalled lots or product is unlikely to cause adverse effects in people.

As a pharmacy technician, you will likely be called on to find the affected lots of recalled drug products. These recalls are announced by the companies and publicized by the FDA on its website at https://www .fda.gov/drugs/drug-safety-and-availability/drug-recalls. If an investigational drug or a radiopharmaceutical is recalled, special conditions may apply to the return, handling, or destruction of these medications. In such cases, be sure to follow the policies and procedures of your workplace.

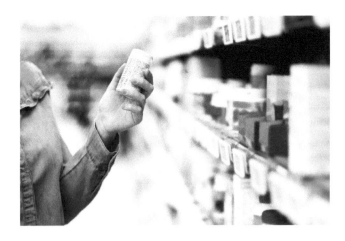

> **Tip:** Product recalls are one of the reasons that state boards of pharmacy require strict documentation of the lot number, manufacturer, expiration date, and other details when a drug product is stored on pharmacy shelves outside of its original container. For example, an identification issue can occur when a prescription is returned to stock if the patient does not pick it up. In the event of a product recall, it is imperative to be able to identify all units of a drug from a specific lot or batch, even if they are not stored in the original manufacturer's packaging.

Dietary Supplement Health Education Act

Because consumers are bombarded by false, misleading information about health foods, alternative medicines, and dietary supplements, pharmacists and pharmacy technicians play an important role in helping patients sort out legitimate, useful products from those that are just quackery. The first step in providing this assistance is to understand the rules governing the available products and the role the FDA plays in the system.

In 1994, the US Congress passed an important bill, the Dietary Supplement Health and Education Act of 1994 (DSHEA), that governs the sale and marketing of dietary supplements. Also known as alternative medicines, vitamins, minerals, herbs, medical foods, or amino acids, these products are in a gray area between regular foods and medications.

As a result of this bill, products labeled as dietary supplements may make 3 types of claims on their labels:

- **Nutrient-content claims** describe the amount of nutrients contained in the product. Examples include "High in calcium" or "Excellent source of vitamin C."
- **Disease claims** are based on established scientific evidence and describe well-established links between diet and health. Examples include prevention of some birth defects by folic acid supplements and prevention of osteoporosis by calcium supplements.
- **Nutrition support claims** describe relationships between dietary intake and disease or health, such as the use of vitamin C in preventing scurvy. They may include "structure-function claims," such as "calcium builds strong bones" or "antioxidants maintain cell integrity."

The FDA (Figure 3-2), in implementing DSHEA, required that dietary supplements carry a "Supplement Facts" panel, similar to the "Nutrition Facts" panel you see on most foods. The supplement's panel includes the following:

- Appropriate serving size.
- Information on 14 nutrients, when present at significant levels, including sodium, vitamin A, vitamin C, calcium, and iron.
- The presence of other vitamins and minerals if they are added or are part of the product's nutritional claims.
- Dietary ingredients for which no Reference Daily Intakes have been established.
- For proprietary blends of ingredients (for example, a mixture of herbs for the liver), the names of the ingredients and the total amount of ingredients. The specific amount of each ingredient is not required.

A key point regarding dietary supplements is that they are not reviewed and regulated by the FDA in the same way as drugs. For a drug to be marketed in the United States, a sponsoring company must prove to the FDA that the drug is both safe and effective. In contrast, dietary supplement companies must merely notify the FDA at least 75 days before a product is to go on the market. The FDA can only stop the company from marketing the product if the agency can prove that the product is not safe. Efficacy is not considered with dietary supplements. So, in terms of both FDA process and the onus of responsibility, dietary supplements are the opposite of drugs. With drugs, manufacturers must convince the FDA that new medications are safe and effective before they are allowed to market products containing that agent. With dietary supplements, the FDA must prove lack of safety, within 75 days, in order to stop a manufacturer from marketing a product. In addition, manufacturing processes are more loosely regulated with dietary supplements as compared with drug products.

Risk Evaluation and Mitigation Strategies

Pharmacists and pharmacy technicians are at the front lines of the health care system and have a unique role in communicating drug risks to patients at the dispensing point. In the 1970s, the FDA began requiring **patient package inserts** to be dispensed with oral contraceptives and estrogen-containing drug products to standardize information that was provided to patients about these products. These inserts were one of the FDA's first formal efforts to communicate specific drug risks to patients through added labeling.

During the 1990s, the FDA began employing "restricted distribution," or "restricted access," programs to limit availability of selected drug products that were thought to be of significant risk if used inappropriately. These drug products included clozapine (Clozaril—Novartis), thalidomide (Thalomid—Celgene), isotretinoin products (Accutane—Roche, Amnesteem—Mylan, others), and dofetilide (Tikosyn—Pfizer). Drugs included in these programs had special requirements for physicians and other prescribers, patients, and pharmacies. For example, pharmacy registration and documentation of laboratory monitoring with a national registry are required to dispense clozapine to help prevent and detect life-threatening agranulocytosis, serious low white blood cell counts, and other cardiovascular and respiratory effects.

In addition, the FDA ruled in 1999 that it could require manufacturer-produced **medication guides** for any drug product under certain conditions in which a drug has serious risks and adverse effects that may be prevented by dispensing information to patients. In these cases, patient adherence to provided directions is crucial for a drug's safety. This process was formalized in 2007 with passage of the Food and Drug Administration Amendments Act. This granted the FDA broad authority to require **Risk Evaluation and Mitigation Strategies (REMS)** for certain medications with serious safety concerns to help ensure the benefits of the medication outweigh its risks. Required REMS components may include:

- a medication guide;
- elements to ensure safe use, for example, a patient registry;
- a communication plan; and/or
- an implementation system, such as prescriber and pharmacist training.

Figure 3-2 | Nutrition Facts Label

What's New With the Nutrition Facts Label?

The U.S. Food and Drug Administration (FDA) has updated the Nutrition Facts label on packaged foods and drinks. FDA is requiring changes to the Nutrition Facts label based on updated scientific information, new nutrition research, and input from the public. This is the first major update to the label in over 20 years. The refreshed design and updated information will make it easier for you to make informed food choices that contribute to lifelong healthy eating habits. So, what's changed?

Original Label

Nutrition Facts

Serving Size 2/3 cup (55g)
Servings Per Container 8

Amount Per Serving

Calories 230	Calories from Fat 72

	% Daily Value*
Total Fat 8g	**12%**
Saturated Fat 1g	**5%**
Trans Fat 0g	
Cholesterol 0mg	**0%**
Sodium 160mg	**7%**
Total Carbohydrate 37g	**12%**
Dietary Fiber 4g	**16%**
Sugars 12g	
Protein 3g	

Vitamin A	10%
Vitamin C	8%
Calcium	20%
Iron	45%

* Percent Daily Values are based on a 2,000 calorie diet. Your daily value may be higher or lower depending on your calorie needs.

	Calories:	2,000	2,500
Total Fat	Less than	65g	80g
Sat Fat	Less than	20g	25g
Cholesterol	Less than	300mg	300mg
Sodium	Less than	2,400mg	2,400mg
Total Carbohydrate		300g	375g
Dietary Fiber		25g	30g

New Label

Nutrition Facts

8 servings per container

Serving size	**2/3 cup (55g)**

Amount per serving

Calories	**230**

	% Daily Value*
Total Fat 8g	**10%**
Saturated Fat 1g	**5%**
Trans Fat 0g	
Cholesterol 0mg	**0%**
Sodium 160mg	**7%**
Total Carbohydrate 37g	**13%**
Dietary Fiber 4g	**14%**
Total Sugars 12g	
Includes 10g Added Sugars	**20%**
Protein 3g	

Vitamin D 2mcg	10%
Calcium 260mg	20%
Iron 8mg	45%
Potassium 235mg	6%

* The % Daily Value (DV) tells you how much a nutrient in a serving of food contributes to a daily diet. 2,000 calories a day is used for general nutrition advice.

1. The serving size now appears in larger, bold font and some serving sizes have been updated.

2. Calories are now displayed in larger, bolder font.

3. Daily Values have been updated.

4. Added sugars, vitamin D, and potassium are now listed. Manufacturers must declare the amount in addition to percent Daily Value for vitamins and minerals.

— The New —
Nutrition Facts Label
What's in it for you?

March 2020 — 1

(figure continues on next page)

Figure 3-2 (continued)

1 Serving Sizes Get Real

Servings per container and serving size information appear in large, bold font. Serving sizes have also been updated to better reflect the amount people typically eat and drink today. NOTE: The serving size is not a recommendation of how much to eat.

- The nutrition information listed on the Nutrition Facts label is usually based on one serving of the food; however some containers may also have information displayed per package.
- One package of food may contain more than one serving.

2 Calories Go Big

Calories are now in larger and bolder font to make the information easier to find and use.

2,000 calories a day is used as a guide for general nutrition advice. Your calorie needs may be higher or lower depending on your age, sex, height, weight, and physical activity level. Check your calorie needs at https://www.choosemyplate.gov/resources/MyPlatePlan.

3 The Lows and Highs of % Daily Value

The percent Daily Value (%DV) shows how much a nutrient in a serving of food contributes to a total daily diet. Daily Values for nutrients have been updated, which may make the percent Daily Value higher or lower on the new Nutrition Facts label. As a general guide:

- **5% DV or less** of a nutrient per serving is considered **low**.
- **20% DV or more** of a nutrient per serving is considered **high**.

The footnote at the bottom of the label has been updated to better explain %DV.

Nutrients: The Updated List

What information is no longer required on the label?

Calories from fat has been removed because research shows the type of fat consumed is more important than the amount.

Vitamin A and C are no longer required on the label since deficiencies of these vitamins are rare today. These nutrients can be included on a voluntary basis.

Learn more about the new Nutrition Facts label at: www.FDA.gov/NewNutritionFactsLabel

March 2020 — **2**

Figure 3-2 (continued)

Nutrients: The Updated List (Continued)

What information was added to the label?

Added sugars have been added to the label because consuming too much added sugars can make it hard to meet nutrient needs while staying within calorie limits. Added sugars include sugars that are added during the processing of foods (such as sucrose or dextrose), foods packaged as sweeteners (such as table sugar), sugars from syrups and honey, and sugars from concentrated fruit or vegetable juices.

Vitamin D and potassium are now required to be listed on the label because Americans do not always get the recommended amounts. Diets higher in vitamin D and potassium can reduce the risk of osteoporosis and high blood pressure, respectively.

What vitamins and minerals stayed the same?

Calcium and iron will continue to be listed on the label because Americans do not always get the recommended amounts. Diets higher in calcium and iron can reduce the risk of osteoporosis and anemia, respectively.

Make The Label Work For *You*

Use the label to support your personal dietary needs—choose foods that contain more of the nutrients you want to get more of and less of nutrients you may want to limit.

More often, choose foods that are:

- Higher in dietary fiber, vitamin D, calcium, iron, and potassium.
- Lower in saturated fat, sodium, and added sugars.

Choosing healthier foods and beverages can help reduce the risk of developing some health conditions, such as high blood pressure, cardiovascular disease, osteoporosis, and anemia.

Learn more about the new Nutrition Facts label at: www.FDA.gov/NewNutritionFactsLabel

March 2020 — **3**

Source: US Food and Drug Administration.

Medication Guides

Medication guides are the most frequently used mechanism to meet REMS requirements. The FDA can require a medication guide as part of a REMS program if 1 or more of the following circumstances exists:

1. Patient labeling could help prevent serious adverse effects related to the drug.
2. The drug poses serious risks relative to benefits that could affect patients' decisions to use, or continue to use, the product.
3. Patient adherence to directions for the drug's use is crucial to the drug's effectiveness and the patient's health.

If a medication guide is required as part of a REMS program, the guide must be dispensed to the patient, or the patient's representative, upon request or each time that a drug is dispensed in an outpatient setting and will be used without the supervision of a health care professional. A medication guide may also be required in other circumstances, such as after a significant change to the medication guide or if the REMS requires a review of the medication guide with the patient to ensure safe use.

A complete listing of drugs that require medication guides is available on the FDA's website (https://www.fda.gov/drugs/drug-safety-and-availability/medication-guides).

Individual REMS Requirements

Most of the drugs previously classified as restricted distribution have been transitioned to individual REMS requirements. This means that the requirement is limited to a single drug in a given category or class. Drug products with significant individual REMS requirements include the following:

- Epoetin alfa injection (Epogen—Amgen, Procrit—Janssen)
- Thalidomide
- Alosetron (Lotronex—Prometheus)

Shared System REMS Requirements

Some drug categories or classes have shared system REMS. This means that all agents in the class have the same REMS requirements. Drug products with

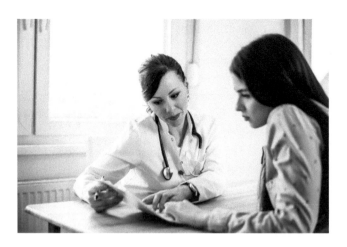

significant shared system REMS requirements include the following:

- Isotretinoin products
- Extended-release and long-acting opioid products
- Transmucosal immediate-release fentanyl products (Actiq—Cephalon, Fentora—Cephalon, others)

It is important to follow these REMS requirements and document dispensing of these agents exactly as specified. As a pharmacy technician, you have an important role in ensuring compliance with these programs.

Centers for Medicare and Medicaid Services

The CMS administers federal coverage of health care in the United States. It was previously known as the Health Care Financing Administration (HCFA) from its inception in 1965, during the Great Society phase of the Lyndon B. Johnson administration, until it was renamed in 2001 during the George W. Bush administration.

Although the Medicare and Medicaid programs sound similar in name, there are some key differences. Medicare pays for acute hospital care for those aged 65 years and older and for those who are disabled. Medicaid provides coverage for indigent patients, meaning those without insurance or enough money to pay for care on their own.

Prescription Drug Coverage: Medicare Part D Versus Medicaid

Since the 2006 implementation of a federal drug benefit, Medicare Part D has also provided prescription drug coverage for all beneficiaries. Before this legislation, Medicare paid for prescription drugs only when they were used in an acute-care institution, such as a hospital, or in conjunction with certain medical devices, such as indwelling catheters, which are tubes that go into very large veins of the body. Chapter 9 offers more background on the emergence of this benefit.

In contrast, Medicaid pays for outpatient prescription drugs and other care for indigent patients in community pharmacies, nursing homes, or hospitals. Some people may qualify for both Medicare and Medicaid and are termed "dual eligibles."

It is important to note that the Medicaid program is financed jointly by the federal and state governments, with each contributing about one-half of the funds. Although Medicaid is a federal program, pharmacists' and pharmacy technicians' interactions are usually with the state government's agency that coordinates the program.

Health Care Reform

In 2010, the Affordable Care Act was passed with the intention of increasing benefits and lowering costs for consumers, providing new funding for public health and disease prevention, boosting the health care workforce and infrastructure, and fostering innovation and quality in the health care system. Although the health care reform implementation process continues at the state and federal regulatory level, numerous provisions within the final law impacted pharmacy practice. Specifically, an emphasis on ways that payment and service delivery models could affect expenditures and quality of care led to new opportunities for pharmacists to have significant roles in transitions of care, medication reconciliation, expanded medication therapy management services, value-based care, and other models of health care delivery.

Prescription Drug Plans

Medicare Part D is a federal program that is administered through dozens of private prescription drug plans (PDPs). Every PDP has its own formulary, and Medicare beneficiaries can choose any PDP operating in their geographic area, which is usually a state. When it comes to obtaining reimbursement for prescriptions and getting approval for nonformulary medications, pharmacists' and pharmacy technicians' interactions are generally with these intermediaries. In most cases, Medicare patients present a prescription insurance card and these claims are processed electronically in the same way that Medicaid or other third-party claims are handled.

> Medicare is the program that pays for acute care for those aged 65 years or older and for those who are disabled. Medicaid-covered individuals include those without insurance or who do not have enough money to pay for care on their own.

Medication Therapy Management

As outlined in Figure 3-3, the Medicare Part D program covers medication therapy management (MTM) services for certain patients. The conditions under which PDPs must provide MTM services are

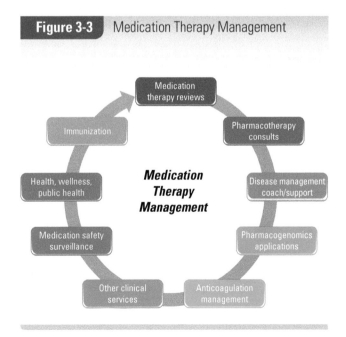

Figure 3-3 Medication Therapy Management

updated annually. These conditions include the use of multiple medications for multiple diseases and an expected total cost of drug therapy in the $3000 range. Currently, pharmacists provide MTM services in all care settings in which patients take medications, via face-to-face or telephone encounters.

Conditions of Participation

In addition to the requirements associated with submitting a claim and processing individual prescriptions, pharmacies must comply with other requirements mandated by CMS and/or state agencies. Broad requirements are referred to as "conditions of participation" because providers—including hospitals, physicians, nursing homes, and pharmacies—must agree to them in order to participate in the Medicare and Medicaid programs. Conditions for participation specify many operational, procedural, and outcome details.

Fraud, Waste, and Abuse

Fraud, waste, and abuse are major issues in the Medicare and Medicaid programs. They occur when health care providers submit false claims or take other actions to get paid more by the programs than they are legitimately due. The federal and state governments pay out billions of dollars each year to providers based on such claims. To counter this, CMS requires fraud, waste, and abuse training for participating pharmacies. This training ensures that pharmacists, technicians, and PDPs have procedures in place to identify and report activities that result in fraud, waste, or abuse of the Medicare and Medicaid systems.

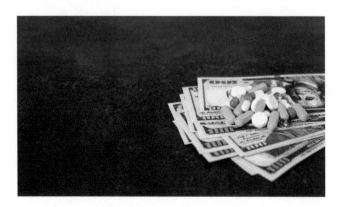

Federal Requirements

Other federal requirements affect pharmacies at the level of dispensing. The Medicaid Tamper-Resistant Prescription Act requires that all handwritten prescriptions for drugs covered by Medicaid include industry-recognized features on prescription blanks that are designed to prevent the following:

- Unauthorized copying of a completed or blank form
- Erasure or modification of information written on the prescription pad by the prescriber
- Use of counterfeit prescription forms

Due to the joint funding of Medicaid programs by state and federal dollars, some states may have additional requirements for processing Medicaid prescriptions.

Drug Enforcement Administration

All medications are dangerous enough to merit special approval by the FDA, but some agents require even more scrutiny and control. Drugs or chemicals with a potential for abuse, physical or psychological addiction, or dependency are called **controlled substances**. These medications can produce physical or psychological withdrawal symptoms if the person discontinues them abruptly. Controlled substances are regulated by the DEA, which is part of the US Department of Justice. Some of these drugs are illegal in the United States. Other controlled substances that have accepted medical uses can be marketed, but their label must prominently display a large letter C and a Roman numeral indicating their class to show that they are subject to special regulations. These drug classes are outlined below.

History

In 1970, the Comprehensive Drug Abuse Prevention and Control Act and the Controlled Substances Act were passed, which created the DEA and gave it responsibility for both regulating the medical use of controlled substances and combating illicit drug trafficking.

Controlled Substance Regulations

The DEA has the authority to specify which drugs need special controls. These drugs are defined in 5 categories of controlled substances:

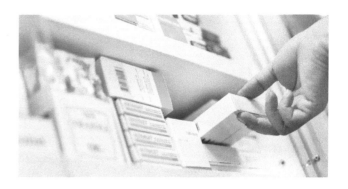

- **Schedule I** drugs have high abuse and addiction potential and have no accepted medical use in the United States. Examples include heroin, LSD, marijuana, and mescaline.
- **Schedule II** drugs have high abuse and addiction potential but do have medical applications. Examples include cocaine, Dilaudid (hydromorphone), Ritalin (methylphenidate), Seconal (secobarbital), and several types of amphetamines.
- **Schedule III** drugs have abuse and addiction potential but not as much as those in Schedule II. Examples include some combination hydrocodone or codeine products.
- **Schedule IV** drugs have a low potential for abuse. Examples include Valium (diazepam) and Halcion (triazolam).
- **Schedule V** drugs have relatively low abuse potential and consist mainly of preparations containing very limited amounts of a controlled substance in each dose. Examples include Lomotil (diphenoxylate and atropine) and some cough syrups containing codeine.

Pharmacy Regulations for Schedule II Substances

The DEA requires that pharmacies, wholesalers, and distributors keep accurate and meticulous records for controlled substances. All entities that prepare, handle, or distribute controlled substances must register with the DEA using **DEA Form 224** (available online at https://www.deadiversion.usdoj.gov/drugreg/reg_apps/224/224_instruct.htm). Through the pharmacist in charge, the pharmacy must be able to account for every dose of Schedule II controlled substances and keep a **perpetual inventory**, an ongoing record, that the DEA can inspect at any time. In addition, the DEA requires that a manual inventory—physically counting each tablet, capsule, and injection in the pharmacy—be performed every 2 years, usually on May 1st of odd-numbered years. Similar records based on approximate counts of Schedule III, IV, and V drugs must also be kept.

Pharmacy technicians often assist with ordering and maintaining controlled substances inventory. **DEA Form 222**, as shown in Figure 3-4, is used for ordering Schedule II controlled substances. The DEA Form 222 is supplied in triplicate, or pharmacies may use the Controlled Substance Ordering System (CSOS), which allows for secure electronic transmission of Schedule I-V controlled substance orders without the supporting paper DEA Form 222. Paper forms and the online submission portal can be found on the DEA website: https://www.deadiversion.usdoj.gov/online_forms_apps.html. In pharmacies using only the paper copy of DEA Form 222, the 3 copies are processed as follows:

- Copies 1 and 2 are sent to the supplier, usually a drug wholesaler but sometimes the drug manufacturer.
- Copy 3 is filed at the pharmacy.

When the pharmacy receives the order from the supplier, copy 3 of DEA Form 222 is pulled. The pharmacist processing the order should record on copy 3 the date and amount of drug product received. Copy 3 is then refiled and kept for 2 years.

The CSOS to order controlled substances online has been designed to ensure confidentiality of communications, authentication of the sending party, integrity of communications (the recipient can tell if the order was changed in transit), and nonrepudiation (using DEA-supplied electronic signatures that are difficult to forge). Electronic records supporting each transaction

Figure 3-4 DEA Order Form

See Reverse of PURCHASER'S Copy for Instructions	No order form may be issued for Schedule I and II substances unless a completed application form has been received. (21 CFR 1305.04).	OMB APPROVAL No. 1117-0010

TO: *(Name of Supplier)* | **STREET ADDRESS**

			TO BE FILLED IN BY PURCHASER	
CITY and STATE	**DATE**	**NATIONAL DRUG CODE**	**No. of Packages Received**	**Date Received**

Line No.	No. of Packages	Size of Packages	Name of Item		No. of Packages Received	Date Received
			TO BE FILLED IN BY PURCHASER			
1						
2						
3						
4						
5						
6						
7						
8						
9						
10						

◄ **LAST LINE COMPLETED** *(MUST BE 10 OR LESS)* | **SIGNATURE OF PURCHASER OR ATTORNEY OR AGENT**

Date Issued	DEA Registration No.	Name and Address of Registrant
Schedules		
Registered as a	No. of this Order Form	

DEA Form-222
(Oct. 1992)

U.S. OFFICIAL ORDER FORMS - SCHEDULES I & II
DRUG ENFORCEMENT ADMINISTRATION
PURCHASER'S Copy 3

Source: US Dept of Justice Drug Enforcement Administration.

must be retained for 2 years, similar to the paper copies of DEA Form 222, and suppliers are required to report transactions to the DEA within 2 business days.

Requirements for Transferring Schedule III, IV, and V Prescriptions

There are also special requirements for transferring Schedule III, IV, and V controlled substance prescriptions from one pharmacy to another. These requirements are in addition to the documentation and rules required for noncontrolled substance prescription transfers. Controlled substance prescriptions can be transferred only 1 time, and the transfer process must be conducted between 2 licensed pharmacists. For paper prescriptions, the pharmacists must note in writing that the outgoing prescription is "VOID" and the incoming prescription is a "TRANSFER." For electronic prescriptions, the transferring pharmacist must deactivate the voided prescription and the receiving pharmacist should create a new electronic record for the prescription and all its information. Both parties must document the other pharmacist's name and pharmacy DEA number. The receiving pharmacy should also document the name, address, and original prescription number from the transferring pharmacy. Check with your pharmacist to verify specific laws and regulations in your state, as additional rules may apply.

Handling Expired Controlled Substances

A final area of concern about controlled substances is what to do when drugs expire. Because of the need to account for all controlled substances to the DEA, the pharmacy cannot just dispose of or return these agents in the same manner used for noncontrolled medications.

Always follow company or pharmacy policy regarding the disposal of controlled substances. Generally, DEA Form 222 is used for returning controlled substances to the manufacturer. The physical return is usually processed through a **reverse distributor**, a type of company that can legally transport controlled substances and provide an appropriate monetary credit to the pharmacy. If outdated or damaged controlled substances are destroyed, **DEA Form 41** must be completed with 2 or more licensed individuals who must witness the destruction of the controlled substances. Similar procedures may apply in hospitals or nursing homes when controlled substances are returned to the pharmacy after patients are discharged or die. In the case of controlled substance theft, **DEA Form 106** must be completed after the local DEA diversion office and police are notified.

Preventing Drug Diversion

Pharmacy technicians should take special care when processing or handling orders or prescriptions for controlled substances, especially those in Schedule II. Most forged prescriptions are for controlled substances. When receiving a prescription for one of these agents, the technician should first verify the patient's name and get his or her address—these are DEA requirements. If anything about the prescription looks unusual, quietly but immediately alert a pharmacist. Forged prescriptions may:

- Have altered quantities
- Be written on prescription forms that were stolen or photocopied
- Be written on prescription forms from hospitals that do not have a specific physician's name
- Be written on prescription forms from distant cities or even another state

The prescriber's name, address, and DEA number must be on the prescription. DEA numbers should be verified for new prescribers using the following procedure:

- Check DEA number to be sure it has 2 letters and 7 numbers (e.g., AA9999999).
- Add up the first, third, and fifth digits, and record the result as SUM1.
- Add up the second, fourth, and sixth digits. Multiply the result by 2, and record the result as SUM2.
- Add SUM1 to SUM2 to obtain SUM3.

In valid DEA numbers, the seventh digit will be the second digit of SUM3. If it is not, then the DEA number is not valid.

For example, the DEA number AP1857397 can be checked as follows:

- Two letters and 7 digits are present.
- The sum of the first, third, and fifth digits is 9 (SUM1).
- The sum of the second, fourth, and sixth digits is 24. Twice this amount is 48 (SUM2).
- The sum of 48 and 9 is 57 (SUM3: second digit is 7).
- The seventh digit of the DEA number is 7, so the number is legitimate.

Patient Information Initiatives

An important role of pharmacists is to ensure that patients understand what drugs they are taking, what each drug is for, and how each drug is to be taken. Some drugs taken by mouth should be taken on an empty stomach, whereas others must be taken with food. Patients often need to learn how to use specialized administration devices like inhalers or to give injections of drugs, such as insulin.

> An important role of pharmacists is to ensure that patients understand what drugs they are taking, what each drug is for, and how each drug is to be taken.

Because pharmacists play a key role in educating patients, the federal government has taken specific measures to ensure that this information is conveyed to patients consistently, access to a pharmacist is provided, and patient confidentiality is ensured.

Omnibus Budget Reconciliation Act of 1990

In 1990, Congress passed the Omnibus Budget Reconciliation Act (OBRA '90). Among its other provisions, the bill required that pharmacists offer to counsel patients whose prescriptions were being paid for under Medicaid—1 of 2 major federal health reimbursement plans. The bill also required state Medicaid administrators, who oversee the programs, to conduct reviews of drug use in each state to ensure drugs are being optimally used.

The implications of OBRA '90 for technicians are 2-fold. First, because the counseling requirement was added to state regulations by most state boards of pharmacy, all patients should be offered pharmacist counseling. If a patient asks for counseling, notify a pharmacist. Under OBRA '90, the pharmacist is required to discuss with the patient or caregiver the following information:

- Name and description of the medication
- Dosage form, dose, route of administration, and duration of drug therapy
- Special directions and precautions for preparation, administration, and use of the medication
- Common or severe side effects, adverse reactions, or interactions and therapeutic contraindications that may be encountered, including ways to avoid them and the action required if they occur
- Techniques for self-monitoring of drug therapy
- Proper storage
- Prescription refill information
- Action to be taken in the event of a missed dose

In addition, the pharmacist is required under OBRA '90 to record and maintain the following information:

- Patient's name, address, telephone number, date of birth (or age), and sex
- Patient's individual history when important, including diseases, known allergies and drug reactions, and a comprehensive list of medications and relevant medical devices
- Pharmacist's comments about the individual's drug therapy

Second, the drug utilization review (DUR) requirement is typically done in real time by computer. This means that while technicians are entering prescription orders into the pharmacy's computer, various alerts may pop up on the computer screen notifying the pharmacist of drug interactions, clinical problems, or reimbursement problems. You will need to refer many of these alerts to the pharmacist for a decision about whether to dispense the prescription, talk with the patient, or contact the prescriber.

Americans with Disabilities Act

Disabilities are diverse and may include severe physical problems that confine people to wheelchairs and learning disabilities that must be compensated for in classrooms and testing situations. Whatever the nature of the disability, the Americans with Disabilities Act (ADA) mandates various actions that must be taken by employers and businesses throughout the United States.

Within pharmacies, ADA requirements may be as simple as the elimination of barriers such as steps, narrow doors, or aisles that cannot be navigated by people in wheelchairs. Or they may include providing accommodations for an employee with a speech, hearing, or visual disability. Talk with the pharmacists and managers in your pharmacy about what steps have

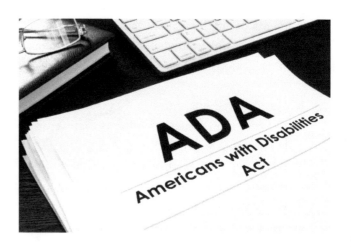

been taken in the dispensing process to comply with the ADA and about any areas that can be improved in this regard. ADA modifications may extend beyond drugs to medical devices available in some pharmacies. For example, many blood glucose meters are often marketed for patients with disabilities, such as visually impaired patients. Check with your pharmacy wholesaler or the product manufacturer about availability of medical devices with accessibility features. You may also be able to order assistive devices such as pill bottle openers, automatic dispensers, or pill alarms to help patients with disabilities adhere to their medication regimen. More information about ADA is available from www.ada.gov; 800-514-0301 (voice); 800-514-0383 (TTY).

Health Insurance Portability and Accountability Act

The Health Insurance Portability and Accountability Act of 1996 (HIPAA) requires that all health care providers ensure that patient confidentiality is maintained in all communications with patients. HIPAA defines under federal law what constitutes "protected health information" (PHI), including documents kept on paper, documents in electronic form, and oral communications. Health care providers must not disclose PHI unless treatment, payment, or health care operations are involved or they have patient permission to disclose information outside these areas.

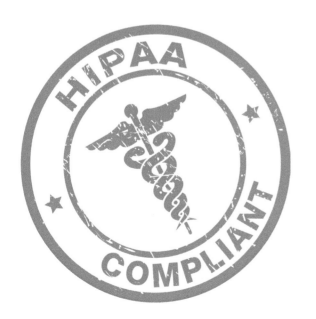

Health care providers, including most pharmacies, must give patients a written Notice of Privacy Practices. The notice must describe how the Privacy Rule allows providers to use and disclose PHI and state that a patient's permission is necessary before their health records are shared for any other reason. The notice must summarize the organization's duties to protect PHI and communicate patients' privacy rights, including the right to complain to the Department of Health and Human Services and to the organization if an individual believes their privacy rights have been violated. Finally, this notice should include instructions for contacting the organization for more information and to make a complaint.

Pharmacies and other health providers must appoint a **privacy officer** who is responsible for ensuring that all policies and procedures are followed, documentation and filing is performed correctly, and patient requests for PHI are responded to in a timely fashion. In addition, the privacy officer monitors for changes to HIPAA regulations and ensures continued compliance. The privacy officer may be any member of the pharmacy staff, including a pharmacy technician.

Pharmacies should ensure that PHI is disposed of correctly and not disclosed incorrectly but also provide patients with access to their own PHI. Your pharmacy will have specific training and procedures to comply with HIPAA that you should follow carefully. State attorneys general can impose fines up to $250,000 for violations that are of the same type and occur in a single year or up to $1.5 million per violation category per year in the event of a pharmacy HIPAA violation.

Pseudoephedrine

The Combat Methamphetamine Act of 2005 subjected products containing ephedrine, pseudoephedrine, and phenylpropanolamine to sales restrictions, storage limits, and recordkeeping requirements to help prevent diversion of these substances for the production of "crystal meth." This act limited sales to 3.6 grams per day or 90 grams per 30 days of the base products. Pharmacies must store products behind the counter and keep a written or electronic logbook of name and quantity of product sold, names and addresses of purchasers, and date and time of sales.

State Boards of Pharmacy

The division of responsibilities between the state and federal governments follows the line of reasoning known as states' rights: all responsibilities not specifically assigned to the federal government by the US Constitution are reserved for the states. Drug and pharmacy regulations are not mentioned in the Constitution and therefore are delegated to the states. However, this has been an area in which the federal government has creatively enlarged its role when it believed that public health was at risk. But, for now, states remain the main regulatory authority for pharmacies, pharmacists, and technicians. However, in any case where there is disagreement between federal and state law, you should follow the more restrictive of the 2 laws.

States regulate professions through boards composed largely of members of the profession with a smaller number of consumer members. Federal laws do not specifically deal with regulation of the professions. As mentioned earlier, the FDA's legend drugs do not specify what types of practitioners may legally prescribe these drugs. Federal law often depends heavily on the framework present in individual states.

State boards of pharmacy were developed around 1900 based on the recommendations of the American Pharmacists Association in its model pharmacy laws. Pharmacy organizations and pharmacy laws have often grown together, and the organization of the state boards followed this trend. State boards of pharmacy, based on authority granted to them by the various state legislatures, promulgate the specific regulations that govern the practice of pharmacy on a day-to-day basis. Boards issue licenses to pharmacists and pharmacies, and many register technicians.

The National Association of Boards of Pharmacy (NABP) was formed in 1904. It has grown to hold a powerful position in coordinating activities among the state boards. It now provides a national examination, called the NAPLEX (North American Pharmacist Licensure Examination), for administration in all states. NABP coordinates the reciprocation of pharmacist licenses between states. The association develops model pharmacy practice acts that state legislatures can consider when updating state laws to incorporate changes in pharmacy. NABP also certifies Internet pharmacies as having met minimum criteria that their activities are within federal and state laws.

The NABP defines pharmacy technicians as "personnel registered with the Board who may, under the supervision of the pharmacist, assist in the pharmacy and perform such functions as assisting in the dispensing process; processing medical coverage claims; stocking medications; cashiering, but excluding drug regimen review; clinical conflict resolution; prescriber contact concerning prescription drug order clarification or therapy modification; patient counseling; dispensing process validation; prescription transfer; and receipt of new prescription drug orders."

It is impossible to convey the specifics of each state's pharmacy board regulations in a national text. Instead, you will need to become familiar with the rules for the states in which you work. Talk with your employer or the pharmacists with whom you work about what you need to know. In addition, the addresses and telephone numbers of the state boards of pharmacy are available from the NABP (https://nabp.pharmacy/about/boards-of-pharmacy/). You may contact your state board directly for information.

Voluntary Accreditation

In addition to legal requirements for practicing pharmacy, pharmacists and pharmacies often voluntarily participate in other types of oversight programs. For instance, pharmacists may choose to train pharmacy residents. This opens up the pharmacy to inspection by national accrediting bodies for residency programs.

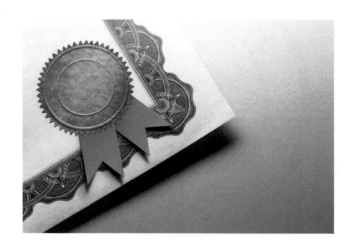

A hospital may want to be reimbursed through certain federal or private payers, and these organizations may require accreditation through CMS or voluntary alternatives. In all of these situations, surveyors visit the hospital or pharmacy and assess its compliance with certain standards of practice, care, and quality. Opportunities for accreditation now exist for pharmacies, pharmacy resident and technician training, schools of pharmacy, hospitals, and many other health care entities.

The major accrediting body in health care is The Joint Commission (https://www.jointcommission.org/), a nongovernmental body. The Joint Commission accredits and certifies more than 22,000 health care organizations and programs in the United States, including hospitals and health care organizations that provide ambulatory and office-based surgery, behavioral health, home health care, laboratory, and nursing care center services. Because The Joint Commission accreditation can take the place of visits by CMS officials for providers such as hospitals and clinical laboratories, accreditation is a major focus of health systems and pharmacies offering long-term care services.

Other accreditation processes exist for pharmacy settings outside of health systems. The NABP's Community Pharmacy Accreditation is a 3-year accreditation targeted toward community pharmacies providing an advanced level of services that are looking to (1) demonstrate compliance to a set of practice standards and (2) exhibit consistency in delivering optimal patient care programs and services. The application process and criteria for accreditation, as well as a link to download the accreditation standards, are available at https://nabp.pharmacy/programs/accreditations-inspections/community-pharmacy/. The American Society of Health-Systems Pharmacists (ASHP) has developed accreditation standards for specialty pharmacies, telehealth pharmacies, community and outpatient pharmacies, and international pharmacy services. The ASHP accreditation standards focus on optimal care delivery through evaluation of:

- Effective patient care plans to achieve desired medication therapy outcomes
- Patient-specific assessments and optimal collection, use, and documentation of information

- Inclusion of specialty drug-specific assessment and disease state-specific assessment requirements
- Comprehensive review of the patient's medication history and medication list prior to each fill
- Documentation of all pharmacy case management activities
- Patient consultation and education
- Quality metrics and quality improvement plans

More information on ASHP accreditation is available at https://www.ashp.org/Products-and-Services/ASHP-Accreditation-Programs.

Pharmacy Facilities and Equipment Requirements

Legal and regulatory requirements also exist for pharmacy facilities themselves. Some of these requirements depend on the type of products or services available at the pharmacy. Examples include storing Schedule II controlled substances in a locked cabinet or keeping refrigerated drugs at the appropriate temperature. Storage requirements for medications and expiration dating are reviewed in Chapter 4.

In many cases, state boards of pharmacy regulate equipment or facilities that are required to operate a pharmacy. Generally, a pharmacy should possess basic equipment for measuring and mixing, such as a Class A balance, pharmacy weights, graduated cylinder, mortar and pestle, adequate counter space, separate refrigerator for medications, lockable cabinet for Schedule II medications, a sink with hot and cold water, and an alarm system. Equipment must be clean and in good operating condition. Pharmacy areas should be clean and uncluttered.

If your pharmacy provides compounding services, additional equipment and procedures will be needed. The USP, which sets standards for the quality and purity of many products and processes, provides guidelines for sterile and nonsterile compounding in pharmacies in 2 of its standards. USP <797> provides procedures and quality assurance requirements for facilities involved in the preparation, storage, or dispensing of sterile products to help ensure product sterility and decrease contamination. USP <795> provides procedures and quality assurance requirements for nonsterile compounding. Chapters 12 and 13 contain more information on implementing these standards and guidelines in the pharmacy.

Technicians should check with their pharmacist or state board of pharmacy for information on requirements that are specific to their state or the type of services provided in the pharmacy.

Safety Data Sheets

The Occupational Safety and Health Administration (OSHA), under the 2012 Hazard Communication Standard, requires that chemical manufacturers, distributors, or importers provide Safety Data Sheets (SDSs) (formerly Material Safety Data Sheets [MSDSs]) for each hazardous chemical to communicate information on these hazards (Figure 3-5). OSHA, a unit in the US Department of Labor, requires that work sites where hazardous chemicals are used or stored do the following:

- Identify and list hazardous chemicals.
- Obtain information, in the form of SDSs, about hazardous chemicals from manufacturers, importers, or distributors of the chemicals.
- Develop and implement a written hazard communication program, including labels on the products, SDSs, and employee training.
- When necessitated by spills or employee exposure, communicate hazard information to employees.

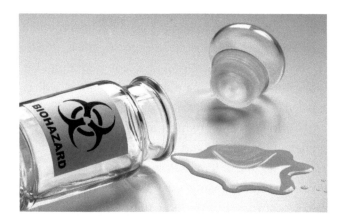

| Figure 3-5 | OSHA Quick Card: Hazard Communication Safety Data Sheets |

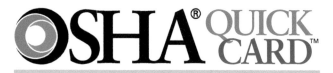

Hazard Communication Safety Data Sheets

The Hazard Communication Standard (HCS) requires chemical manufacturers, distributors, or importers to provide Safety Data Sheets (SDSs) (formerly known as Material Safety Data Sheets or MSDSs) to communicate the hazards of hazardous chemical products. The HCS requires new SDSs to be in a uniform format, and include the section numbers, the headings, and associated information under the headings below:

Section 1, Identification includes product identifier; manufacturer or distributor name, address, phone number; emergency phone number; recommended use; restrictions on use.

Section 2, Hazard(s) identification includes all hazards regarding the chemical; required label elements.

Section 3, Composition/information on ingredients includes information on chemical ingredients; trade secret claims.

Section 4, First-aid measures includes important symptoms/effects, acute, delayed; required treatment.

Section 5, Fire-fighting measures lists suitable extinguishing techniques, equipment; chemical hazards from fire.

Section 6, Accidental release measures lists emergency procedures; protective equipment; proper methods of containment and cleanup.

Section 7, Handling and storage lists precautions for safe handling and storage, including incompatibilities.

(Continued on other side)

For more information:

OSHA® Occupational Safety and Health Administration
www.osha.gov (800) 321-OSHA (6742)

OSHA 3493-01R 2016

Figure 3-5 (continued)

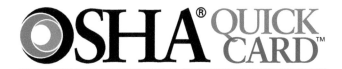

Hazard Communication Safety Data Sheets

Section 8, Exposure controls/personal protection lists OSHA's Permissible Exposure Limits (PELs); ACGIH Threshold Limit Values (TLVs); and any other exposure limit used or recommended by the chemical manufacturer, importer, or employer preparing the SDS where available as well as appropriate engineering controls; personal protective equipment (PPE).

Section 9, Physical and chemical properties lists the chemical's characteristics.

Section 10, Stability and reactivity lists chemical stability and possibility of hazardous reactions.

Section 11, Toxicological information includes routes of exposure; related symptoms, acute and chronic effects; numerical measures of toxicity.

Section 12, Ecological information*
Section 13, Disposal considerations*
Section 14, Transport information*
Section 15, Regulatory information*

Section 16, Other information, includes the date of preparation or last revision.

*Note: Since other Agencies regulate this information, OSHA will not be enforcing Sections 12 through 15 (29 CFR 1910.1200(g)(2)).

Employers must ensure that SDSs are readily accessible to employees.
See Appendix D of 29 CFR 1910.1200 for a detailed description of SDS contents.

For more information:

 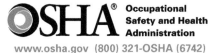 **Occupational Safety and Health Administration**
U.S. Department of Labor   www.osha.gov (800) 321-OSHA (6742)

OSHA defines hazardous chemicals as those that can cause physical damage and those that pose a danger to health. Chemicals used or stored in pharmacies may be flammable or explosive, falling into the first category. Several drugs fall into the latter category, including many agents used to treat cancer.

As a pharmacy technician, you will need to know how these OSHA requirements have been addressed in your pharmacy and what to do if an emergency occurs. Talk with your supervisor if this information was not covered in orientation sessions when you were first hired. More information on OSHA requirements is available at: https://www.osha.gov/.

Conclusion

This chapter summarized some of the most important things for you to understand as a practicing pharmacy technician. It may seem like an overwhelming number of rules and laws to remember every day, but you will be surprised how quickly these will all come to mind when you are using them on a daily basis in the pharmacy. Remember that each of the rules and regulations put in place by the FDA, CMS, DEA, state boards of pharmacy, and others exist to ensure that your patients are consistently safe and receiving the appropriate care, drug products, and patient information. When it comes to medications, many of which are very specialized and have powerful effects on the human body, these rules are absolutely necessary.

REFERENCES

1. DiMasi JA, Grabowski HG, Hansen RW. Innovation in the pharmaceutical industry: new estimates of R&D costs. *J Health Econ*. 2016;47:20-33.
2. US Food and Drug Administration. Available at: https://www.fda.gov/. Accessed December 6, 2020.
3. Diversion Control Division, Drug Enforcement Administration. Available at: https://www.deadiversion.usdoj.gov/. Accessed December 6, 2020.

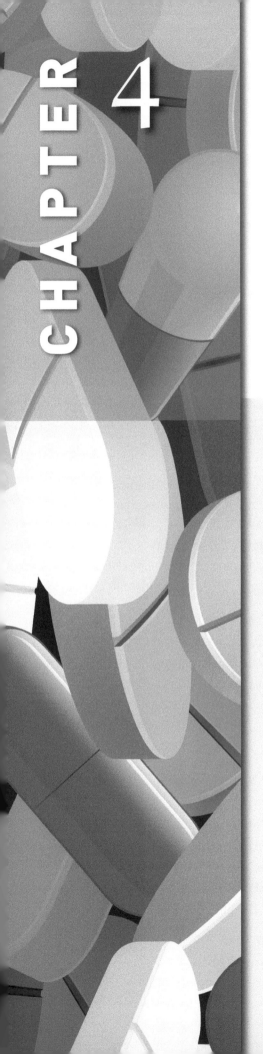

CHAPTER 4

Inventory Control and Management

In many pharmacies, technicians assist with the purchase of pharmaceuticals and other needed products. This chapter provides background on legal, regulatory, and business considerations for ordering and inventory procedures.

Introduction

The job of any manager in the business sector is to create an environment in which the financial and human resources of the firm are used to generate a profit. Even in a small pharmacy, considerable financial resources are invested in the goods for sale. With drug prices being as high as they are, several hundred thousand dollars are tied up in the inventory, equipment, and fixtures of each pharmacy.

> As an employee whose job involves handling your pharmacy's inventory, you can help make the best use of this investment.

As an employee whose job involves handling your pharmacy's inventory, you can help make the best use of this investment. In hospital pharmacies and larger community stores, some technicians specialize in purchasing—they spend the majority of their time checking inventory levels, placing orders, and following up on items not received. To learn about this process, let's start by first exploring the way that drug products are identified and tracked within the supply chain.

Identifying Drug Products for Inventory Tracking

> No matter where a drug product is in the supply chain, it is essential that everyone— pharmacist, technician, patient, or manufacturer— is able to identify it easily.

No matter where a drug product is in the supply chain, it is essential that everyone—pharmacist, technician, patient, or manufacturer—is able to identify it easily. Without a clear way to do this, it would be impossible to keep track of inventory counts and ordering needs. It would also be difficult to determine which patients might be affected in the event of a drug recall. The **National Drug Code (NDC) number** as a drug product identifier is the key piece of information that helps keep track of drug products in the supply chain.

The NDC is a unique 3-segment, 10-digit identification number assigned to each drug product. Each human drug must have an NDC number as a unique product identification number. Further, all NDCs follow a distinct pattern and the numbers correspond to translatable codes.

NDCs follow one of the following numeric sequence configurations to make up the total 10 digits: 4-4-2, 5-3-2, or 5-4-1. For example, the NDC number for a 30-count bottle of Lexapro 10-mg tablets labeled by Physicians Total Care, Inc., is 54868-4700-1, which follows the 5-digit–4-digit–1-digit numeric sequence configuration.

You can "decode" these numbers using the following information:

- The first segment—or the **labeler code**—is assigned by the US Food and Drug Administration (FDA) and identifies the manufacturer or distributor.
- The second segment—or the **product code**—is assigned by the manufacturer, or distributor, and identifies the drug product, including its strength and dosage form.
- The third segment—or the **package code**—is also assigned by the manufacturer, or distributor, and identifies the package size and type.

So, in the Lexapro 10 mg (NDC = 54868-4700-1) example above, the numeric segments tell us the following information:

54868	Labeler code — indicates Physicians Total Care, Inc.
4700	Product code — indicates product is Lexapro 10-mg tablets
1	Package code — indicates package type and size is a bottle of 30

You will not always know what the individual codes translate to, but it's helpful to know that they have a meaning when pulling drugs from the shelf. For example, if you are verifying inventory received from an invoice and a drug package has the incorrect package code in the NDC, this quickly tells you that you have the right drug from the intended manufacturer but in the wrong package size.

> **Tip:** A mismatched NDC in the dispensing process is often the first indicator of a medication error. Stay alert for an NDC that differs from what you expect at any point in the dispensing process—this could indicate that the wrong drug, formulation, strength, or quantity has been pulled or entered.

You also need to know when the drug expires, and in some cases, you may even be able to identify and track a specific production batch. The **manufacturer's expiration date** is printed on the label. This is the date until which the manufacturer can guarantee the full potency and safety of the drug, provided it is stored under required conditions. See Chapter 5 for more on drug storage. The expiration date differs from the beyond-use date that is set for compounds (see Chapters 12 and 13).

Let's look at an example. If you have a bottle of amoxicillin powder for reconstitution on your pharmacy shelf, its expiration date is printed on the bottle by the manufacturer. You can dispense that bottle up to the expiration date—usually up to 1-2 years out—as long as it is stored under the required conditions. Once you add water to mix the suspension, though, you have changed the original powdered product. At this point, a **beyond-use date**—usually 10-14 days—is assigned to indicate how long the mixed suspension is stable for use, regardless of the original product's expiration date.

Manufacturers also assign a **lot number** to each drug. This identifies the drug's internal product batch and is essential in tracing specific products that require recall or removal from inventory. We'll learn more about drug recalls and how to handle them in Chapter 5.

Managing Inventory

To understand the principles behind inventory management and control, think of a newspaper rack in front of your neighborhood coffee shop. During the night, the newspaper carrier puts 10 morning newspapers into the rack. When that carrier returns the next day, what is the ideal number of newspapers that should be remaining?

If sales are to be maximized, then obviously the carrier would like to see an empty rack—all the newspapers sold. However, the carrier would then wonder how many sales had been lost because the rack was empty. In this situation, it is better for the carrier to find 1 newspaper remaining in the rack because that means that as many newspapers as possible were sold without losing any sales.

Inventory management in the pharmacy is similar to this newspaper analogy. In the pharmacy, **inventory management** is the system of ordering, storing, repackaging, and disposing of pharmacy products and merchandise. Pharmacies must have an inventory management system to ensure that needed drugs are available; unexpected shortages of drugs are minimally disruptive to patient care; products get purchased at the best price; and drugs are ordered and disposed of efficiently.

Outlining Inventory Costs

To effectively manage inventory, pharmacies never want to run out of any drug, but they want to keep as little as possible on hand so that **inventory costs** are minimized. Inventory costs encompass the following:

- The **cost of the space**—including rent or mortgage payments, electricity and other utilities, and pharmacy shelving used for product displays or storage. The greater the inventory, the higher the costs.
- The **cost of the drug products**—which can be several hundred dollars for 1 small container.
- The **value of the money**—including finance charges if the inventory was purchased on credit or with borrowed money, or revenue that could have been generated if the money had been put in a savings account or invested in stocks or bonds.

Defining Basic Inventory Terminology

To understand approaches to managing pharmacy inventory, you must first be familiar with basic inventory terminology. Table 4-1 shows key inventory-related terms and definitions.

Table 4-1 Inventory Terminology and Definitions

Term	Definition
Inventory turnover rate	The number of times pharmacies purchase, sell, and replace a product during a specific accounting period.
Periodic automatic replacement (PAR) value or level	The inventory level at which a drug is automatically reordered, or the amount of drug that is automatically reordered. For example, when 2 stock bottles of sertraline 50-mg tablets remain on the shelf, pharmacies may automatically reorder 2 stock bottles of the drug.
Stock rotation	A strategy to manage inventory costs by first using drug products that will expire soonest. So, in the above example, if 2 bottles of sertraline 50 mg are on the shelf, dispense the one that will expire first. This will help to minimize the risk of a product expiring and needing to be returned to the wholesaler for partial credit.
Automated inventory systems	Pharmacy-based computer systems that reconcile actual drug inventory levels in the pharmacy computer when drugs get dispensed, using barcode or other technology. When a drug reaches a predetermined PAR level, it is automatically added to the daily order list or ordered electronically.
Perpetual inventory	A method of inventory control in which the actual quantity of drugs on hand is always maintained in real time via a paper or electronic log, with counts that are updated with each prescription dispensed.

Understanding the Pharmaceutical Supply Chain

Next, you must understand how pharmacies obtain the products they sell and where they send products they no longer need. The major entities in the pharmaceutical supply chain include the following:

- **Manufacturers**—Companies or entities that manufacture, distribute, market, and sell drug products directly to pharmacies. Pharmacies can often get lower prices when they purchase products directly from manufacturers, but they also must order certain minimum quantities.
- **Wholesalers (also referred to as suppliers or distributors)**—These are the "middlemen" in the pharmaceutical supply chain. Wholesalers stock many thousands of items that are generally found in pharmacies, from health and beauty aids to nonprescription agents to the most expensive prescription drugs. As wholesalers have become heavily computerized, they have helped pharmacies to improve their business, financial, and sales analyses based on purchasing patterns.

- **Purchasing groups**—Both hospital and community pharmacies have aligned with each other to increase their purchasing power. By committing to the use of certain common items—such as intravenous fluids and administration sets or specific drugs in commonly used therapeutic categories—members of these purchasing groups can negotiate very favorable prices with manufacturers, wholesalers, or both.
- **Prime vendors**—Many pharmacies also enter into contracts that promise wholesalers a large percentage of the pharmacy's business. In return, these wholesalers—or prime vendors—give special pricing and assist pharmacies in managing inventory levels and costs.
- **Other pharmacies**—When one pharmacy runs out of an item or needs a product they do not usually stock, the staff often borrows from another pharmacy. Ask your pharmacist what other pharmacies in your area to contact for this purpose.
- **Reverse distributors**—Think of these as opposite of wholesalers. When drug products expire and can no longer be dispensed, pharmacies

need to dispose of them in a way that complies with federal and state regulations. In many cases, expired drugs can be returned to the manufacturer or wholesaler for partial credit. Many pharmacies use reverse distributors to facilitate this process. They assist in returning expired or unusable products, help maintain compliance with manufacturers' return policies, and receive and process return credits for the pharmacy.

Calculating Order Quantities

Many pharmacies calculate an **economic order quantity (EOQ)** to help them determine how much of a product to order, as follows:

$$EOQ = \sqrt{\frac{2LM}{W}}$$

L = annual purchases of the item in dollars

M = dollar cost of reordering or issuing a purchase order

W = cost of capital or carrying inventory (interest rate on borrowed funds)

As illustrated in Figure 4-1, the EOQ system creates 3 critical numbers. First, the EOQ is the **ideal amount of inventory** that should be ordered so that the costs of carrying the inventory and the costs of reordering and stocking the inventory are minimized. Next, a **reorder level** must be determined, based on how fast the product is selling and how long it takes to get a new order in. Finally, an **emergency level** is designated so that special actions—such as telephone calls, ordering from a different source, or borrowing—can be taken if the inventory gets too low before the order comes in.

Many pharmacy managers use a "just-in-time" inventory system. As the name suggests, this system is designed to have inventory arrive just as the previous supply is exhausted. For items whose usage and delivery are predictable, this system helps pharmacies minimize inventory costs and stocking levels.

> Many pharmacy managers use a "just-in-time" inventory system designed to have inventory arrive just as the previous supply is exhausted.

Placing Orders

The process of placing orders for pharmaceuticals has become very streamlined with computer and barcode technology (Figure 4-2). In the early days of barcode

---

Figure 4-1   Application of the Economic Order Quantity in Inventory Management

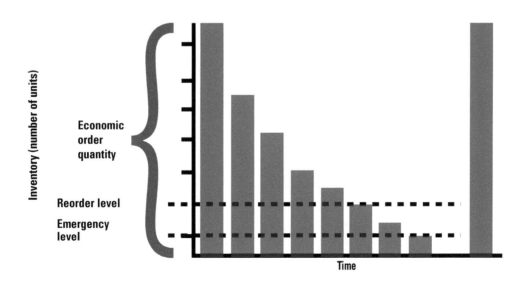

technology, the ordering process was improved by allowing the pharmacist or technician to use a hand-held device to scan labels on pharmacy shelves rather than manually entering order numbers from a hand-written list of items accumulated throughout the day. However, as automation has become more widespread and sophisticated and applications of barcode and scanning technology have been further integrated into pharmacies, the ordering process has become more precise and automatic. In some pharmacy systems, every prescription or medication order dispensed is linked to the pharmacy system through barcode technology. This technology enables the pharmacy computer to track the amount of each drug dispensed daily, track the amount of each drug remaining in stock, maintain a perpetual inventory count, and automatically reorder the amount of each drug that is needed based on preset inventory levels. Alternatively, a list of items and quantities can be generated in a supplier/distributor order form and then edited by the pharmacist or technician to adjust quantities, select substitution items, or add products (Figure 4-3).

Even though the process is becoming increasingly simplified, that does not mean it is any less critical. Whatever role you are asked to play in ordering medications or related products, you should approach the task with the same accuracy and care that you use in filling patients' prescriptions. Make sure you understand what the pharmacist or owner expects, what their views are on inventory management, and how often orders are normally placed.

In addition to computerized systems, pharmacies may still have some vestige of a manual "want book" for making notes about special items that customers have asked for or unusual products that are needed. The **want book**—once the major method of recording needed merchandise—is generally a spiral-bound notebook that all employees use for making notes of orders to be placed. The person who places orders will go through the list, reconcile the items with those already ordered electronically or automatically, and add needed products to the order.

When you are placing special orders for patients or providers, research the information you will likely need for ordering ahead of time:

- Drug name and manufacturer
- Drug strength and dosage form
- Type of packaging (unit-dose or bulk packaging)

Figure 4-2 Barcode Scanning and Computer Technology Streamline Inventory Processes

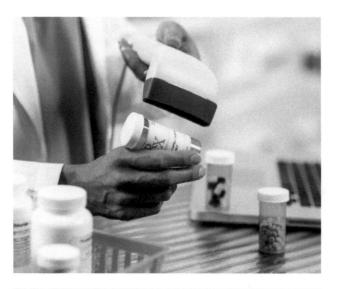

Figure 4-3 Maintaining a Perpetual Inventory Count Requires Manually Counting Some Drugs in the Pharmacy

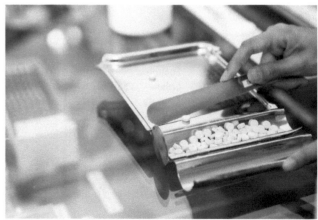

- Quantity contained in the desired unit (eg, 100s, 500 mL)
- Number of units

Keep in mind that ordering procedures for **controlled substances** may differ, depending on the drug you are ordering and state-specific rules. For example, Schedule II controlled substances are ordered using Drug Enforcement Administration (DEA) Form 222 (see next section and Chapter 3, Pharmacy Law and Regulation).

Receiving Orders

When orders arrive from either the manufacturer or the wholesaler, they should be accompanied by an invoice or a packing slip that lists the charges to the pharmacy. As you remove the items from the box and place them into inventory, it is critical that you check the items against this list—otherwise, the pharmacy will not know whether they have received all the items on the invoice and whether all of the charges to the pharmacy are valid.

Be sure to follow any internal pharmacy procedures concerning the receipt of inventory. For example, you may need to confirm the order receipt in the pharmacy computer system, either through manual entry or by barcoding the incoming items. Unless you let the computer know that the order has been received, it will reflect an incorrect inventory level and may keep trying to order more products—even though adequate amounts are on hand.

If your order contains controlled substances, you will need to follow special procedures to check these in. As mentioned in Chapter 3, Pharmacy Law and Regulation, **DEA Form 222**—supplied in triplicate—is used for ordering Schedule II controlled substances. Recall from Chapter 3 that copies 1 and 2 of the form are sent to the supplier, usually a drug wholesaler. The third copy is filed at the pharmacy when the order is placed. When the order is received, copy 3 of DEA Form 222 is pulled from the pharmacy files, and on that copy, the person processing the order records the date and amount of drug product received. Copy 3 is then refiled and kept for 2 years. This process can now also be documented electronically in many states, but pharmacies still may be required to maintain both physical and electronic documentation. Additional inventory requirements exist for controlled substances (Table 4-2).

Repackaging Inventory

In some practice settings, you will be called on to repackage finished dosage forms for dispensing, such as unit-dose packaging. Most drugs may be ordered in unit-dose packaging, but technicians may need to repackage some products

> In some practice settings, you will be called on to repackage finished dosage forms for dispensing.

Table 4-2	Inventory Requirements for Scheduled Drugs

Because scheduled drugs have a higher potential for abuse and diversion (see also Chapter 5), additional inventory practices are required to ensure the accuracy of controlled substance drug inventory, as follows:

- The pharmacy must completely and accurately record the initial inventory of all scheduled drugs before the pharmacy opens for business the first time and when the pharmacist-in-charge or pharmacy director changes.
- The pharmacy must conduct a biennial inventory every 2 years after that. The biennial inventory includes an exact count of Schedule II drugs and an estimate of Schedule III, IV, and V drugs.
- The pharmacy must maintain a perpetual inventory for scheduled drugs, although exact requirements may vary by state. A perpetual inventory for Schedule II drugs shows the actual number of units of each drug on hand at any time.
- The pharmacy must maintain inventories and records for scheduled drugs separately from those of other nonscheduled drugs, in a readily retrievable manner, for at least 2 years.

that are not commercially available as prepackaged unit doses or when commercially available products need to fit into automated dispensing machines, specialized drug delivery systems, or unit-dose delivery systems, such as blister cards.

Documenting repackaged items may require entering specific information into inventory records, or a repackaging log, including the following:

- Date the drug was removed from bulk inventory into repackaged form
- Drug name, strength, dosage form, and quantity used
- Lot number
- Manufacturer's expiration date and assigned expiration date
- Initials of technician and supervising pharmacist
- Other information as required by pharmacy policies

The expiration date assigned to a repackaged item cannot be longer than 6 months and may not exceed 25% of the remaining time on the manufacturer's original expiration date. It is also important that repackaged medications can be traced back to their original source, if needed, in case of a recall. To help facilitate this, labeling for repackaged drugs should include the manufacturer's name and lot number—in addition to the drug name, strength, dosage form, and expiration date.

Returning Inventory

When drug products expire, are discontinued, are recalled, or are otherwise unusable, you will need to have a method to return or dispose of them. Most manufacturers have policies and procedures about (1) whether the pharmacy can get credit for the expired drug products and (2) how much credit is allowed and what the pharmacy must do to get the credit. For example, the pharmacy must give the expired drugs to a sales representative or destroy the expired drugs and sign a statement attesting to the type and quantity. Some vendors, wholesalers, or manufacturers may accept outdated or expired products for a partial credit on return. As discussed earlier, many pharmacies use reverse distributors to return outdated or recalled medications to the manufacturer. **Reverse distributors** help pharmacies maintain compliance with the manufacturer's return policies and assist with receiving and processing return credits.

Items that cannot be returned to the vendor or wholesaler include compounded or reconstituted products and, in some cases, partially used bottles of medicine. Follow your pharmacy's procedures for identifying and returning outdated, discontinued, or recalled drug products.

If the expired products are controlled substances as scheduled by DEA, then other rules and regulations apply to the drugs. Be sure to work with your pharmacist in handling expired drug products so that the pharmacy can recoup these costs and comply with all legal and regulatory requirements. Chapter 5 reviews more details of drug recalls, expiration dating, and disposal of unneeded medications.

Conclusion

Inventory management is an important part of pharmacy practice, and technicians play key roles in managing this valuable asset of the pharmacy business. However, ordering, receiving, and dispensing inventory is only part of the story. Chapter 5 reviews how drugs are stored, steps for handling drug recalls, and what happens when drugs must be returned to the manufacturer or when they are stolen.

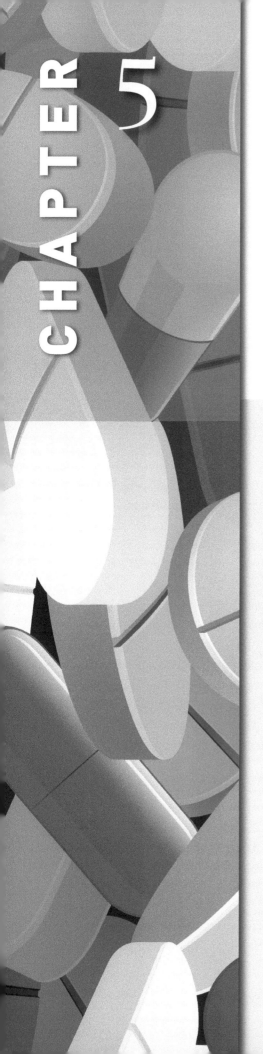

Drug Formularies, Storage, Recalls, Shortages, and Diversion

Chapter 5 describes ways that manufacturers, regulatory agencies, managed care organizations, third-party payers, and the pharmacy interact to effectively manage the drug supply chain. In covering drug formularies, medication-storage requirements, shortages, product recalls, and the need to protect against theft or diversion of controlled substances, this chapter helps us view pharmacy practice in a perspective beyond what you may see in a single location.

Introduction

As noted in the last chapter, a well-maintained and well-managed pharmacy inventory is critical to commercial success in pharmacy. Without access to the right drug product at the time that a patient needs it, the pharmacist's value is considerably diminished.

In this chapter, we consider several advanced aspects of inventory management, including the following:

- Management of the drug formulary
- Proper storage of pharmaceuticals
- Manufacturer or Food and Drug Administration (FDA) recall of pharmaceuticals
- Drug shortages
- Diversion and theft of drug products

Drug Formularies and Policies

> Formularies specify which medications or drug products are to be used for patients in a particular health care system.

In health care systems and in the Medicare Part D program, physicians and financial managers working in concert with pharmacists have established lists of preferred drug products. The lists, called **formularies**, specify which medications or drug products are to be used for patients in the system. In institutions and many managed care organizations, formulary decisions are made by a committee composed primarily of health care providers. This committee includes representatives from health system administration or management, physicians, pharmacists, and nurses.

Medications and products are selected for inclusion on the formulary by using 4 criteria to compare them with other available products:

- Better effectiveness for treating or preventing the disease in question
- Fewer side effects
- Better pharmacokinetic profiles, including fewer drug interactions with food or other drugs, or fewer number of daily doses
- Lower costs

By shifting pharmaceutical use toward formulary agents, the health system enjoys several benefits. First, in many cases, patients are treated with more effective and/or safer medications and have better outcomes. The health system is able to eliminate other medications and drug products from its inventory, saving on the inventory and related costs. Second, the system also purchases larger quantities of the formulary agents, which may enable it to receive larger discounts from the manufacturer or wholesaler. Third, if the health system is dominant enough in a given geographic area, it may be able to negotiate even larger discounts based on its ability to guarantee certain usage levels of the product to the manufacturer.

Occasionally, a health system will add a drug to its formulary but place it in a restricted category. Usually this is done because the drug has serious side effects, is difficult to use properly, or is very expensive. Once a drug is given restricted status, it requires specific conditions, often referred to as "criteria for use," to be met for that drug to be prescribed, or prescribing may be limited to certain types of physician specialists or general practitioners with special permission from physician specialists. For example, an effective medication that is used to stop bleeding but is associated with a very high risk of serious blood clots may be limited to use only in patients with the most serious bleeding cases.

Another common formulary policy involves automatic stop orders. In this case, physicians instruct the pharmacy to automatically stop therapy with certain medications unless the prescribing physician reorders them or asks for the agents to be continued. This is most commonly done with antibiotics, which need to be reassessed a few days after they are begun when certain laboratory tests become available.

While the utility and effectiveness of drug formularies is not universally supported, they have definitely proven useful for limiting pharmacy inventories and directing physician prescribers toward preferred agents. You are sure to see formularies used in hospital and large health care systems, and outpatient pharmacies routinely must deal with formularies of various managed care plans and third-party payers. Chapter 14, Pharmacy Billing and Reimbursement, provides more information on formulary issues in outpatient pharmacies.

Storage of Pharmaceutical Products

Medications are often sensitive to changes in temperature, light, humidity, or other environmental factors. Because of their delicate nature, medications must be stored under specified conditions so that they do not lose their potency.

Storage conditions are defined when a drug is first approved for marketing in the United States. The FDA approves the storage conditions for drug products based on clinical trial and research data. The official categories for drug storage are listed in Table 5-1.

The manufacturer combines FDA and US Pharmacopeial Convention considerations about its drug to calculate an **expiration date** for the product based on studies that show how quickly the drug loses potency under approved storage conditions. Use of the drug product beyond this date is not allowed under federal and state laws in the United States.

Your pharmacy will have a process in place for personnel to regularly monitor the **shelf-life** of medication inventory and pull expired medications from pharmacy shelves. Many pharmaceutical manufacturers use every-6-month dating, meaning that expiration dates are set in June and December of each

year. For these products, you will need to go through the inventory of the pharmacy only twice a year to check for expired drugs. However, other companies assign expiration dates based on the actual month a product is expected to drop below the allowable limit, and these must be removed monthly. Your pharmacy may also have expiration dates in the computer system, so that you can work from an expired drugs list in pulling old products. Whatever method you use, expired medications should be systematically and regularly pulled from pharmacy shelves and discarded or returned to the manufacturer.

> Medications must be stored under specified conditions so that they do not lose potency.

Pharmacy computer systems generally put a 1-year expiration date on prescription labels; the patient is instructed to throw the medication away after 1 year regardless of the original manufacturer's date. Several factors should be remembered about this type of dating:

- The reason for the arbitrary 1-year date is that many consumers do not store the drug product under FDA-defined conditions. For instance, many people store their medications throughout their house. For example, the bathroom is the most humid room in most homes, and humidity is the most important factor in degradation for many drugs. Thus, even if the manufacturer's original expiration date is several years away, a 1-year expiration date is used for prescriptions at the time of dispensing.
- In areas with especially hot or humid climates, you should advise patients to keep their prescription medications in locations where the temperature and humidity are controlled. In particular, advise patients not to expose prescription drugs to excessive heat by leaving them in hot automobiles on warm days.
- If you are dispensing a prescription drug product with less than 1 year remaining in the company's expiration date, then you must place that date on the patient's prescription label instead of the standard 1-year date.

Table 5-1	Temperature Definitions for Storage of Pharmaceuticals

Temperature definitions as they pertain to storage of drug products are set by the US Pharmacopeia (USP). Although further detail is provided by USP, definitions for basic storage areas are provided below. Technicians should follow temperature monitoring and documentation requirements for your pharmacy.

- **Freezer**—a place in which the temperature is maintained thermostatically between −25°C and −10°C (−13°F and 14°F).
- **Refrigeration**—a cold place in which the temperature is maintained thermostatically between 2°C and 8°C (36°F and 46°F).
- **Controlled room temperature**—a temperature maintained thermostatically that encompasses the usual and customary working environment of 20°C-25°C (68°F-77°F).

US Pharmacopeia issues standards that govern the conditions under which medications should be stored as they move through distribution channels, from manufacturer to wholesaler to pharmacy to patient.

The US Pharmacopeial Convention issues standards that govern the conditions under which medications should be stored as they move through distribution channels, from manufacturer to wholesaler to pharmacy to patient. These requirements sometimes mean that products must be placed on ice or otherwise refrigerated during shipment.

Recalls of Drug Products

Sometimes, despite FDA's and manufacturers' best efforts, drug products must be recalled from the market. FDA places recalls into 3 categories based on the seriousness of the problem and the relative risk to public health in general. Refer to Chapter 3, Pharmacy Law and Regulation, for a description of the 3 categories.

As with expired medications, you must follow specific instructions from the manufacturer so that the pharmacy can be refunded for recalled products. In addition, pharmacies must contact patients whose prescriptions were dispensed using recalled drug products (or, when the pharmacy can track this, nonprescription drug products that consumers have purchased over the counter; Figure 5-1). Follow the policies and procedures in your pharmacy for how these notifications are to be handled (for example, mail, phone, fax, or e-mail), considering the relative seriousness of the recall.

Follow your pharmacy's policies and procedures for monitoring drug supply and handling shortages.

Shortages of Drug Products

In extreme cases, a voluntary recall can lead to drug shortages. But recalls are not the only cause of shortages. Shortages can be influenced by many factors, including unavailability of raw materials

Figure 5-1 Medication Recalls. For full resolution of this image, please see the complementary supplemental files posted on PharmacyLibrary.com/updates.

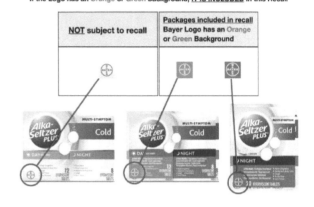

HOW TO IDENTIFY ALKA-SELTZER PLUS PACKAGES SUBJECT TO THIS RECALL
View the front panel of any Alka-Seltzer Plus product purchased after Feb 9, 2018, and locate the Bayer Logo on the lower left corner. If the Logo has an Orange or Green background, IT IS INCLUDED in this Recall

When prescription drugs or other medications are recalled, pharmacies must notify patients of the need to stop taking the drugs and explain the procedure for returning unused product for credit.

to make drug products, natural disasters, manufacturing difficulties, formulation changes, and unexpected increases in demand (Figure 5-2). Some shortages are predictable, such as generic availability of a product that causes the manufacturer of the brand-name agent to decrease supply. Other shortages remain unpredictable, and sometimes, the cause may not even be known.

No matter what brings it about, though, a shortage can wreak havoc in the pharmacy, especially in an inpatient environment where drug products may only be available from a single source and are used in acute or life-threatening situations.

When a drug product is in short supply, it usually falls to the pharmacy to take the lead on developing a plan for getting needed drug products to patients. Your pharmacy will have a process in place for monitoring medication supply trends, tracking your current inventory on hand, and anticipating the potential effect on patient care of a shortage. Once a shortage is confirmed, pharmacists and technicians will need to explore alternative suppliers, prioritize patients to ensure that drug use is appropriate, and identify potential therapeutic alternatives.

Follow your pharmacy's policies and procedures for monitoring drug supply and handling shortages.

Figure 5-2 Causes of Drug Shortages

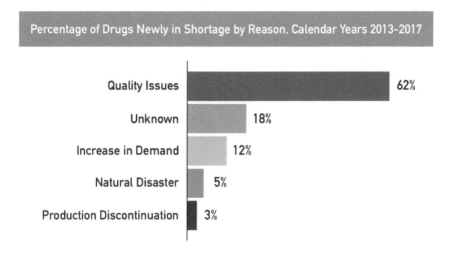

If a shortage occurs, avoid stockpiling inventory as a response—this can further worsen the shortage overall, and costly inventory may be wasted if the shortage unexpectedly resolves.

Be aware of risks associated with "gray-market" vendors or secondary wholesalers that may not be able to adequately assure the source or quality of their products. Sterility concerns have also been raised with products obtained from some high-volume compounding pharmacies in times of drug shortages.

For more information in the event of a shortage, contact the manufacturer or check online drug shortage websites maintained by FDA (https://www.fda.gov/drugs/drug-safety-and-availability/drug-shortages) and the American Society of Health-System Pharmacists (https://www.ashp.org/Drug-Shortages/Current-Shortages).

Theft and Diversion of Drugs

All pharmacies must have precautions in place to guard against the theft of money or drugs through burglary, robbery, or shoplifting. But an equally important concern is internal theft of money and diversion of medications by employees of the pharmacy or other personnel in institutions such as hospitals and nursing homes.

As a technician, you need to be familiar with the actions expected of you if a crime is taking place. Some medications have abuse potential, and it is possible for employees to become addicted to controlled substances that are scheduled by the Drug Enforcement Administration (DEA) or to become involved in diverting drugs to illegal markets for personal profit.

The presence of **controlled substances**—strong opioids for pain, amphetamines, benzodiazepines and other sleep agents, and sometimes even cocaine—makes pharmacies a target for addicts looking for their preferred substance of abuse or criminals who want to sell the drugs on illicit markets. Health system pharmacies have even been targeted for robberies and burglaries because of the quantities and types of controlled substances stored there. Some pharmacies intersperse Schedule III, IV, and V controlled substances in the general medication storage areas, but Schedule II drugs are kept in locked cabinets (Figure 5-3), vaults, or safes.

Because of these dangers, pharmacies must have action plans in place for employees to follow if they know or believe that a crime is in progress. You should talk with the management of your pharmacy if you have not been told what to do in the event of robbery,

> All pharmacies must have precautions in place to guard against the theft of money or drugs through burglary, robbery, or shoplifting.

Figure 5-3 Storing Controlled Substances

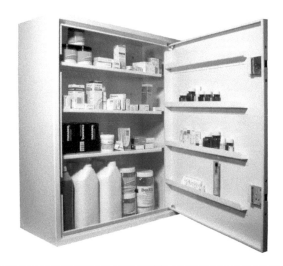

Locked cabinets such as this one are used in some pharmacies for storage of controlled substances.

burglary, or shoplifting. If you are not comfortable with the action being requested, you should talk with your supervisor about your feelings.

Potential situations and possible measures you may be asked to take include the following:

- **Robbery.** Robbery usually involves threats by criminals brandishing firearms or other weapons. It is usually the most dangerous situation that can occur in a pharmacy. Especially when the perpetrator is an addict seeking drugs, pharmacy personnel are facing a desperate person who may harm or kill anyone who does not comply with his or her demands. The most common recommendation is to give the robber whatever is requested. Many pharmacies have buttons located near cash registers and in the prescription department that will alert the police to the crime in progress.
- **Burglary.** Burglaries occur when the pharmacy is closed. Thus, the situation you might encounter is finding the results of a burglary when you come to work to open the pharmacy. Another common scenario could occur when the pharmacy's security system is activated; if you are a contact person for the pharmacy,

you might be called by the security company or the police to check the pharmacy to see if anything is wrong. If you discover a burglary, it is best to not enter the pharmacy or to leave if you have already entered. Caution is needed in case the burglar is still in the pharmacy, and it is essential that you do not change the crime scene until after the police have investigated and possibly taken fingerprints.

- **Shoplifting.** The theft of merchandise is undoubtedly the most common crime in the pharmacy (Figure 5-4). In larger community stores, several antishoplifting devices may be in use, including cameras, reflectors, 1-way mirrors, or even security officers. Your job as a pharmacy technician generally will not involve watching for shoplifters, but you should be very familiar with the policies and procedures of the pharmacy so that you will know what is expected when you encounter a shoplifting situation. Pharmacy owners and managers take shoplifting very seriously, and most prosecute those involved. First, because most pharmacies only clear a small profit on each sale, they need to generate many dollars in sales to recoup the theft of even $1 worth of merchandise. Second,

Figure 5-4 Preventing Shoplifting

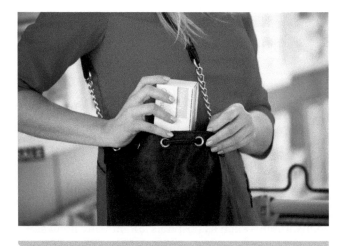

Mirrors or other monitoring technology may be used in pharmacies to help identify a person shoplifting a medicine.

failure to prosecute shoplifters sends the message that there is little risk in trying—if shoplifters are not caught, they get the merchandise; if they are caught, they just give the goods back and walk out.

While often not given the same emphasis as external thefts, internal theft of money, merchandise, and medications is an equally serious concern for the pharmacy owner and manager. Pharmacy managers may ask you to become bonded (a type of insurance) if your job involves handling money. Be careful when handling money, and be sure you understand the pharmacy's policies and procedures about how cash should be handled. Even if you become one of the most trusted employees in the pharmacy, you must still be watched. Do not be insulted if your supervisor or the pharmacy owner or manager asks you questions or double-checks your activities when it comes to money.

Likewise, theft of merchandise by employees is a serious situation. It has the same effect on the pharmacy's financial performance as does shoplifting. Owners and managers must deal with the attitude of some employees that one of the "benefits" of employment is taking items from the workplace for their own personal use. This is not true, and the consequences of bending the rules in this area can be termination from employment and even prosecution for theft.

When the items taken from the pharmacy are prescription medications, the situation becomes even more serious. Not only is theft involved, but the federal law requiring a prescription order has been violated. In hospitals and nursing homes, medications may be diverted by nurses, physicians, and other personnel (including nonprofessional staff such as housekeepers) who have access to drugs in patient care areas. Prescriptions are required for these medications because their use needs to be monitored by a qualified prescriber, usually a physician.

The most serious situation involving internal diversion of prescription medications is the theft of controlled substances (those in Schedules II, III, IV, and V, as defined in Chapter 3, Pharmacy Law and Regulation).

If you or someone you work with becomes addicted to prescription medications or alcohol, help is available. Most state pharmacy associations have programs for impaired pharmacists and technicians. While most people enter these programs after recommendation of a state board of pharmacy or other authority, some agree to enter treatment because their medication dependence is affecting their work performance. In addition, if the state board of pharmacy becomes aware of the problem, the person's professional license may be revoked, and a condition of reinstatement may be successful completion of therapy in an impaired-health-professional program. Contact your state pharmacy association or the American Pharmacists Association at (800) 237-APHA or www.pharmacist.com for more information.

> Theft of merchandise by employees is a serious situation. It has the same effect on the pharmacy's financial performance as does shoplifting.

> The most serious situation involving internal diversion of prescription medications is the theft of controlled substances.

Conclusion

Formularies, storage, recalls, shortages, and diversion are concepts important to understanding contemporary pharmacy practice. The information in this chapter will provide you with useful background information about each of these topics that you will find valuable in your job as a pharmacy technician.

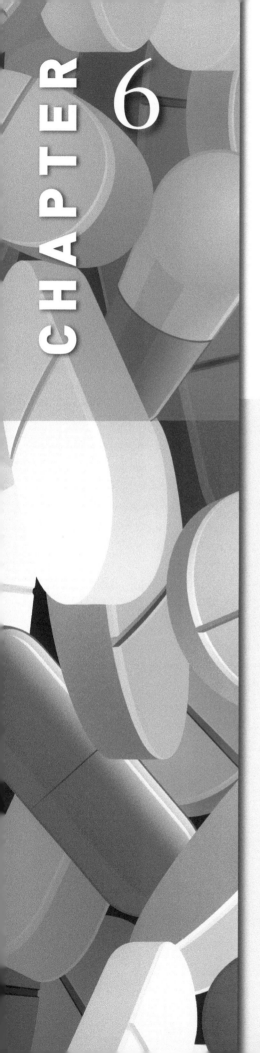

CHAPTER 6

Role and Advancement of the Pharmacy Technician in Pharmacy Practice

This chapter introduces you to the most common activities and responsibilities of the pharmacy technician practicing in the first part of the 21st century. It reviews certification and credentialing opportunities for pharmacy technicians for career advancement through the Pharmacy Technician Certification Board.

Introduction

As pharmacy has advanced throughout the years to allow pharmacists to take on increasingly advanced roles in clinical practice, pharmacy technicians' roles and responsibilities have expanded tremendously. Along with this expansion, technicians have more opportunities for credentialing and career advancement than ever before. This chapter reviews the role of the technician, licensure, certification, and advanced credentialing opportunities for technicians.

Pharmacy Technician Certification, Credentialing, and Advancement

Over the past 50 years, the role of the pharmacy technician has been established as an essential element of pharmacy practice. In the 1950s and 1960s, hospitals began incorporating an identifiable group of pharmacy assistants into daily operations, and during the 1980s, the Michigan Pharmacists Association (MPA) and later the Illinois Council of Hospital (now Health-System) Pharmacists (ICHP) developed a certification examination for pharmacy technicians. These voluntary programs involved written examinations that sought to recognize a minimum level of knowledge thought to be needed by those working as pharmacy technicians. The examinations were so successful in Michigan and Illinois that both groups began marketing their certification processes to other state organizations. In the mid-1990s, more than one-half of the states in the United States were offering either the Michigan or the Illinois examination to pharmacy technicians. By 2005, the American Pharmacists Association (APhA) and the American Society of Health-System Pharmacists (ASHP) joined with MPA and ICHP to form the Pharmacy Technician Certification Board (PTCB; https://www.ptcb.org/).

> The clinical pharmacy movement sought to create a role for pharmacists who would provide patient-specific drug information or advice to physicians and other members of the health care team.

Before going on to discuss certification in more detail, it is important to point out some differences in licensure-related terms that can be confusing. The process and requirements for becoming a practicing pharmacy technician are regulated at the state level, and throughout your career, you may need to register or become licensed or certified to be eligible to practice, depending on your role and state and/or employer requirements.

Registration occurs to keep track of who is a technician and where they work or live, and in some states, to document background checks. In most cases, registration is not linked to specific education or training requirements, but some states do require technicians to complete continuing pharmacy education (CPE) to maintain their registration.

Licensure is the process by which permission is granted for someone to practice an occupation after they have met a minimum level of practice competency. Licensure may require registration, certification by exam, or completion of other education and training, depending on the state.

Certification is the process by which a nongovernmental organization recognizes an individual who meets predetermined qualifications specified by that organization. At least 50% of states include certification in their regulations.

The remainder of this section will focus on certification and credentialing of pharmacy technicians, which are offered nationally to all pharmacy technicians. Soon after it was founded in the early 2000s, PTCB began administering a national certification exam, the **Pharmacy Technician Certification Exam (PTCE)**. Technicians who successfully pass the certification exam are referred to as certified pharmacy technicians (CPhTs).

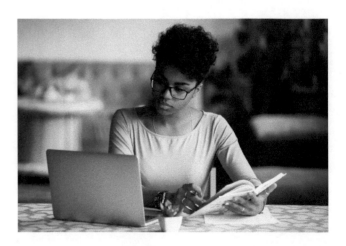

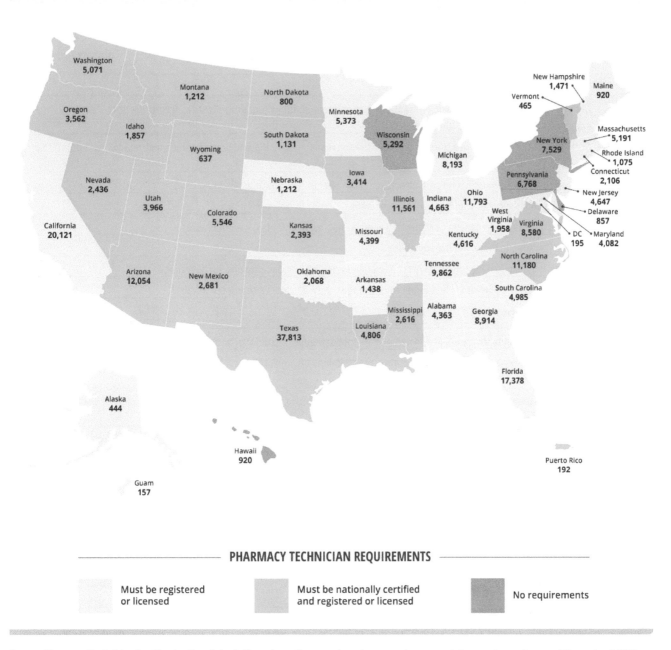

PHARMACY TECHNICIAN REQUIREMENTS

Must be registered or licensed

Must be nationally certified and registered or licensed

No requirements

Source: Pharmacy Technician Certification Board. Available at: https://www.ptcb.org/resources/state-regulations-and-map. Accessed December 5, 2020.

As of December 2019, there were nearly 300,000 active PTCB CPhTs in the United States (Figure 6-1). The PTCE is divided into 4 domains (Table 6-1). Beginning in January 2020, technicians are required to complete a PTCB-recognized education/training program or document equivalent work experience (minimum of 500 hours) to be eligible for certification. All certification should be maintained by completing a minimum number of CPE hours and/or other requirements. Complete information about recertification requirements is available on the PTCB website. If you are unsure of requirements you need to meet, you should contact your state board of pharmacy for state-specific requirements and consult with your employer about any additional rules or conditions within your organization. A complete explanation of eligibility requirements and list of recognized training programs is available on the PTCB website (https://www.ptcb.org/guidebook/).

| Table 6-1 | Pharmacy Technician Certification Examination (PTCE) Content Outline[a] |

1.	**MEDICATIONS**	**40%**
1.1	Generic names, brand names, and classifications of medications	
1.2	Therapeutic equivalence	
1.3	Common and life-threatening drug interactions and contraindications (eg, drug-disease, drug-drug, drug-dietary supplement, drug-laboratory, drug-nutrient)	
1.4	Strengths/dose, dosage forms, routes of administration, special handling and administration instructions, and duration of drug therapy	
1.5	Common and severe medication side effects, adverse effects, and allergies	
1.6	Indications of medications and dietary supplements	
1.7	Drug stability (eg, oral suspensions, insulin, reconstitutables, injectables, vaccinations)	
1.8	Narrow therapeutic index (NTI) medications	
1.9	Physical and chemical incompatibilities related to nonsterile compounding and reconstitution	
1.10	Proper storage of medications (eg, temperature ranges, light sensitivity, restricted access)	
2.	**FEDERAL REQUIREMENTS**	**12.5%**
2.1	Federal requirements for handling and disposal of nonhazardous, hazardous, and pharmaceutical substances and waste	
2.2	Federal requirements for controlled substance prescriptions (ie, new, refill, transfer) and DEA controlled substance schedules	
2.3	Federal requirements (eg, DEA, FDA) for controlled substances (ie, receiving, storing, ordering, labeling, dispensing, reverse distribution, take-back, and loss or theft of)	
2.4	Federal requirements for restricted drug programs and related medication processing (eg, pseudoephedrine, Risk Evaluation and Mitigation Strategies [REMS])	
2.5	FDA recall requirements (eg, medications, devices, supplies, supplements, classifications)	
3.	**PATIENT SAFETY AND QUALITY ASSURANCE**	**26.25%**
3.1	High-alert/risk medications and look-alike/sound-alike (LASA) medications	
3.2	Error prevention strategies (eg, prescription or medication order to correct patient, Tall Man lettering, separating inventory, leading and trailing zeros, barcode usage, limit use of error-prone abbreviations)	
3.3	Issues that require pharmacist intervention (eg, drug utilization review [DUR], adverse drug event [ADE], OTC recommendation, therapeutic substitution, misuse, adherence, postimmunization follow-up, allergies, drug interactions)	
3.4	Event reporting procedures (eg, medication errors, adverse effects, and product integrity, MedWatch, near miss, root-cause analysis [RCA])	
3.5	Types of prescription errors (eg, abnormal doses, early refill, incorrect quantity, incorrect patient, incorrect drug)	
3.6	Hygiene and cleaning standards (eg, handwashing, personal protective equipment [PPE], cleaning counting trays, countertop, and equipment)	

Table 6-1   (continued)

4.	ORDER ENTRY AND PROCESSING	21.25%
4.1	Procedures to compound nonsterile products (eg, ointments, mixtures, liquids, emulsions, suppositories, enemas)	
4.2	Formulas, calculations, ratios, proportions, alligations, conversions, Sig codes (eg, b.i.d., t.i.d., Roman numerals), abbreviations, medical terminology, and symbols for days supply, quantity, dose, concentration, dilutions	
4.3	Equipment/supplies required for drug administration (eg, package size, unit dose, diabetic supplies, spacers, oral and injectable syringes)	
4.4	Lot numbers, expiration dates, and National Drug Code (NDC) numbers	
4.5	Procedures for identifying and returning dispensable, nondispensable, and expired medications and supplies (eg, credit return, return to stock, reverse distribution)	

Abbreviations: DEA, Drug Enforcement Administration; FDA, Food and Drug Administration; OTC, over the counter.
ªAdapted from information supplied by the Pharmacy Technician Certification Board, available at https://www.ptcb.org/. Accessed December 5, 2020. [Editor's note: An alternative to the PTCB, the Exam for the Certification of Pharmacy Technicians (ExCPT), was established in 2005 as an alternative to the PTCB certification. PTCB certification is the only certification endorsed by the major national pharmacy organizations and the National Association of Boards of Pharmacy.]

Over time, PTCB has continued to develop new professional advancement pathways for pharmacy technicians to increase their roles and responsibilities. In 2017, PTCB launched a mechanism for technicians to become certified as a **compounded sterile preparation technician (CSPT)**. To be eligible to apply for the exam, a technician must be a PTCB CPhT in good standing and have completed a PTCB-recognized sterile compounding education/training program and have 1 year of continuous full-time compounded sterile preparation work experience or 3 years of continuous full-time compounded sterile preparation work experience. Once a technician is deemed eligible for CSPT certification, they must pass the CSPT exam and undergo a competency attestation by a qualified supervisor. Table 6-2 summarizes the CSPT exam content; a complete explanation of eligibility requirements is available on the PTCB website.

PTCB also offers specialized pathways for **advanced credentialing** (eg, Medication History Certificate) that technicians can achieve by completing a variety of **assessment-based certificate programs**. This process offers a mechanism for technicians to demonstrate specialized knowledge and expertise in a specific area of practice. According to PTCB, the certifications and certificate programs serve different purposes: "Certifications [eg, CPhT]

assess an individual's mastery of job knowledge, require Continuing Education, and award an acronym after one's name. Certificate programs [eg, advanced credentialing] evaluate learning outcomes from a PTCB-Recognized Education/Training Program, do not expire or require maintenance, and do not award an acronym after the name."

PTCB currently has 6 certificate programs for pharmacy technician advanced credentialing:

1. Technician Product Verification ("Tech-Check-Tech") Certificate
2. Medication History Certificate
3. Controlled Substance Diversion Prevention Certificate
4. Billing and Reimbursement Certificate

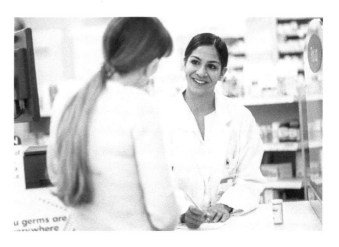

Table 6-2	Compounded Sterile Preparation Technician (CSPT) Certification Examination Content Outline[a]

1.	**MEDICATIONS AND COMPONENTS**	**17%**
1.1	Generic names, brand names, indications, side effects, and therapeutic classifications of medications used in sterile compounding	
1.2	Types of high-alert/narrow therapeutic index (NTI) medications used in sterile compounding (eg, insulin, heparin, concentrated electrolytes, chemotherapy)	
1.3	Dosage (eg, strength, dosage forms) and administration (eg, routes, instructions) of compounded sterile preparations (CSPs)	
1.4	Drug-specific factors affecting stability of compounded sterile preparations (CSPs; eg, containers, light, concentration, closure, temperature, agitation)	
1.5	Type, purpose, and use of technical and clinical references for sterile compounding (eg, package inserts, Safety Data Sheets [SDSs])	
1.6	Factors (eg, temperature, microbial limits of sterility, storage time, complexity of preparation, location of preparation) that influence the assignment of beyond-use dates (BUD) for compounded sterile preparations (CSPs)	
1.7	Physical and chemical compatibility criteria for components (eg, medications, ingredients, base solutions, filters, tubing, closures)	
2.	**FACILITIES AND EQUIPMENT**	**22%**
2.1	Types and uses of primary engineering controls (PECs; eg, laminar airflow workbenches [LAFW] and systems [LAFS], biological safety cabinets [BSC], compounding aseptic isolators [CAI], compounding aseptic containment isolators [CACI])	
2.2	Types of secondary engineering controls (SECs; eg, anteroom, buffer area, segregated compounding areas [SCAs], containment segregated compounding areas [C-SCAs])	
2.3	Features of secondary engineering controls (SECs; eg, air pressure differentials, HEPA filtration, ISO classification, air changes per hour [ACPH])	
2.4	Temperature, pressure, and humidity parameters and/or tolerances for facilities and controlled environments	
2.5	Procedures and requirements for conducting different types of environmental monitoring	
2.6	Action levels and parameters for assessing environmental monitoring results (eg, surface sampling, viable air sampling, nonviable air sampling)	
2.7	Common factors contributing to out of specification environmental monitoring results	
2.8	Operational standards (eg, food and drink restrictions, facility access) for maintaining the safety and sterility of sterile compounding environments	
3.	**STERILE COMPOUNDING PROCEDURES**	**53%**
3.1	Types, purpose, and procedures for conducting required personnel training and competency assessments (eg, gloved fingertip sampling, media fill) and the minimum frequency with which they must occur	
3.2	Equations and calculations used to prepare compounded sterile preparations (CSPs; eg, infusion times, percent solutions, dilutions, alligations, dispensing quantities, days supply, ratios and proportions, quantities, doses, concentrations, conversions)	
3.3	Personal health and hygiene requirements for sterile compounding (eg, no active respiratory infections, rashes, weeping sores, visible jewelry, long or artificial nails, cosmetics)	
3.4	Hand hygiene procedures	
3.5	Types of garb and personal protective equipment (PPE)	
3.6	Procedures for donning, doffing, and disposal of garb and personal protective equipment (PPE) for nonhazardous and/or hazardous drugs	

Table 6-2 (continued)

3.	**STERILE COMPOUNDING PROCEDURES**	**53%**
3.7	Properties and usage indications for deactivating, decontaminating, cleaning, and disinfecting agents	
3.8	Procedures and requirements for cleaning and disinfecting compounding equipment, primary engineering controls (PECs), and secondary engineering controls (SECs) for nonhazardous compounded sterile preparations (CSPs)	
3.9	Procedures and requirements for deactivating, decontaminating, cleaning, and disinfecting compounding equipment, primary engineering controls (PECs), and secondary engineering controls (SECs) for hazardous compounded sterile preparations (CSPs)	
3.10	Principles of aseptic manipulation and procedures for operating within horizontal and vertical air flow equipment (eg, first air, zone of turbulence)	
3.11	Types of and requirements for cleaning and disinfecting critical sites of components (eg, vials, ampules, ports)	
3.12	Safety procedures for handling sharps	
3.13	Documentation and record-keeping requirements for sterile compounding (eg, master formulation record, compounding record)	
3.14	Procedures to accurately weigh and measure components; principles of volumetric and gravimetric accuracy	
3.15	Procedures for compounding parenteral nutrition (PN)	
3.16	Procedures for preparing specialized compounded sterile preparations (CSPs; eg, epidurals, intrathecals, cassettes, ophthalmics, irrigations)	
3.17	Procedures for compounding hazardous drugs (eg, negative pressure technique, using closed system drug-transfer devices [CSTDs])	
3.18	Procedures for compounding sterile preparations from nonsterile components (eg, presterilization, terminal sterilization, filtration, aseptic preparation)	
3.19	Potential signs of defective compounded sterile preparations (CSPs; eg, discoloration, particulates, leaks, turbidity)	
3.20	Conditions under which sterility, potency, and endotoxin testing are required	
3.21	Procedures for interpreting results of sterility, potency, and endotoxin testing	
4.	**HANDLING, PACKAGING, STORAGE, AND DISPOSAL**	**8%**
4.1	Handling, labeling, packaging, storage, and disposal requirements for nonhazardous medications, components, sharps, and finished compounded sterile preparations (CSPs)	
4.2	Handling, labeling, packaging, storage, and disposal requirements for hazardous medications, components, sharps, and finished compounded sterile preparations (CSPs)	
4.3	Types of and requirements for supplies used in packaging and repackaging (eg, bags, syringes, glass, PVC, latex-free, DEHP-free)	

Abbreviations: DEHP, diethylhexyl phthalate; HEPA, high-efficiency particulate air; ISO, International Organization for Standardization; PVC, polyvinyl chloride.
[a]Adapted from information supplied by the Pharmacy Technician Certification Board, available at https://www.ptcb.org/. Accessed December 5, 2020.

5. Hazardous Drug Management Certificate
6. Immunization Administration Certificate (in development as of December 2020)

To be eligible to complete a certificate program and earn an advanced credential, technicians must hold an active PTCB CPhT certification and meet specific requirements. Eligibility requirements differ by credential and may include completion of a PTCB-recognized education/training program or state board–approved validation program in that practice area, demonstration of on-the-job experience practicing in the specialized area for up to 1 year, or other requirements. For example, to be eligible to apply for the Controlled Substances Diversion Certificate, pharmacy technicians must hold an active PTCB CPhT and either complete a PTCB-recognized Technician Product Verification education/training program or complete their state board-approved validation program. Additional information about PTCB certificate programs and eligibility requirements is available in the Credentialing section of the PTCB website (https://www.ptcb.org/credentials/).

Active PTCB CPhTs with advanced knowledge and experience can further their professional achievement through the Advanced Certified Pharmacy Technician (CPhT-Adv) certification. CPhTs who earn the CPhT-Adv credential are recognized for their expertise and experience and demonstrate an unwavering commitment to advancing medication safety. The CPhT-Adv certification may be associated with additional technician roles, responsibilities, and advancement opportunities within an organization. Technicians are eligible to submit an application for the CPhT-Adv certification if they have at least 3 years of work experience as a pharmacy technician within the past 8 years and have completed at least 4 PTCB certificate programs (must include Technician Product Verification and/or Medication History) or 3 certificate programs (must include Technician Product Verification and/or Medication History) plus the Compounded Sterile Preparation Technician® (CSPT®) certification.

Additional CPE requirements must be met for technicians to maintain their CPhT-Adv. Complete information about the CPhT-Adv certification is available on the PTCB website.

As pharmacists have taken on more responsibilities in patient-centered care, certified and credentialed pharmacy technicians are also expanding their responsibilities through these professional development pathways or on-the-job training. A technician's career path looks very different today than it looked 50 years ago. Some roles that you may be involved in as a technician include reviewing medication histories, technician product verification, hazardous drug management, billing and reimbursement, immunization assistance, supply chain management, financial assistance, medication therapy management, patient care transitions, training, leadership, and supervisory roles.

Codes of Ethics

At the individual level, the actions of pharmacists and technicians are guided by codes of ethics. These statements, approved by national organizations of pharmacists and technicians, help guide behaviors that are not necessarily illegal but that nonetheless may bring harm to the patient.

The Code of Ethics of the American Pharmacists Association and the Code of Ethics for Pharmacy Technicians are shown in Figures 6-2 and 6-3, respectively. Read these documents and talk with your colleagues about them. They are important statements of what you, as a pharmacy technician, should and should not do in your workplace.

Pharmacy Technicians Today

Pharmacy technicians are very diverse and range from career employees who have worked in the field for decades to student pharmacists who are employed as pharmacy technicians while they pursue a pharmacy degree. According to the Bureau of Labor Statistics, in 2019, pharmacy technicians held about 422,300 jobs, with slightly more than half (51%) employed in community pharmacies and nearly 20% employed in the hospital setting. The median wage at that time was $16.32 per hour, or $33,950 per year.

Figure 6-2 Code of Ethics of the American Pharmacists Association

PREAMBLE: Pharmacists are health professionals who assist individuals in making the best use of medications. This Code, prepared and supported by pharmacists, is intended to state publicly the principles that form the fundamental basis of the roles and responsibilities of pharmacists. These principles, based on moral obligations and virtues, are established to guide pharmacists in relationships with patients, health professionals, and society.

I. A pharmacist respects the covenantal relationship between the patient and pharmacist.

Considering the patient-pharmacist relationship as a covenant means that a pharmacist has moral obligations in response to the gift of trust received from society. In return for this gift, a pharmacist promises to help individuals achieve optimum benefit from their medications, to be committed to their welfare, and to maintain their trust.

II. A pharmacist promotes the good of every patient in a caring, compassionate, and confidential manner.

A pharmacist places concern for the well-being of the patient at the center of professional practice. In doing so, a pharmacist considers needs stated by the patient as well as those defined by health science. A pharmacist is dedicated to protecting the dignity of the patient. With a caring attitude and a compassionate spirit, a pharmacist focuses on serving the patient in a private and confidential manner.

III. A pharmacist respects the autonomy and dignity of each patient.

A pharmacist promotes the right of self-determination and recognizes individual self-worth by encouraging patients to participate in decisions about their health. A pharmacist communicates with patients in terms that are understandable. In all cases, a pharmacist respects personal and cultural differences among patients.

IV. A pharmacist acts with honesty and integrity in professional relationships.

A pharmacist has a duty to tell the truth and to act with conviction of conscience. A pharmacist avoids discriminatory practices, behavior or work conditions that impair professional judgment, and actions that compromise dedication to the best interests of patients.

V. A pharmacist maintains professional competence.

A pharmacist has a duty to maintain knowledge and abilities as new medications, devices, and technologies become available and as health information advances.

VI. A pharmacist respects the values and abilities of colleagues and other health professionals.

When appropriate, a pharmacist asks for the consultation of colleagues or other health professionals or refers the patient. A pharmacist acknowledges that colleagues and other health professionals may differ in the beliefs and values they apply to the care of the patient.

VII. A pharmacist serves individual, community, and societal needs.

The primary obligation of a pharmacist is to individual patients. However, the obligations of a pharmacist may at times extend beyond the individual to the community and society. In these situations, the pharmacist recognizes the responsibilities that accompany these obligations and acts accordingly.

VIII. A pharmacist seeks justice in the distribution of health resources.

When health resources are allocated, a pharmacist is fair and equitable, balancing the needs of patients and society.

Adopted by the membership of the American Pharmaceutical (now Pharmacists) Association, October 27, 1994.

To promote your success as a pharmacy technician, the remaining chapters in this book provide an overview of topics most relevant to your daily activities, aligned with the PTCB certification exam domains. Although you must learn many facts to properly and safely assist with the practice of pharmacy, your position as a pharmacy technician can offer you a lifetime of rewarding experiences as you support the activities of "the world's second-oldest profession."

Figure 6-3 Code of Ethics for Pharmacy Technicians

PREAMBLE: Pharmacy technicians are health care professionals who assist pharmacists in providing the best possible care for patients. The principles of this code, which apply to pharmacy technicians working in any and all settings, are based on the application and support of the moral obligations that guide the pharmacy profession in relationships with patients, health care professionals, and society.

PRINCIPLES

A pharmacy technician's first consideration is to ensure the health and safety of the patient and to use knowledge and skills to the best of his/her ability in serving others.

A PHARMACY TECHNICIAN

- supports and promotes honesty and integrity in the profession, which includes a duty to observe the law, maintain the highest moral and ethical conduct at all times, and uphold the ethical principles of the profession;
- assists and supports the pharmacist in the safe, efficacious, and cost-effective distribution of health services and health care resources;
- respects and values the abilities of pharmacists, colleagues, and other health care professionals;
- maintains competency in his/her practice and continually enhances his/her professional knowledge and expertise;
- respects and supports the patient's individuality, dignity, and confidentiality;
- respects the confidentiality of a patient's records and discloses pertinent information only with proper authorization;
- never assists in the dispensing, promoting, or distribution of medications or medical devices that are not of good quality or do not meet the standards required by law;
- does not engage in any activity that will discredit the profession and will expose, without fear or favor, illegal or unethical conduct in the profession; and
- associates with and engages in the support of organizations which promote the profession of pharmacy through the utilization and enhancement of pharmacy technicians.

Adopted by the American Association of Pharmacy Technicians. Reprinted with permission. Available at: https://www.pharmacytechnician.com/. Accessed December 5, 2020.

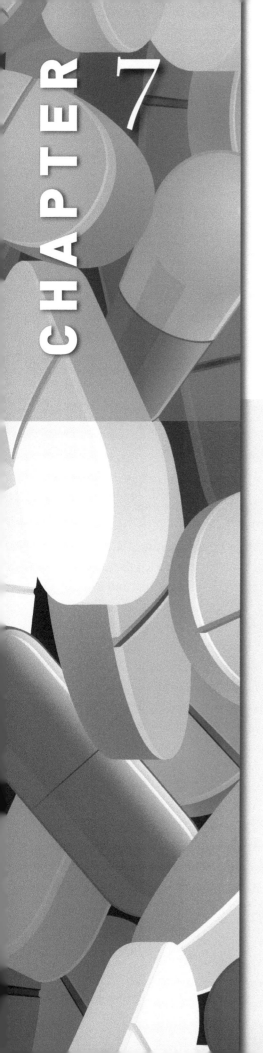

CHAPTER 7

Pharmacy Quality Assurance and Medication Safety

Pharmacy technicians play an important role in the overall operation and management of pharmacies and ensuring patient safety. Chapter 7 will detail some of your roles and responsibilities in quality control, quality assurance, and medication safety.

Introduction

Within pharmacy and other parts of health care, customers—who might be physicians, nurses, or patients—have a wide variety of expectations regarding the products involved and the services they expect. For pharmacy, products are usually medications and related devices. Services include the speed with which medications are provided, information that is provided along with the product, and clinical services, such as providing drug information to physicians and nurses, checking for drug interactions, monitoring for effectiveness and side effects, and referring patients to other providers when necessary.

Testing for variances in prescriptions and other work performed in the pharmacy falls under the broad framework known as **quality assurance**. Specific quality control tests are used to assess quality assurance. You will also hear people using the term **quality improvement**. As a pharmacy technician, it is not enough to ensure quality—you should always seek to improve processes and systems so that quality continually improves. While not discussed specifically in this chapter, quality improvement is a desirable goal for both prescription processing and other more subjective measures of quality important to the "customers" of the pharmacy.

Table 7-1 reviews common terms associated with the quality assurance process. Keep in mind that the voluntary accreditation processes through The Joint Commission and other organizations discussed in Chapter 3, Pharmacy Law and Regulation, are part of pharmacy's efforts to continually improve the quality of pharmacy care.

> Testing for variances in prescriptions and other work performed in the pharmacy falls under the broad framework known as quality assurance.

Principles of Quality Assurance and Control

Imagine that you own a factory that makes toy balls. Inside each ball is a small doll, but the balls are sealed inside plastic wrapping when they come off the conveyor belt. Because children want to be able to pick out the ball with the correct doll inside, it is critically important that the package labeling matches the contents of the ball. However, to check if the packaging has been matched correctly with the ball and its contents, you would have to open the package—thereby destroying the marketable product. How would you ensure the quality of the manufacturing process in this situation?

You could take several approaches. Various checks could be put into the manufacturing process. Quality assurance of this process would start with only having the correct packaging and dolls present on the manufacturing line during production. Employees would double-check one another when the packaging, balls, and dolls are placed into the machine that combines them. Then, as a final check, a small percentage of the finished packages would be opened and checked to make sure they are correct. If any incorrect dolls or packages were found, then more packages would be opened to see if the problem was widespread. If more incorrect products were found, then the entire batch of products might be opened and repackaged correctly.

These are the precise elements used in many pharmacies as means of quality assurance. If you review

Table 7-1	Common Terminology in Pharmacy Quality Assurance
TERM	**DEFINITION**
Quality assurance	All factors that influence the quality of medication and related products, pharmacy services, and patient care in the medication use process.
Quality improvement	Achieved by defining specific outcomes that are measured and monitored for improvement over time as changes are made in the system.
Continuous quality improvement	The philosophy of continually improving the processes associated with providing any good or service.
Quality indicator	The measure of a particular process or outcome, such as the number of medication errors that occur after implementation of new patient safety processes.

Chapter 10, Processing Prescriptions and Medication Orders, and think about all the things that could go wrong at each step, you will have a good idea of the task confronting anyone seeking to ensure quality in the pharmacy. Errors in this process can occur in all pharmacy settings and with any type of medication—oral tablets and injectable, compounded, or other drugs.

However, there is an important difference between oral and prepared injectable or compounded medications. With an oral medication in a prescription vial, you can check the color and markings on tablets and capsules to see if the correct drug was picked, and you can count the number of tablets. Thus, every prescription for oral medications you prepare can be checked by a pharmacist for accuracy. But with injectable or compounded products, visual inspection can be more difficult. Most injectable products are clear and colorless, regardless of how much drug was put in the solution. A compounded cream or ointment is usually the color and consistency of the base product, regardless of whether too little or too much of the proper amount of the active ingredient was incorporated. To ensure quality for most injectable and compounded products, pharmacists must use similar techniques to those used in the toy factory, such as employing double checks and carefully organizing inventory.

Importance of Training

The basis of any quality assurance system is proper personnel training. For technicians who work in community pharmacies or unit-dose areas of hospitals and long-term care pharmacies, proper quality assurance training ensures that technicians are familiar with the drugs they prepare and that they understand pharmacy procedures. In the admixture room of the hospital, home care, or long-term care pharmacy, technicians must be familiar with the drugs as well as the principles of aseptic technique and sterile product preparation. For compounding, knowledge of the drug properties, available equipment, and correct techniques is required to obtain a high-quality product. All subsequent parts of the quality assurance process rest on a knowledgeable worker performing tasks in which he or she is competent.

Quality Control of Solid Oral Dosage Forms

For solid oral medications, the pharmacist will generally check every prescription or medication order processed by technicians. In most cases, with both liquid and solid dosage forms, you should keep the stock container that you obtained the medication from with the prescription to be checked so the pharmacist can make sure that it is the correct product. As shown in Figure 7-1, the pharmacist will check the directions on the prescription label against the original physician's order.

Most computer systems display a scanned image of the prescription on the screen or use barcode technology to electronically double-check the prescription or medication order as it moves through the dispensing process. These systems may also have a

> The basis of any quality assurance system is proper personnel training.

> Most computer systems display a scanned image of the prescription on the screen or use barcode technology to electronically double-check the prescription or medication order as it moves through the dispensing process.

Figure 7-1 Pharmacist Check

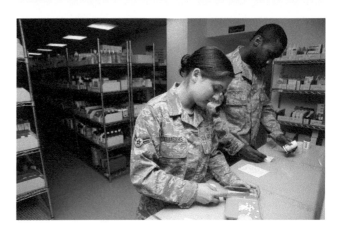

Here, a pharmacist checks the work of a technician before dispensing a prescription.

Table 7-2	Nonsterile Compounding: Selected USP Chapter <795> Quality Control Elements

USP Chapter <795> requires pharmacists and technicians to adhere to these guidelines—among others—to help ensure quality control of nonsterile compounded preparations (see also Chapter 12, Nonsterile and Bulk Compounding):

- When preparing the compound, the pharmacist or technician should follow all instructions exactly as written in the Master Formulation Record and Compounding Record, and document any deviations from these written instructions.

- The pharmacist or technician should check and recheck their work at every step, with a trained second person performing a double-check at critical steps.
- The pharmacist or technician should follow the pharmacy's established written procedures for describing any tests or processes they use to verify the uniformity and integrity of the compounded product.
- The pharmacist or technician should use established control procedures to document and verify consistency and performance of any compounding equipment.

Source: United States Pharmacopeia and National Formulary (USP34-NF 29). *Pharmaceutical Compounding—Nonsterile Preparations.* Rockville, MD: United States Pharmacopeial Convention; 2011:330-336.

picture of the correct tablet or capsule on the screen for the pharmacist to check against the product inside the vial. In some pharmacies such as mail service centers or very high-volume operations, computer systems use a small camera to electronically check the product inside the vial to make sure it matches the image stored in its files. The pharmacist will also look at any auxiliary labels that were placed on the bottle. If everything is correct, the pharmacist dispenses (or authorizes dispensing of) the prescription to the patient and provides any needed counseling about proper use of the medication. In hospitals where solid oral dosage forms are placed into patient carts, a similar checking process is used. Many larger hospitals have robotic devices for cart fills, and the barcoding process used with robots ensures virtually 100% accuracy.

Quality Control of Sterile and Nonsterile Compounded Products

As with procedures for preparing compounds, Chapters <795>, <797>, and <800> of the United States Pharmacopeia (USP) provide standards for quality control procedures required for compounding nonsterile and sterile preparations (Tables 7-2 and 7-3).

Table 7-3	Sterile Compounding: Selected USP Chapter <797> Quality Control Elements

USP Chapter <797> requires pharmacies to follows these steps to help ensure quality control of sterile compounded preparations (see also Chapter 13, Sterile Compounding):

- For all personnel involved in sterile compounding, pharmacy management must provide written descriptions of their training, written performance evaluations, and documentation that each person assigned to the aseptic area has completed specialized training.
- To ensure the quality, identity, accuracy, and appropriateness of ingredients, pharmacists and technicians must review all vendor labels, pharmacy labeling, certificates of analysis, direct chemical analyses, and compounding facility storage conditions.

- To ensure sterility is maintained, pharmacists and technicians must follow inspection procedures for all commercially manufactured sterile components (eg, drug products and devices), and document these steps in writing.
- To ensure the accuracy and precision of all compounding devices, pharmacy management must establish and implement written procedures for inspection, calibration, maintenance, and monitoring of any necessary equipment, apparatus, or devices used in sterile compounding, including any automated compounding devices.

Source: United States Pharmacopeia and National Formulary. *Pharmaceutical Compounding—Sterile Preparations.* Rockville, MD: United States Pharmacopeial Convention; 2008.

In addition to specific elements of quality control listed in these tables, the standard operating procedures detailed by USP and described further in Chapters 12 and 13 of this textbook also provide an element of quality control—such as the requirement for **personal protective equipment (PPE)** when compounding with hazardous drugs.

In intravenous admixture, sterile, and nonsterile compounding areas, there should be nothing in the laminar flow hood or preparation area except those items you are using to prepare the specific product. Pharmacists will check prescriptions individually, but the appearance of the product is not as helpful as with solid oral dosage forms. Rather, you should keep all injectable product vials—empty or not—for inspection by the pharmacist, generally with the syringe pulled back to the amount you put into the admixture. For certain types of admixtures—such as chemotherapy, total parenteral nutrition (TPN), and heparin—another technician or the pharmacist must check all calculations to be sure they are correct. Similar processes are used to check compounded prescriptions, including retaining all bulk containers and indicating how much of each ingredient you used.

Finally, the quality assurance system requires further checking of a small percentage of admixtures and compounded products, similar to opening the packages in the toy factory. For instance, to check for sterility of intravenous admixtures, a 2% sample of the outgoing products may be randomly chosen each day to test for bacterial or fungal **contamination**. Because the tests often destroy the product, these units must sometimes be made again. If any contaminated samples are detected in this 2% sample, the percentage of sampled units may be increased temporarily to 5% or more. If further contaminated units are found, then the system may be declared "out of control," leading to a process of decontaminating the preparation area, checking the technique of personnel, and retraining employees as needed. This process and increased sampling would be continued until the system is back "in control," after which the 2% sampling would resume.

Similarly, TPN admixtures are sometimes chemically tested. Samples of prepared units can be sent to the laboratory for analysis of pH (hydrogen ion concentration) and dextrose (sugar), amino acid, sodium, potassium, calcium, phosphate, and chloride content. With this type of testing, the units are not destroyed, so a higher percentage of units can be sampled—even up to 100% of units, if needed—at times when problems are occurring with product quality. If problems persist, pharmacy managers might correlate inaccurate units with certain personnel, products, or work shifts in an attempt to correct the system. However, they also need to check with laboratory managers because errors can be made there as well.

Quality processes should also be in place to ensure compliance with legal and regulatory standards for environmental safety when disposing of nonhazardous and hazardous pharmaceutical waste products. As detailed in Chapter 13, Sterile Compounding, these processes generally include sanitation management, hazardous waste handling, and infection control.

> Quality processes should be in place to ensure compliance with legal and regulatory standards for environmental safety when disposing of nonhazardous and hazardous pharmaceutical waste products.

Medication Safety

A **medication error** is defined by the National Coordinating Council for Medication Error Reporting and Prevention as "any preventable event that may cause or lead to inappropriate medication use or patient harm, while the medication is in the control of the health care professional, patient, or consumer. Such events may be related to professional practice, health care products, procedures, and systems including: prescribing; order communication; product labeling, packaging, and nomenclature; compounding; dispensing; distribution; administration; education; monitoring; and use." In the same way that prescription processes need quality control steps to ensure the integrity of the final product, measures also need to be in place to prevent errors.

Table 7-4 — Major Areas in Which Errors Occur During Prescription Processing

- Incorrect interpretation of the prescription or medication order
- Incorrect entry of the order into the computer
- Incorrect medication, dosage form, or strength picked from storage shelves or bins
- Incorrect amount of medication placed in container
- Incorrect label attached to vial or product
- Incomplete or improper auxiliary labels attached to vial or product
- Prescription given to wrong patient

Source: Used with permission from the Institute for Safe Medication Practices. Report medication errors or near misses to the ISMP Medication Errors Reporting Program (ISMP MERP) at 1-800-FAIL-SAF(E) or online at www.ismp.org.

Table 7-4 lists the areas where errors most often occur during prescription processing. In many cases, a medication error will be detected using the individual steps listed above for ensuring quality in the dispensing processes of manufactured and compounded drug preparations. In the same way, paying close attention to at-risk elements of the dispensing process is very important for preventing medication errors.

Common Causes of Medication Errors

There are several categories of medication errors (Table 7-5). Research has shown that nearly three-fourths of errors occur from prescribing errors, omission errors, and wrong dose errors. It is important to take as many preventive steps as possible in the dispensing process to stop an error before it has a chance to occur. The first step in doing that is identifying common causes of error that the pharmacy dispensing system can minimize to lower patient safety risk.

Medication errors may result from the use of **abbreviations** that are easily misinterpreted. The Institute for Safe Medication Practices (ISMP) maintains a list of error-prone abbreviations, symbols, and dose designations (Figure 7-2). Organizations accredited by The Joint Commission must maintain a "Do Not Use" list of abbreviations to help promote safe communication. ISMP recommends avoiding the use of error-prone abbreviations on all types of pharmacy communications, including written telephone/verbal prescriptions, computer-generated labels, labels for drug storage bins, and medication administration records, as well as in pharmacy and prescriber computer order entry screens.

Table 7-5 — Causes of Medication Errors

Prescribing error	When any action during the writing or dispensing of a prescription causes either a decrease in the efficacy of treatment or an increased risk of harming the patient compared with the general accepted use of the drug
Omission error	Prescribed dose is not administered as ordered
Wrong time error	Prescribed dose is not administered at the correct time
Unauthorized drug error	Wrong drug is administered to the patient
Improper dose error	Patient receives a lower, higher, or more than prescribed dose of the drug than was originally prescribed
Wrong dosage form error	Prescribed route of administration of a drug is incorrect
Wrong drug preparation error	Drug is not prepared as prescribed
Wrong administration technique error	Mistakes occur in administering the drug, which may be caused by improperly following protocols, performance deficit, or lack of knowledge
Deteriorated drug errors	Expired drug is used or the chemical or physical potency and integrity of the drug have been compromised

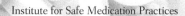

Institute for Safe Medication Practices

ISMP's List of *Error-Prone Abbreviations, Symbols,* and *Dose Designations*

The abbreviations, symbols, and dose designations found in this table have been reported to ISMP through the ISMP National Medication Errors Reporting Program (ISMP MERP) as being frequently misinterpreted and involved in harmful medication errors. They should **NEVER** be used when communicating medical information. This includes internal communications, telephone/verbal prescriptions, computer-generated labels, labels for drug storage bins, medication administration records, as well as pharmacy and prescriber computer order entry screens.

Abbreviations	Intended Meaning	Misinterpretation	Correction
μg	Microgram	Mistaken as "mg"	Use "mcg"
AD, AS, AU	Right ear, left ear, each ear	Mistaken as OD, OS, OU (right eye, left eye, each eye)	Use "right ear," "left ear," or "each ear"
OD, OS, OU	Right eye, left eye, each eye	Mistaken as AD, AS, AU (right ear, left ear, each ear)	Use "right eye," "left eye," or "each eye"
BT	Bedtime	Mistaken as "BID" (twice daily)	Use "bedtime"
cc	Cubic centimeters	Mistaken as "u" (units)	Use "mL"
D/C	Discharge or discontinue	Premature discontinuation of medications if D/C (intended to mean "discharge") has been misinterpreted as "discontinued" when followed by a list of discharge medications	Use "discharge" and "discontinue"
IJ	Injection	Mistaken as "IV" or "intrajugular"	Use "injection"
IN	Intranasal	Mistaken as "IM" or "IV"	Use "intranasal" or "NAS"
HS	Half-strength	Mistaken as bedtime	Use "half-strength" or "bedtime"
hs	At bedtime, hours of sleep	Mistaken as half-strength	
IU**	International unit	Mistaken as IV (intravenous) or 10 (ten)	Use "units"
o.d. or OD	Once daily	Mistaken as "right eye" (OD-oculus dexter), leading to oral liquid medications administered in the eye	Use "daily"
OJ	Orange juice	Mistaken as OD or OS (right or left eye); drugs meant to be diluted in orange juice may be given in the eye	Use "orange juice"
Per os	By mouth, orally	The "os" can be mistaken as "left eye" (OS-oculus sinister)	Use "PO," "by mouth," or "orally"
q.d. or QD**	Every day	Mistaken as q.i.d., especially if the period after the "q" or the tail of the "q" is misunderstood as an "i"	Use "daily"
qhs	Nightly at bedtime	Mistaken as "qhr" or every hour	Use "nightly"
qn	Nightly or at bedtime	Mistaken as "qh" (every hour)	Use "nightly" or "at bedtime"
q.o.d. or QOD**	Every other day	Mistaken as "q.d." (daily) or "q.i.d. (four times daily) if the "o" is poorly written	Use "every other day"
q1d	Daily	Mistaken as q.i.d. (four times daily)	Use "daily"
q6PM, etc.	Every evening at 6 PM	Mistaken as every 6 hours	Use "daily at 6 PM" or "6 PM daily"
SC, SQ, sub q	Subcutaneous	SC mistaken as SL (sublingual); SQ mistaken as "5 every;" the "q" in "sub q" has been mistaken as "every" (e.g., a heparin dose ordered "sub q 2 hours before surgery" misunderstood as every 2 hours before surgery)	Use "subcut" or "subcutaneously"
ss	Sliding scale (insulin) or ½ (apothecary)	Mistaken as "55"	Spell out "sliding scale;" use "one-half" or "½"
SSRI	Sliding scale regular insulin	Mistaken as selective-serotonin reuptake inhibitor	Spell out "sliding scale (insulin)"
SSI	Sliding scale insulin	Mistaken as Strong Solution of Iodine (Lugol's)	
i/d	One daily	Mistaken as "tid"	Use "1 daily"
TIW or tiw	3 times a week	Mistaken as "3 times a day" or "twice in a week"	Use "3 times weekly"
U or u**	Unit	Mistaken as the number 0 or 4, causing a 10-fold overdose or greater (e.g., 4U seen as "40" or 4u seen as "44"); mistaken as "cc" so dose given in volume instead of units (e.g., 4u seen as 4cc)	Use "unit"
UD	As directed ("ut dictum")	Mistaken as unit dose (e.g., diltiazem 125 mg IV infusion "UD" misinterpreted as meaning to give the entire infusion as a unit [bolus] dose)	Use "as directed"
Dose Designations and Other Information	**Intended Meaning**	**Misinterpretation**	**Correction**
Trailing zero after decimal point (e.g., 1.0 mg)**	1 mg	Mistaken as 10 mg if the decimal point is not seen	Do not use trailing zeros for doses expressed in whole numbers
"Naked" decimal point (e.g., .5 mg)**	0.5 mg	Mistaken as 5 mg if the decimal point is not seen	Use zero before a decimal point when the dose is less than a whole unit
Abbreviations such as mg. or mL. with a period following the abbreviation	mg mL	The period is unnecessary and could be mistaken as the number 1 if written poorly	Use mg, mL, etc. without a terminal period

(figure continues on next page)

Figure 7-2 (continued)

Institute for Safe Medication Practices

ISMP's List of *Error-Prone Abbreviations, Symbols,* and *Dose Designations* (continued)

Dose Designations and Other Information	Intended Meaning	Misinterpretation	Correction
Drug name and dose run together (especially problematic for drug names that end in "l" such as Inderal40 mg; Tegretol300 mg)	Inderal 40 mg Tegretol 300 mg	Mistaken as Inderal 140 mg Mistaken as Tegretol 1300 mg	Place adequate space between the drug name, dose, and unit of measure
Numerical dose and unit of measure run together (e.g., 10mg, 100mL)	10 mg 100 mL	The "m" is sometimes mistaken as a zero or two zeros, risking a 10- to 100-fold overdose	Place adequate space between the dose and unit of measure
Large doses without properly placed commas (e.g., 100000 units; 1000000 units)	100,000 units 1,000,000 units	100000 has been mistaken as 10,000 or 1,000,000; 1000000 has been mistaken as 100,000	Use commas for dosing units at or above 1,000, or use words such as 100 "thousand" or 1 "million" to improve readability

Drug Name Abbreviations	Intended Meaning	Misinterpretation	Correction
To avoid confusion, do not abbreviate drug names when communicating medical information. Examples of drug name abbreviations involved in medication errors include:			
APAP	acetaminophen	Not recognized as acetaminophen	Use complete drug name
ARA A	vidarabine	Mistaken as cytarabine (ARA C)	Use complete drug name
AZT	zidovudine (Retrovir)	Mistaken as azathioprine or aztreonam	Use complete drug name
CPZ	Compazine (prochlorperazine)	Mistaken as chlorpromazine	Use complete drug name
DPT	Demerol-Phenergan-Thorazine	Mistaken as diphtheria-pertussis-tetanus (vaccine)	Use complete drug name
DTO	Diluted tincture of opium, or deodorized tincture of opium (Paregoric)	Mistaken as tincture of opium	Use complete drug name
HCl	hydrochloric acid or hydrochloride	Mistaken as potassium chloride (The "H" is misinterpreted as "K")	Use complete drug name unless expressed as a salt of a drug
HCT	hydrocortisone	Mistaken as hydrochlorothiazide	Use complete drug name
HCTZ	hydrochlorothiazide	Mistaken as hydrocortisone (seen as HCT250 mg)	Use complete drug name
MgSO4**	magnesium sulfate	Mistaken as morphine sulfate	Use complete drug name
MS, MSO4**	morphine sulfate	Mistaken as magnesium sulfate	Use complete drug name
MTX	methotrexate	Mistaken as mitoxantrone	Use complete drug name
PCA	procainamide	Mistaken as patient controlled analgesia	Use complete drug name
PTU	propylthiouracil	Mistaken as mercaptopurine	Use complete drug name
T3	Tylenol with codeine No. 3	Mistaken as liothyronine	Use complete drug name
TAC	triamcinolone	Mistaken as tetracaine, Adrenalin, cocaine	Use complete drug name
TNK	TNKase	Mistaken as "TPA"	Use complete drug name
ZnSO4	zinc sulfate	Mistaken as morphine sulfate	Use complete drug name

Stemmed Drug Names	Intended Meaning	Misinterpretation	Correction
"Nitro" drip	nitroglycerin infusion	Mistaken as sodium nitroprusside infusion	Use complete drug name
"Norflox"	norfloxacin	Mistaken as Norflex	Use complete drug name
"IV Vanc"	intravenous vancomycin	Mistaken as Invanz	Use complete drug name

Symbols	Intended Meaning	Misinterpretation	Correction
℥	Dram	Symbol for dram mistaken as "3"	Use the metric system
ℳ	Minim	Symbol for minim mistaken as "mL"	
x3d	For three days	Mistaken as "3 doses"	Use "for three days"
> and <	Greater than and less than	Mistaken as opposite of intended; mistakenly use incorrect symbol; "< 10" mistaken as "40"	Use "greater than" or "less than"
/ (slash mark)	Separates two doses or indicates "per"	Mistaken as the number 1 (e.g., "25 units/10 units" misread as "25 units and 110" units)	Use "per" rather than a slash mark to separate doses
@	At	Mistaken as "2"	Use "at"
&	And	Mistaken as "2"	Use "and"
+	Plus or and	Mistaken as "4"	Use "and"
°	Hour	Mistaken as a zero (e.g., q2° seen as q 20)	Use "hr," "h," or "hour"
Ø or ∅	zero, null sign	Mistaken as numerals 4, 6, 8, and 9	Use 0 or zero, or describe intent using whole words

**These abbreviations are included on The Joint Commission's "minimum list" of dangerous abbreviations, acronyms, and symbols that must be included on an organization's "Do Not Use" list, effective January 1, 2004. Visit www.jointcommission.org for more information about this Joint Commission requirement.

© ISMP 2013. Permission is granted to reproduce material with proper attribution for internal use within healthcare organizations. Other reproduction is prohibited without written permission from ISMP. Report actual and potential medication errors to the ISMP National Medication Errors Reporting Program (ISMP MERP) via the Web at www.ismp.org or by calling 1-800-FAIL-SAF(E).

ISMP
INSTITUTE FOR SAFE MEDICATION PRACTICES
www.ismp.org

As the number of approved drugs has exploded over the past half century, the process of coming up with unique generic and brand names has become more challenging. As a result, many names are similar in the way they are spelled and/or pronounced. In some cases, this leads to a drug name change. For example, in 2010, Takeda Pharmaceuticals changed the brand name of its acid reflux drug dexlansoprazole from Kapidex to Dexilant in response to dispensing errors that were occurring between the brand-name products Kapidex, Casodex (bicalutamide), and Kadian (morphine sulfate extended-release).

To help avoid medication errors that result from **look-alike, sound-alike drug names**, manufacturers often put the unique parts of generic names in uppercase letters, known as "tall-man lettering," as shown in Figure 7-3. Most pharmacists and technicians also take added precautions in the pharmacy to avoid confusion, such as separating look-alike, sound-alike products from each other on pharmacy shelves or using shelf tags or stickers as an extra alert when 2 similar products are shelved close to one another. The ISMP maintains lists of drug products that are commonly confused with one another and those for which tall-man lettering is recommended to highlight name similarities in the "Tools" area of its website (www.ismp.org/tools). It may be helpful to post medications from these lists that are commonly used in your pharmacy as a reminder to pharmacy staff. This can help to avoid medication errors caused when the wrong bottle of medication is retrieved from pharmacy shelves or storage areas.

A **narrow therapeutic index** drug is one where small differences in dose or blood concentration may lead to dose- and blood-concentration-dependent, serious therapeutic failures or adverse drug reactions. Some of these narrow therapeutic index drugs are designated as **high-alert** medications by ISMP (Figures 7-4 and 7-5) because a single medication error can cause significant patient harm. The blood thinner warfarin is an example of a high-alert, narrow therapeutic index drug—accidentally dispensing 10-mg tablets in place of 1-mg tablets would lead to a 10-fold dose increase and the possibility for a serious and potentially fatal bleeding event. When you are dispensing high-alert medications, pay special attention to ensure that you have retrieved the exact strength the prescriber is asking for, whether it's 100 mcg or 100 mg; 0.1 mg or 1 mg; 1% or 10%; or 125 mg/5 mL or 250 mg/5 mL.

System-Based Causes of Errors

It is also important to step back and look at the bigger picture when thinking of quality assurance for patient safety. To return to our manufacturing example of dolls inside a toy ball, a defect in the manufacturing equipment as the cause of a problem might never be detected if you only focused on individual steps or the final verification to identify if a problem existed. To repair quality issues, sometimes it is necessary to address the overall system.

The same is true with patient safety and medication errors—these may result from system-based causes or factors common to a specific health care or pharmacy system that increase the likelihood of an error. Common system-based causes of errors include lack of information about the patient or the medication, unsafe drug storage or distribution, unsafe staffing patterns or work environment, inadequate staff orientation or competency validation, and inadequate

| Figure 7-3 | Look-Alike Generic Names |

The product labels show unique portions of names in uppercase letters.

Institute for Safe Medication Practices

ISMP's **List of *High-Alert Medications***

H igh-alert medications are drugs that bear a heightened risk of causing significant patient harm when they are used in error. Although mistakes may or may not be more common with these drugs, the consequences of an error are clearly more devastating to patients. We hope you will use this list to determine which medications require special safeguards to reduce the risk of errors. This may include strategies such as standardizing the ordering, storage,

preparation, and administration of these products; improving access to information about these drugs; limiting access to high-alert medications; using auxiliary labels and automated alerts; and employing redundancies such as automated or independent double-checks when necessary. (Note: manual independent double-checks are not always the optimal error-reduction strategy and may not be practical for all of the medications on the list).

Classes/ Categories of Medications
adrenergic agonists, IV (e.g., **EPINEPH**rine, phenylephrine, norepinephrine)
adrenergic antagonists, IV (e.g., propranolol, metoprolol, labetalol)
anesthetic agents, general, inhaled and IV (e.g., propofol, ketamine)
antiarrhythmics, IV (e.g., lidocaine, amiodarone)
antithrombotic agents, including: ■ anticoagulants (e.g., warfarin, low-molecular-weight heparin, IV unfractionated heparin) ■ Factor Xa inhibitors (e.g., fondaparinux) ■ direct thrombin inhibitors (e.g., argatroban, bivalirudin, dabigatran etexilate, lepirudin) ■ thrombolytics (e.g., alteplase, reteplase, tenecteplase) ■ glycoprotein IIb/IIIa inhibitors (e.g., eptifibatide)
cardioplegic solutions
chemotherapeutic agents, parenteral and oral
dextrose, hypertonic, 20% or greater
dialysis solutions, peritoneal and hemodialysis
epidural or intrathecal medications
hypoglycemics, oral
inotropic medications, IV (e.g., digoxin, milrinone)
insulin, subcutaneous and IV
liposomal forms of drugs (e.g., liposomal amphotericin B) and conventional counterparts (e.g., amphotericin B desoxycholate)
moderate sedation agents, IV (e.g., dexmedetomidine, midazolam)
moderate sedation agents, oral, for children (e.g., chloral hydrate)
narcotics/opioids ■ IV ■ transdermal ■ oral (including liquid concentrates, immediate and sustained-release formulations)
neuromuscular blocking agents (e.g., succinylcholine, rocuronium, vecuronium)
parenteral nutrition preparations
radiocontrast agents, IV
sterile water for injection, inhalation, and irrigation (excluding pour bottles) in containers of 100 mL or more
sodium chloride for injection, hypertonic, greater than 0.9% concentration

Specific Medications
epoprostenol (Flolan), IV
magnesium sulfate injection
methotrexate, oral, non-oncologic use
opium tincture
oxytocin, IV
nitroprusside sodium for injection
potassium chloride for injection concentrate
potassium phosphates injection
promethazine, IV
vasopressin, IV or intraosseous

Background
Based on error reports submitted to the ISMP National Medication Errors Reporting Program, reports of harmful errors in the literature, and input from practitioners and safety experts, ISMP created and periodically updates a list of potential high-alert medications. During October 2011-February 2012, 772 practitioners responded to an ISMP survey designed to identify which medications were most frequently considered high-alert drugs by individuals and organizations. Further, to assure relevance and completeness, the clinical staff at ISMP, members of our advisory board, and safety experts throughout the US were asked to review the potential list. This list of drugs and drug categories reflects the collective thinking of all who provided input.

www.ismp.org

Source: Used with permission from the Institute for Safe Medication Practices. Report medication errors or near misses to the ISMP Medication Errors Reporting Program (ISMP MERP) at 1-800-FAIL-SAF(E) or online at www.ismp.org.

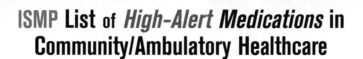

ISMP List of *High-Alert Medications* in Community/Ambulatory Healthcare

High-alert medications are drugs that bear a heightened risk of causing significant patient harm when they are used in error. Although mistakes may or may not be more common with these drugs, the consequences of an error are clearly more devastating to patients. We hope you will use this list to determine which medications require special safeguards to reduce the risk of errors and minimize harm.

This may include strategies like providing mandatory patient education; improving access to information about these drugs; using auxiliary labels and automated alerts; employing automated or independent double checks when necessary; and standardizing the prescribing, storage, dispensing, and administration of these products.

Classes/Categories of Medications
antiretroviral agents (e.g., efavirenz, lami**VUD**ine, raltegravir, ritonavir, combination antiretroviral products)
chemotherapeutic agents, oral (excluding hormonal agents) (e.g., cyclophosphamide, mercaptopurine, temozolomide)
hypoglycemic agents, oral
immunosuppressant agents (e.g., aza**THIO**prine, cyclo**SPORINE**, tacrolimus)
insulin, all formulations
opioids, all formulations
pediatric liquid medications that require measurement
pregnancy category X drugs (e.g., bosentan, **ISO**tretinoin)

Specific Medications
car**BAM**azepine
chloral hydrate liquid, for sedation of children
heparin, including unfractionated and low molecular weight heparin
met**FORMIN**
methotrexate, non-oncologic use
midazolam liquid, for sedation of children
propylthiouracil
warfarin

Background
Based on error reports submitted to the ISMP Medication Errors Reporting Program (ISMP MERP), reports of harmful errors in the literature, and input from practitioners and safety experts, ISMP created a list of potential high-alert medications. During June-August 2006, 463 practitioners responded to an ISMP survey designed to identify which medications were most frequently considered high-alert drugs by individuals and organizations. In 2008, the preliminary list and survey data as well as data about preventable adverse drug events from the ISMP MERP, the Pennsylvania Patient Safety Reporting System, the FDA MedWatch database, databases from participating pharmacies, public litigation data, literature review, and a small focus group of ambulatory care pharmacists and medication safety experts were evaluated as part of a research study funded by an Agency for Healthcare Research and Quality (AHRQ) grant. This list of drugs and drug categories reflects the collective thinking of all who provided input. This list was created as part of the AHRQ funded project "Using risk models to identify and prioritize outpatient high-alert medications" (Grant # 1P20HS017107-01).

ISMP
INSTITUTE FOR SAFE MEDICATION PRACTICES
www.ismp.org

patient education. In addition to encouraging individuals to minimize at-risk behaviors in the dispensing processes, most organizations and institutions have adopted a **systems approach** to preventing medication errors and improving patient safety. These systems may be as simple as having precise written procedures for programming and using automated dispensing cabinets or as complex as adoption of an electronic medical record with computerized physician order entry to improve patient safety throughout the health system.

> Always follow your pharmacy's policies and procedures to minimize risk in the dispensing processes and facilitate patient safety in everything you do.

As a pharmacy technician, you may not work directly to make changes in these systems, but you will certainly have a role in their everyday functioning. Always follow your pharmacy's policies and procedures to minimize risk in the dispensing processes and facilitate patient safety in everything you do. In most cases, the systems approach is being used every day to create the safest environment possible. Additional resources for medication safety are available at the ISMP website (www.ismp.org/).

Reporting a Medication Error

If a medication error occurs, follow the reporting and risk management procedures of your institution or pharmacy to the letter. Error reporting will be conducted both internally within your organization and externally through national reporting processes. National organizations track medication errors and adverse events to help increase awareness and implement changes to prevent future problems.

The **ISMP Medication Errors Reporting Program (MERP)** is a confidential voluntary external program that works to analyze medication errors, identify trends or potential safety issues, and communicate these to patients and health care providers nationally. Health care practitioners or patients can report medication errors anonymously to the ISMP MERP system at https://www.ismp.org/report-medication-error.

The **Food and Drug Administration (FDA) MedWatch** program tracks information on serious adverse drug events, potential and actual product use errors, and product quality problems that are reported through the FDA MedWatch Form (Figure 7-6). Individuals can access the FDA MedWatch program to report an adverse event at www.accessdata.fda.gov/scripts/medwatch/.

Other organizations also track medication error reporting data—including subscription-based systems such as USP MEDMARX (https://psnet.ahrq.gov/issue/medmarxr)—to allow for internal documentation and data tracking of errors and adverse events within a health system. Additionally, some state boards of pharmacy require a documented continuous quality improvement process within each pharmacy—including community pharmacies—to ensure that all personnel are monitoring, reporting, and learning from medication errors and from those "near-miss" situations when an error is narrowly avoided.

Other Elements of Quality Assurance

Many other areas of quality assurance will affect your daily activities and workflow as a pharmacy technician. Although an in-depth review of these areas is beyond the scope of this chapter, information is provided below to help you understand the impact of each one in your pharmacy.

Productivity, Efficiency, and Customer Satisfaction Measures

Quality assurance measures may include tracking customer wait times, improving efficiency in prescription or medication order processing, using customer satisfaction surveys, and analyzing communication practices within the pharmacy. In the case of health system technicians, the pharmacy's "customers" may include persons in other institutional departments that directly interact with the pharmacy, such as nurses or physicians.

Figure 7-6 FDA MedWatch Adverse Event Reporting Form

Reset Form

U.S. Department of Health and Human Services
Food and Drug Administration
MEDWATCH

For VOLUNTARY reporting of adverse events, product problems and product use/medication errors

Form Approved: OMB No. 0910-0291, Expires: 11-30-2021
See PRA statement on reverse.

FDA USE ONLY
Triage unit sequence #
FDA Rec. Date

FORM FDA 3500 (2/20)
The FDA Safety Information and Adverse Event Reporting Program

Page 1 of 2

Note: For date prompts of "dd-mmm-yyyy" please use 2-digit day, 3-letter month abbreviation, and 4-digit year; for example, 01-Jul-2018.

A. PATIENT INFORMATION

1. **Patient Identifier**
In Confidence

2. **Age**
☐ Year(s) ☐ Month(s)
☐ Week(s) ☐ Day(s)
or Date of Birth (e.g., 08 Feb 1925)

3. **Gender** (check one)
☐ Female
☐ Male
☐ Intersex
☐ Transgender
☐ Prefer not to disclose

4. **Weight**
☐ lb
☐ kg

5. **Ethnicity** (check one)
☐ Hispanic/Latino
☐ Not Hispanic/Latino

6. **Race** (check all that apply)
☐ Asian ☐ American Indian or Alaskan Native
☐ Black or African American ☐ White
☐ Native Hawaiian or Other Pacific Islander

B. ADVERSE EVENT, PRODUCT PROBLEM

1. **Type of Report** (check all that apply)
☐ Adverse Event ☐ Product Problem (e.g., defects/malfunctions)
☐ Product Use/Medication Error ☐ Problem with Different Manufacturer of Same Medicine

2. **Outcome Attributed to Adverse Event** (check all that apply)
☐ Death   Date of death (dd-mmm-yyyy):
☐ Life-threatening   ☐ Disability or Permanent Damage
☐ Hospitalization (initial or prolonged)   ☐ Congenital Anomaly/Birth Defects
☐ Other Serious or Important Medical Events
☐ Required Intervention to Prevent Permanent Impairment/Damage

3. **Date of Event** (dd-mmm-yyyy)   4. **Date of this Report** (dd-mmm-yyyy)

5. **Describe Event, Problem or Product Use/Medication Error**

(Continue on page 2)

6. **Relevant Tests/Laboratory Data**   Date (dd-mmm-yyyy)

(Continue on page 2)

7. **Other Relevant History, Including Preexisting Medical Conditions** (e.g., allergies, pregnancy, smoking and alcohol use, liver/kidney problems, etc.)

(Continue on page 2)

C. PRODUCT AVAILABILITY

1. **Product Available for Evaluation?** (Do not send product to FDA)
☐ Yes ☐ No ☐ Returned to Manufacturer on (dd-mmm-yyyy)

2. **Do you have a picture of the product?** (check yes if you are including a picture) ☐ Yes

D. SUSPECT PRODUCTS

1. **Name, Strength, Manufacturer/Compounder** (from product label). #1 ☐ Yes
Does this report involve cosmetic, dietary supplement or food/medical food? #2 ☐ Yes

#1 – Name and Strength	#1 – NDC # or Unique ID
#1 – Manufacturer/Compounder	#1 – Lot #
#2 – Name and Strength	#2 – NDC # or Unique ID
#2 – Manufacturer/Compounder	#2 – Lot #

2. **Dose or Amount**   **Frequency**   **Route**
#1
#2

3. **Treatment Dates/Therapy Dates** (give best estimate of length of treatment (start/stop) or duration.)
#1 Start
#1 Stop
Is therapy still on-going? ☐ Yes ☐ No
#2 Start
#2 Stop
Is therapy still on-going? ☐ Yes ☐ No

4. **Diagnosis for Use** (Indication)
#1
#2

5. **Product Type** (check all that apply)
#1 ☐ OTC   #2 ☐ OTC
☐ Compounded   ☐ Compounded
☐ Generic   ☐ Generic
☐ Biosimilar   ☐ Biosimilar

6. **Expiration Date** (dd-mmm-yyyy)
#1
#2

7. **Event Abated After Use Stopped or Dose Reduced?**
#1 ☐ Yes ☐ No ☐ Doesn't apply
#2 ☐ Yes ☐ No ☐ Doesn't apply

8. **Event Reappeared After Reintroduction?**
#1 ☐ Yes ☐ No ☐ Doesn't apply
#2 ☐ Yes ☐ No ☐ Doesn't apply

E. SUSPECT MEDICAL DEVICE

1. **Brand Name**

2a. **Common Device Name**   2b. **Procode**

3. **Manufacturer Name, City and State**

4. **Model #**   **Lot #**   5. **Operator of Device**
Catalog #   Expiration Date (dd-mmm-yyyy)   ☐ Health Professional
Serial #   Unique Identifier (UDI) #   ☐ Patient/Consumer
☐ Other

6a. **If Implanted, Give Date** (dd-mmm-yyyy)   6b. **If Explanted, Give Date** (dd-mmm-yyyy)

7a. **Is this a single-use device that was reprocessed and reused on a patient?** ☐ Yes ☐ No
7b. **If Yes to Item 7a, Enter Name and Address of Reprocessor**

8. **Was this device serviced by a third party servicer?** ☐ Yes ☐ No ☐ Unknown

F. OTHER (CONCOMITANT) MEDICAL PRODUCTS

1. **Product names and therapy dates** (Exclude treatment of event)

(Continue on page 2)

G. REPORTER (See confidentiality section on back)

1. **Name and Address**

Last Name:	First Name:
Address:	
City:	State/Province/Region:
ZIP/Postal Code:	Country:
Phone #:	Email:

2. **Health Professional?** ☐ Yes ☐ No
3. **Occupation**
4. **Also Reported to:**
☐ Manufacturer/Compounder
☐ User Facility
☐ Distributor/Importer

5. **If you do NOT want your identity disclosed to the manufacturer, please mark this box:** ☐

FORM FDA 3500 (2/20)   Submission of a report does not constitute an admission that medical personnel or the product caused or contributed to the event.
* Please see instructions

(figure continues on next page)

Figure 7-6 (continued)

Reset Form

U.S. Department of Health and Human Services
Food and Drug Administration

MEDWATCH

FORM FDA 3500 (2/20) *(continued)*
The FDA Safety Information and
Adverse Event Reporting Program

(CONTINUATION PAGE)
For VOLUNTARY reporting of
adverse events, product problems
and product use/medication errors

Page 2 of 2

B.5. **Describe Event or Problem** *(continued)*

Back to Item B.5

B.6. **Relevant Tests/Laboratory Data** *(continued)*

Date *(dd-mmm-yyyy)*   Relevant Tests/Laboratory Data   Date *(dd-mmm-yyyy)*

Additional comments

Back to Item B.6

B.7. **Other Relevant History** *(continued)*

Back to Item B.7

F.1. **Concomitant Medical Products and Therapy Dates** *(Exclude treatment of event)* *(continued)*

Back to Item F.1

Source: https://www.fda.gov/media/76299/download.

Inventory Control

This important area of pharmacy is discussed in much more detail in Chapter 4, Inventory Control and Management. Quality processes in inventory control systems help to contain pharmacy costs and ensure accurate inventory counts for compliance with federal and state law, when applicable. Examples of these processes include routinely checking received items against invoices and/or packing slips when orders arrive in the pharmacy, examining expiration dates of received products and rotating stock when placing new inventory on pharmacy shelves, and double counting quantities of controlled substance prescriptions.

Communicating Changes in Product Availability

There are many reasons why a drug product may become unavailable, including recalls, formulary changes, product discontinuations, or manufacturer shortages. These are reviewed in more detail in Chapter 5, Drug Formularies, Storage, Recalls, Shortages, and Diversion. For now, keep in mind that maintaining an efficient and effective system for communicating changes in product availability is an important element of a high-quality patient care system. Changes in product availability may be communicated personally (through patient or staff communication) or in writing (through memoranda, pharmacy or institutional newsletters, or other documents).

Understanding Your Role as a Pharmacy Technician

As a pharmacy technician, keep in mind the importance of your role in ensuring quality and patient safety in the pharmacy. From a management perspective, managers and pharmacists attempt to ensure the accuracy of prescriptions and the overall success of the pharmacy through 5 functions:

- **Planning**—setting the mission, short- and long-term goals, processes, and procedures that guide workers in the pharmacy.
- **Organizing**—establishing job descriptions and defining the relationships among various workers.
- **Staffing**—hiring people into positions who have the necessary qualifications for the expected duties.
- **Directing**—communicating with staff about when and how tasks are to be completed and providing the needed motivation and leadership.
- **Controlling**—checking on quality and outcomes to make sure that staff actions and pharmacy processes result in the desired products and services.

Managers, supervisors, and pharmacists that you work with have expected duties they must perform in these 5 areas. To be a successful employee, you will need to understand what you are expected to do (job description), when and how tasks are to be completed (either through verbal instructions from supervisors or policy and procedure manuals), and how you can help gather data to show that the desired quality and outcomes are being attained.

Conclusion

As a pharmacy technician, especially in a hospital or other institutional pharmacy, you may be asked to participate in and help collect data for quality assurance programs. Monitoring and measuring these data are a part of the continuous quality improvement process. If you participate in these processes in your pharmacy, the information in this chapter will help you understand how the data will be used to identify and rectify problems with quality in the pharmacy.

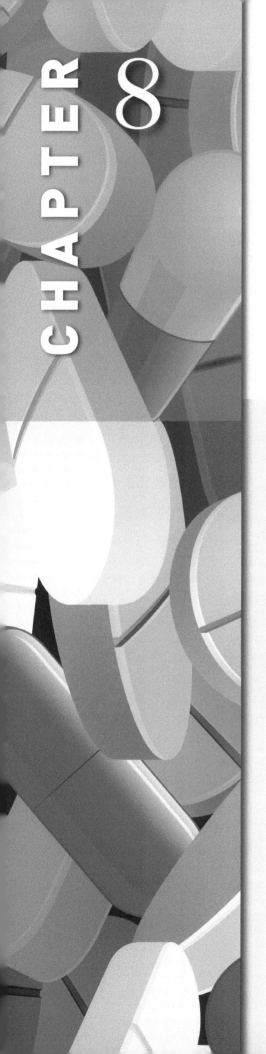

Interacting With Patients

Kimberly Atkinson, PharmD

Katherine Vogel Anderson, PharmD, BCACP

Communicating appropriately and effectively with patients is the theme of Chapter 8, which expands on legally mandated counseling by pharmacists and defines the role of the technician. This chapter briefly describes techniques for handling patients with special communication requirements, including those with terminal illnesses and those who become belligerent. This chapter discusses confidentiality of patient information, summarizes a court case that involved a pharmacy technician, and discusses provisions of a federal law that protects the confidentiality of patients' health information.

Introduction

Regardless of the role you play and the type of pharmacy you are working in, you will interact with other people. In a community pharmacy, most communications will likely be with patients, patients' caregivers, medical office staff, insurance company associates, pharmacy employees at other pharmacies, and coworkers. In a hospital or long-term care facility, you may most commonly communicate with physicians, nurses, social workers, case managers, patients (at the time of admission or discharge, for medication reconciliation), and coworkers. But no matter where you work and what you're doing, these communications with other people will be a major determinant of how well you are viewed as doing your job.

This chapter focuses on communicating with patients. However, think broadly as you read this material because much of it applies to communications with any of the people you encounter during your daily activities as a pharmacy technician. Without positive interactions with other people, your prescription-filling efforts and your contribution to the overall operation of the pharmacy will likely be overlooked. Unless people sense a warm, caring, and empathic attitude, they may disregard how well you are performing or how much you know. As Theodore Roosevelt once said, "No one cares how much you know, until they know how much you care."

> Regardless of the role you play and the type of pharmacy you are working in, you will interact with other people.

Understanding the Definitions and Principles of Communication

In its simplest form, communication is the process of conveying information from one person to another (Figure 8-1). In the case of spoken communication, one person says something (a process called encoding), and someone hears and interprets it (decoding). If the communication has been effective, the second person will have received the same message that the first person sent. The second person may then respond, and the first person uses this information (feedback) to assess whether the correct message was received.

In this process, there is much room for error. You probably have seen what happens to a message when it is passed around among the members of a group—it becomes distorted as people place their own interpretations on what was said and then pass it along in their own words. Based on the feedback the sender of a message receives, the sender may restate the message in other words and ask the recipient to repeat what he or she has heard. This process of encoding, decoding, and feedback can continue until both parties feel they have the same message.

In addition, people interpret **nonverbal clues**—such as facial expressions, hand motions, and the way the body is positioned—as they are decoding messages. For instance, if someone gives off nonverbal clues of being dishonest, such as darting eyes, throat clearing, or leaning backward, the recipient of the message may not believe the person. Or if a person laughs while conveying serious information, the recipient may be confused about what the real message is. Suppose a man just diagnosed with diabetes yawned during a 30-minute patient education session about the disease—you might wonder why he is bored when

Figure 8-1 The Process of Communication

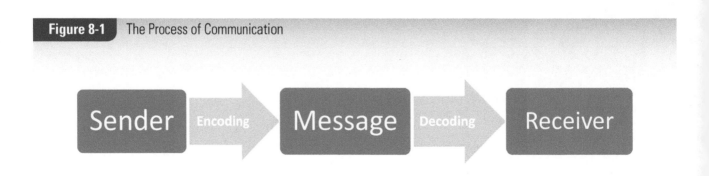

he should be receiving valuable information that could affect his future health.

People also glean a lot of information from the written word and from pictures or graphics that accompany those words. To increase the chance that patients will understand what their medications are used for and how the medications are to be used, pharmacists routinely provide them with informative flyers that explain the medication in both words and diagrams. While the above description of communication is useful from a learning standpoint, the linear process described often seems rare in the real world. Instead, both parties may be trying to communicate with each other simultaneously, ignoring each other's messages as they struggle to get their own messages across. So, what is communication? Here is one brief definition: Communication is the process of interaction between participants who occupy different but overlapping environments and create a relationship by exchanging messages.

Four major principles are associated with the process of communication:

- **Communication can be intentional or unintentional.** When talking with patients, you must be careful not to convey unintentional messages of indifference, anger, or frustration—and these messages can come from the way you stand, look, or behave during the interaction.
- **It is impossible not to communicate.** Even when you stand and listen to someone else, not saying anything, the speaker is reading your face, your hands, and your body for nonverbal clues of agreement or understanding or emotions such as anger or happiness. When dealing with patients, pharmacists and technicians must communicate in a way that imbues trustworthiness and concern so that effective communications can occur.
- **Communication is irreversible.** Once something has been said, it can never be erased. Like an arrow from a bow, you cannot pull back the words once you have released them. You can apologize, but the damage will remain the same. When talking with patients, there is no room for error, unprofessional attitudes, or indifference.
- **Communication is unrepeatable.** Every encounter is completely new. What worked with one patient may not work well with the next. What worked this month may not work when the same patient is counseled next month. Effective communication in health care depends not on a set of standardized words and phrases but on utilizing general guidelines for communication. These guidelines reflect an appreciation for the process of encoding, decoding, and feedback and an understanding of these principles of communication.

> People interpret nonverbal clues—such as facial expressions, hand motions, and the way the body is positioned—as they are decoding messages.

Communicating With Patients

In an encounter with a patient, you must first be aware of the purpose of the interaction. Are you trying to gather information from the patient (name, address, allergies to medications), or are you trying to convey information to the patient (when the prescription will be ready, whether the patient wants to be counseled by the pharmacist)?

When you are trying to gather information from patients, different types of questions are effective in different types of situations:

- **Open-ended questions**—those that cannot be answered with a "yes" or "no" ("Since you began this medicine for high blood pressure last month, how have you been feeling?")
- **Closed-ended questions**—those that can be answered with a "yes" or "no" ("Did you finish all your medication last month?")
- **Direct questions**—those that ask for the desired information in a straightforward manner ("Do you feel better or worse when you're taking this medication?")

■ **Indirect questions**—questions or even statements that disguise the actual information being sought by calling for a general response from the other party ("I'm wondering how you've been doing on this new medication.")

When seeking information from a patient, you must listen carefully. Try to be aware of whether the patient is answering the questions completely and accurately. If the patient appears to be changing the subject or trying to get across information other than what you are asking for, listen to what he or she is saying. Perhaps the patient has an existing relationship with the pharmacist or someone else in the pharmacy; if so, call on that person to help. If the patient is describing some problem other than the one you are asking about, listen to the message, repeat it to the patient, and then take an appropriate action.

> If the patient is describing some problem other than the one you are asking about, listen to the message, repeat it back to the patient, and then take an appropriate action.

Suppose, for example, you are working in the prescription department and a patient in her twenties brings a bottle of liquid cough and cold medication to you. She asks if this product is good for fever, in addition to coughs and head congestion. At this point, you need to know more, perhaps from both the patient and the pharmacist. First, you need to gather information by asking the patient several questions: Who will use the product (the patient herself, an adult family member, a child, or a friend)? What symptoms does the patient have? Is the nose runny or stopped up? How high is the fever? Is the cough productive? How long have these symptoms been present? This information-gathering step is critical to your ability to answer the woman's question. Without it, your response could be inappropriate, incorrect, or just plain meaningless.

When you are giving information to a patient, ask him or her to repeat the information to you. For instance, when counseling a patient, the pharmacist should make sure the patient can state the following accurately:

■ Name of the drug
■ What it is being used for
■ How often the medication is taken
■ How the medication is used (apply, insert, swallow, inject)
■ What to do if a dose is missed

In the given example of the young woman with the cough and cold remedy, suppose she tells you that the medication is for a 3-year-old boy who has had a fever of 103°F for 4 days. You read on the package that the medication is not for use in children younger than 4 years old without the advice of a physician and that it does not contain any drug that would reduce fever. You should at this point consult with the pharmacist, who would likely recommend that the woman take the child to the doctor immediately because of the high fever and his young age. In this example, if you had merely answered the woman's question, perhaps by assuming that she was purchasing the medication for herself, you and the pharmacist would have missed an opportunity to provide valuable information to the woman—with potentially serious results for the young boy.

When patients are buying or seeking information about nonprescription medications, you can use the over-the-counter (OTC) **drug facts label** on the products to guide discussions. These labels list in a standardized way the active ingredient(s), uses, warnings, direction, and other information needed to safely use nonprescription medications (Figure 8-2). Products approved as **dietary supplements** have a similar label (Figure 8-3), but because specific uses cannot be stated for these products, labels will contain structure-function, nutrient-content, or disease claims to guide patients in their purchasing decisions (see the discussion in Chapter 3 of the Dietary Supplement Health and Education Act of 1994 for more information).

Communicating in Special Circumstances

When patients come to the pharmacy to pick up medications, they may be sick, concerned about some aspect of their health, or be in generally good health without

Figure 8-2 The Over-the-Counter "Drug Facts" Label

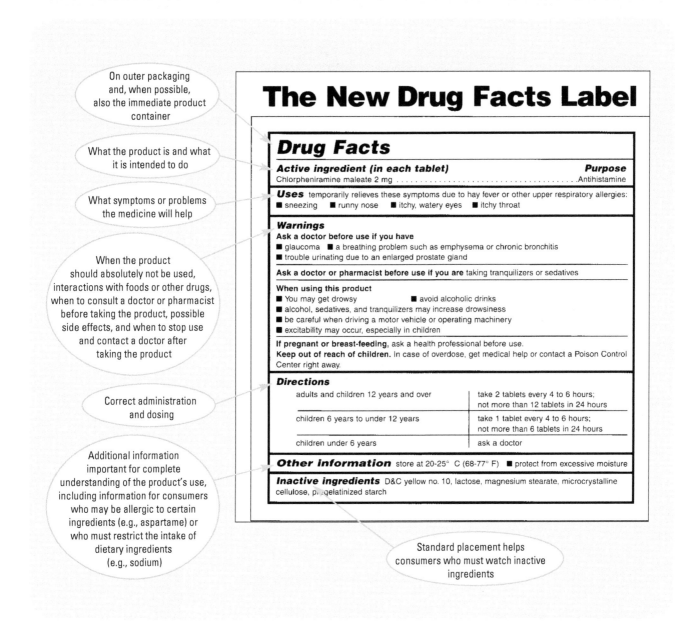

On outer packaging and, when possible, also the immediate product container

What the product is and what it is intended to do

What symptoms or problems the medicine will help

When the product should absolutely not be used, interactions with foods or other drugs, when to consult a doctor or pharmacist before taking the product, possible side effects, and when to stop use and contact a doctor after taking the product

Correct administration and dosing

Additional information important for complete understanding of the product's use, including information for consumers who may be allergic to certain ingredients (e.g., aspartame) or who must restrict the intake of dietary ingredients (e.g., sodium)

Standard placement helps consumers who must watch inactive ingredients

---

any acute concerns. Patients may be facing their own impending death or the passing of a loved one, a life-changing sickness that will require them to take medications for the rest of their lives, or anger about why this disease happened to them. Regardless, when you interact with any patient in the pharmacy, you must be cognizant of and empathic about their health status. In the case of an acutely ill patient, it is inappropriate to close a purchase by saying, "Come back again soon." This comment, while common in other retail stores, has a totally different meaning in a pharmacy.

You should be able to recognize certain patient types and develop strategies that will enable you to communicate with these individuals at a time with other important concerns. These patients might include the following:

- **The dying patient:** While most people who are facing death say there really is little that others can say to help them, they greatly appreciate the chance to say how they are feeling and know that others care enough to listen.

Figure 8-3 Dietary Supplement Label

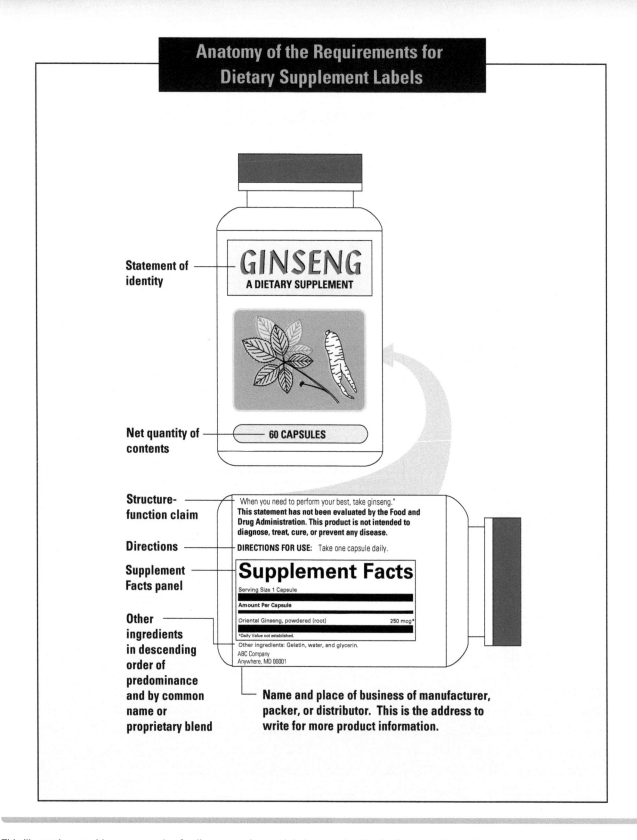

Anatomy of the Requirements for Dietary Supplement Labels

Statement of identity — GINSENG / A DIETARY SUPPLEMENT

Net quantity of contents — 60 CAPSULES

Structure-function claim — When you need to perform your best, take ginseng." This statement has not been evaluated by the Food and Drug Administration. This product is not intended to diagnose, treat, cure, or prevent any disease.

Directions — DIRECTIONS FOR USE: Take one capsule daily.

Supplement Facts panel —

Supplement Facts
Serving Size 1 Capsule

Amount Per Capsule

Oriental Ginseng, powdered (root)	250 mcg*

*Daily Value not established.

Other ingredients in descending order of predominance and by common name or proprietary blend — Other ingredients: Gelatin, water, and glycerin.

ABC Company
Anywhere, MD 00001

Name and place of business of manufacturer, packer, or distributor. This is the address to write for more product information.

This illustration provides an example of a dietary supplement label as required by the Food and Drug Administration.

Dying patients, especially those who have been long-term patients in a pharmacy, should not be ignored when they come to this difficult phase in their lives. Dying patients also need information from the pharmacist, and you should make sure that they have opportunities for these discussions. For example, patients who are taking pain medications need to know how the medications can be used safely, how to manage side effects such as drowsiness and vomiting, and whether they can continue activities such as driving a car. While most interactions will be with the patient, it is also important to be aware that the patient's family may be involved with the dying patient's care. Family members picking up medications for the patient should be treated with care and attention.

- **The angry or uncooperative patient.** Patients may have feelings of anger and frustration when they are diagnosed with an illness (Figure 8-4). They may be facing lifelong disability or life-altering diseases. Involving patients in their treatment plans and showing them how they can treat the disease and its symptoms may help to dissipate some of this frustration. Often, patients want a listening ear to vent their frustrations. By listening and being

| **Figure 8-4** | Angry or Frustrated Patient |

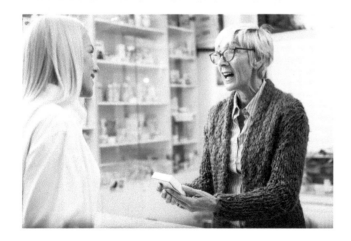

When they are diagnosed with an illness, patients may have feelings of anger and frustration that make them seem uncooperative in the pharmacy.

receptive to patient concerns, the true reason behind their negative emotions may rise to the surface. For example, the patient may be unhappy with the price of their medications. Pharmacists and technicians are in a prime position to be patient advocates and find cost-effective alternatives or coupons that may make the price more affordable for the patient. Even if the outcome is not achieved, putting in the extra effort can build positive rapport with the patient.

- **The stressed patient.** Some people respond to news of disease by becoming withdrawn, anxious, or stressed. You can best help these patients by showing genuine interest in their condition and expressing hope that they will get better. Such interactions may help stressed patients overcome their feelings of helplessness. If possible, try to remember personal details that are gleaned from short conversations with the patient over time. For example, if patients have pets at home, ask how their pets are doing. Patients appreciate this attention to detail, and it can make them feel like they are valued and cared for rather than being "just a customer" or a task that needs to be completed by the end of the day.

Distributing Medications and Providing Patient Counseling and Education

If part of your job is to hand the completed prescription to the patient (and/or collect the money for the prescription), you should be aware of several important issues, including storage of the medication before distribution, helpful information you can provide to the patient, and legal requirements about information the pharmacist must provide to the patient.

> The storage of medications, a very important issue, is the subject of much attention in the pharmacy world.

Medication Storage

The storage of medications, a very important issue, is the subject of much attention in the pharmacy world (see Chapter 5, Drug Formularies, Storage, Recalls, Shortages, and Diversion). An increasing number of medications must be stored at specific temperatures (such as frozen, refrigerated, or room temperature). The medications are generally stored at the specified temperature all the way through the drug distribution system—from manufacturer to wholesaler to pharmacy to patient. However, some medications that are refrigerated in the pharmacy (such as an antibiotic) may be stored at room temperature by the patient if they are only prescribed for a few days.

Because of storage considerations, you should ensure the following:

- Once a prescription is prepared, it should be stored at the appropriate temperature in the pharmacy until it is delivered to the patient. For instance, if a prescription or refill that needs to be stored in the refrigerator is called into the pharmacy but the patient does not pick up the medication for a few hours or days, it should be stored as directed in the refrigerator until the patient arrives.
- When you hand prescriptions to patients, be sure they understand how to store medications when they get home. It may be helpful to distinguish between storing a medicine at freezing temperature ("keep this in your freezer, where your ice is") or refrigerated temperature ("keep this in your refrigerator, where you put your milk").
- If a prescription is being delivered by car, mail, or other carrier, it must not be exposed to extreme temperatures (such as being left in a hot car during the summer) or kept outside its normal storage temperature for more than 24 hours. You may need to pack refrigerated or frozen drugs in an insulated container—perhaps even one containing ice or dry ice (Figure 8-5)—if delicate drug products are being shipped.

Information for the Patient

When you are giving prescriptions to patients, you are required under most state laws and the **Omnibus Budget Reconciliation Act of 1990 (OBRA '90)** to ask whether the person wants the pharmacist to counsel

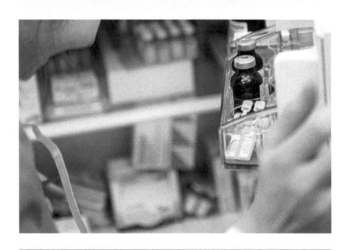

Figure 8-5 Refrigerated or Frozen Medications

The medications stored under refrigeration (2°C-8°C) should be shipped under the same conditions.

them about their prescription. In most pharmacies, the patient's signature is captured electronically when they pick up their prescription, indicating whether or not they are requesting counseling. Alternatively, patients may sign a logbook or a portion of the printed prescription label that is then removed and placed in a pharmacy logbook. When patients sign, make sure they understand what they are signing because many patients think they are simply acknowledging receipt of their medications and do not realize they are declining counseling from the pharmacist.

As was discussed in Chapter 3, Pharmacy Law and Regulation, OBRA '90 requires the pharmacist to offer to discuss with the patient or caregiver the following information:

- Name and description of the medication
- Dosage form, dose, route of administration, and duration of drug therapy
- Special directions and precautions for preparation, administration, and use of the medication by the patient
- Common or severe side effects, adverse reactions or interactions, and therapeutic contraindications that may be encountered, including ways of avoiding them and the action required if they occur

- Techniques for self-monitoring of drug therapy
- Proper storage
- Prescription refill information
- Action to be taken in the event of a missed dose

In addition, the pharmacist is required under OBRA '90 to record and maintain the following information:

- Patient's name, address, telephone number, date of birth (or age), and sex
- Patient's individual history when relevant, including diseases, known allergies and drug reactions, and a comprehensive list of medications and relevant medical devices
- Pharmacist's comments about the individual's drug therapy

If patients decline counseling but then ask you questions about the prescription, be cautious in your responses. As a pharmacy technician, you can easily provide straightforward information such as the name of the drug, how it is taken and stored, and whether it can be refilled. However, the pharmacist will need to respond to queries involving what the drug is for, what side effects or adverse reactions may occur, and what to do if a dose is missed. While you certainly will learn many of these things in your work as a pharmacy technician, these questions are best handled by the pharmacist for legal, ethical, and practical reasons.

Ensuring Confidentiality

Working in health care gives you access to the most private aspects of patients' lives: their medical and social histories, medication lists, financial information, height, weight, and other health-related information. You must keep such information confidential and use it only in the course of your job as a pharmacy technician. You must especially take care in the community pharmacy environment to be aware of individuals in the waiting or shopping areas outside the pharmacy. Avoid talking so loudly that you reveal protected health information to other individuals unintentionally. In the hospital setting, avoid discussing patient questions or situations in elevators or in hallways outside the central

pharmacy. Pharmacies face penalties under the **Health Insurance Portability and Accountability Act (HIPAA)**. Requirements under HIPAA and potential penalties are discussed in Chapter 3, Pharmacy Law and Regulation.

Simply put, there is no acceptable reason to discuss outside your job anything that you learn while working as a pharmacy technician about patients and the medications they are taking.

Social Media

Social media has been defined as "websites and applications that enable users to create and share content or to participate in social networking." Social media platforms include Facebook, Instagram, Twitter, and LinkedIn. In the pharmacy setting, social media may be used to provide patient education regarding medications, to market programs or specials at the pharmacy, or to just engage more with patients. As social networking becomes commonplace in professional environments, it is important that your online interactions are appropriate, are professional when called for, and do not compromise your patients or yourself. When working within any health care system, it is also important to know what your employer's policies are regarding use of social media.

In its Statement on the Use of Social Media by Pharmacy Professionals, the American Society of Health-System Pharmacists (ASHP) defines the responsibilities of professionals as "advancing the well-being and dignity of their patients, acting with integrity and conscience, and collaborating respectfully

> If patients state that they do not want counseling but then proceed to ask you questions about the prescription, be cautious in your responses.

> There is no acceptable reason to discuss outside your job anything that you learn while working as a pharmacy technician about people and the medications they are taking.

with health care colleagues." These responsibilities should be upheld by all of those working within the pharmacy, including technicians and interns.

- **Advancing the well-being and dignity of patients.** Pharmacy technicians should be aware of the benefits and limitations surrounding online communication. Social media can be an excellent way to engage with patients, but it should not become a substitute for other means of communication regarding patients' health, such as a phone consultation or an office visit. Pharmacy professionals should be aware when social media content is inaccurate or misleading and avoid spreading misinformation. It is also important to avoid complaining about patients on social media. This is unprofessional behavior, at baseline, and can be hurtful to the patient. For example, in November 2019, a nurse posted on TikTok, a popular video platform, a 15-second clip mocking patients for allegedly "faking" their ailments. This can be incredibly damaging to a patient who may be struggling with a chronic condition. In addition, it is illegal to post any patient's protected health information on social media, as this would be a violation of HIPAA.
- **Acting with integrity and conscience.** As members of a health care team, it is expected that technicians conduct themselves as professionals, even on social media. Make a conscious effort to keep your personal and professional information separate on social media. What is posted to social media leaves a "digital footprint" that can impact future advancement opportunities.
- **Collaborating respectfully with health care colleagues.** Although social media can be an excellent platform for debate about pharmacy practice and health care in general, it should be conducted in a professional manner. Comments and arguments made during these debates should be done so respectfully and should not mock or otherwise disparage patients or other health care professions, providers, or institutions.

Protecting patient privacy should be at the forefront when posting on social media. Many social media websites include settings to ensure the highest level of protection for personal information; however, these settings still have flaws and loopholes. Privacy settings on your accounts should be checked regularly to ensure they are set to standards with which you are comfortable.

English as a Second Language

As a pharmacy technician, it is very likely that you will encounter a patient at the pharmacy whose first language is not English. According to the Center for Immigration Studies (**https://cis.org/**), the number of US residents who speak a language other than English at home has doubled since 1990 and tripled since 1980. The National Center for Health Statistics (**https://www.cdc.gov/nchs/index.htm**) found that approximately 21.9% of US residents speak a foreign language at home. From 2013 to 2016, nearly 50% of US residents used at least 1 prescription drug within the past 30 days.

The consequences of providing false or inaccurate information about a patient's medications can be dangerous to the patient; therefore, it is essential to know how to communicate this information in an appropriate manner. Using professional interpreters is the gold standard for communicating health information with patients whose first language is not English; however, this is not always feasible. Google Translate (**https://translate.google.com/**) is a popular and accessible resource to help communicate in different languages. However, there are risks to using this tool in regard to accuracy within a health care setting. For example, a study by Patil and colleagues published in the *British Medical Journal* in 2014 examined 10 commonly used medical statements that were translated using Google Translate to 26 languages and then back to English by native speakers of that language. Investigators found that 57.7% of the total translations were correct, whereas 42.3% were wrong, with some serious errors. For example, in Polish, "Your husband has the opportunity to donate his organs" translated to "Your husband can donate his tools." A second alternative to a professional translator is a mobile application. Applications that have been reviewed and scored highly for their effectiveness, quality, and value include Canopy Medical Translator (**https://withcanopy.com/**), Universal Doctor Speaker (**https://www.universaldoctor.com/**), and Vocre Translate (**https://www.vocre.com/**). Use caution with nonmedical translators. They can be beneficial, but they also may not convey the intended message you are trying to communicate.

There may also be times when only a handful of words need to be translated. In these cases, a printed booklet that fits easily within your pocket may suffice. These are widely available and are written specifically for individuals working within pharmacy, such as *Essential Spanish for Pharmacy* written by the American Pharmacists Association. Prescription labels, written information, and medication guides should be provided to patients in their preferred language. Most major pharmacies also have access to translation software built into their electronic pharmacy system. The patient's preferred language should also be documented within the patient's profile to provide continuity of care each time a patient picks up prescriptions. Patients whose first language is not English are at higher risk for experiencing adverse effects with medications. They should be provided with extra time and attention to ensure there are no gaps in knowledge about their medications.

Conclusion

The bottom line when taking care of any patients is to ensure that they are receiving the correct medication, they have a complete understanding of their medications and how to take them appropriately, and all medications are delivered safely. Communicating with patients will be an essential part of most pharmacy technicians' workday. Whether through written or verbal communication, technicians in nearly all practice environments should be prepared to interact with patients in challenging situations. These communications will be a major determinant of how well you are able to execute many aspects of your role as a technician.

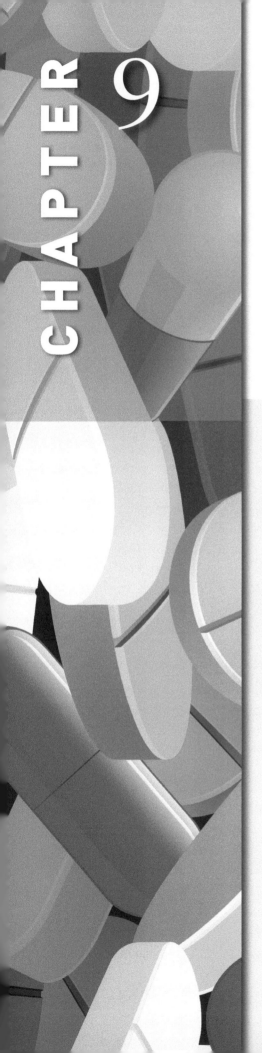

Patient Care Services and the Pharmacy Technician

Chapter 9 describes the pharmacist's emphasis on patient care services such as medication therapy management, immunization, point-of-care testing, and medication reconciliation. It also details ways that technicians can participate in these services and assist in data collection, patient interviews, data entry, documentation, and delivering patient care services.

Introduction

The assistance that pharmacy technicians provide with the dispensing aspect of pharmacy practice has been instrumental in allowing pharmacists to expand into more clinical roles. Technicians are also helping with many of the tasks associated with new and emerging clinical functions of pharmacists. Pharmacy technicians are filling important roles to help pharmacists provide patient-centered care, including medication therapy management services, pharmacy-based immunization delivery, point-of-care testing, and medication reconciliation activities.

Medication Therapy Management

In December 2003, the US Congress passed the Medicare Prescription Drug, Improvement, and Modernization Act (MMA), creating Part D of the Medicare program (see Chapter 3). As a result of the recognition of medication-related problems and the important roles pharmacists could play in preventing and resolving them, this law created a **medication therapy management (MTM)** services benefit for patients who have several chronic diseases, take multiple medications for those diseases, and have expected annual drug costs above a level that is adjusted annually.

The profession of pharmacy has been working since then to incorporate MTM services into everyday practice in a broad variety of settings. Soon after passage of MMA, the American Pharmacists Association convened meetings of key pharmacy organizations to develop a consensus-wide definition of MTM services (Table 9-1).

To fulfill these MTM tasks, the profession also developed a framework for delivering MTM services, referred to as the MTM Core Elements, which was published in the *Journal of the American Pharmacists Association* in 2008. This framework includes the following components:

1. Medication therapy review (MTR)
2. Personal medication record (PMR)
3. Medication-related action plan
4. Intervention and/or referral
5. Documentation and follow-up

Figure 9-1 shows how the MTM Core Elements fit into the patient care process to build the MTM service model. Pharmacists often rely on technicians to participate in these foundational components of MTM services, whether in spearheading the drug preparation phase of the dispensing process, participating in medication histories and patient scheduling, or facilitating patient communication. It will be helpful in your practice to understand each of the core elements of MTM services.

Medication Therapy Review

According to the MTM Core Elements, an MTR is defined as "a systematic process of collecting patient-specific information, assessing medication therapies to identify medication-related problems, developing a prioritized list of medication-related problems, and creating a plan to resolve them." In this step of the framework, the patient presents all of his or her medications to the pharmacist, who assesses each agent and how the patient is taking it—with the goal of identifying problems and potential solutions for the patient. In a traditional MTM service model, patients at risk for adverse events should receive a **comprehensive medication review (CMR)** of their medications at least once each year, with **targeted medication reviews (TMR)** throughout the year (more details are provided on CMRs and TMRs below).

Personal Medication Record

In the PMR step, a record is created of all of the patient's medications, including prescription and non-prescription drugs, herbal products, and dietary supplements (Figure 9-2). The PMR is a written record developed in collaboration with the individual and his or her other health care providers; patients can use the PMR to help keep track of and manage their medications at home.

Medication-Related Action Plan

Once the pharmacist has reviewed the patient's medication list and conducted a thorough assessment of patient complaints or symptoms, he or she can begin

Medication therapy management is a distinct service or group of services that optimize therapeutic outcomes for individual patients. Medication therapy management services are independent of, but can occur in conjunction with, the provision of a medication product.

Medication therapy management encompasses a broad range of professional activities and responsibilities within the licensed pharmacist's, or other qualified health care provider's, scope of practice. These services include but are not limited to the following, according to the individual needs of the patient:

a. Performing or obtaining necessary assessments of the patient's health status

b. Formulating a medication treatment plan

c. Selecting, initiating, modifying, or administering medication therapy

d. Monitoring and evaluating the patient's response to therapy, including safety and effectiveness

e. Performing a comprehensive medication review to identify, resolve, and prevent medication-related problems, including adverse drug events

f. Documenting the care delivered and communicating essential information to the patient's other primary care providers

g. Providing verbal education and training designed to enhance patient understanding and appropriate use of his/her medications

h. Providing information, support services, and resources designed to enhance patient adherence with his/her therapeutic regimens

i. Coordinating and integrating medication therapy management services within the broader health care management services being provided to the patient

A program that provides coverage for medication therapy management services shall include:

a. Patient-specific and individualized services or sets of services provided directly by a pharmacist to the patient.[a] These services are distinct from formulary development and use, generalized patient education and information activities, and other population-focused quality assurance measures for medication use.

b. Face-to-face interaction between the patient[a] and the pharmacist as the preferred method of delivery. When patient-specific barriers to face-to-face communication exist, patients shall have equal access to appropriate alternative delivery methods. Medication therapy management programs shall include structures supporting the establishment and maintenance of the patient–pharmacist relationship.

c. Opportunities for pharmacists and other qualified health care providers to identify patients who should receive medication therapy management services.

d. Payment for medication therapy management services consistent with contemporary provider payment rates that are based on the time, clinical intensity, and resources required to provide services (e.g., Medicare Part A and/or Part B for Current Procedural Terminology [CPT] and Resource-Based Relative Value Scale [RBRVS]).

e. Processes to improve continuity of care, outcomes, and outcome measures.

Approved July 27, 2004, by the Academy of Managed Care Pharmacy, the American Association of Colleges of Pharmacy, the American College of Apothecaries, the American College of Clinical Pharmacy, the American Society of Consultant Pharmacists, the American Pharmacists Association, the American Society of Health-System Pharmacists, the National Association of Boards of Pharmacy,[b] the National Association of Chain Drug Stores, the National Community Pharmacists Association, and the National Council of State Pharmacy Association Executives.

[a]In some situations, medication therapy management services may be provided to the caregiver or other persons involved in the care of the patient.

[b]Organization policy does not allow the National Association of Boards of Pharmacy to take a position on payment issues.

Source: Bluml BM. Definition of medication therapy management: development of professionwide consensus. *J Am Pharm Assoc.* 2005;45:566-572.

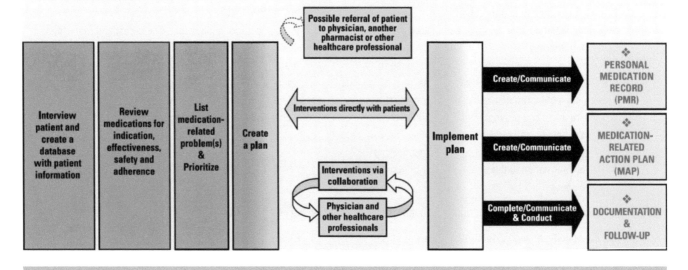

The Medication Therapy Management Core Elements Service Model

The diagram below depicts how the MTM Core Elements (❖) interface with the patient care process to create an MTM Service Model.

Source: American Pharmacists Association and the National Association of Chain Drug Stores Foundation. Medication therapy management in pharmacy practice: core elements of an MTM service model (version 2.0). *J Am Pharm Assoc.* 2008;48:341-353.

to develop a plan to help the patient address concerns and minimize medication-related problems. The medication-related action plan (MAP) contains a list of actions for the patient to use to track progress in self-managing their medications (Figure 9-3). The MAP document, along with specific patient education, is an essential element of the MTM care process.

Intervention and/or Referral

Sometimes patients will need to follow up with another health care provider after their pharmacist MTM visit, such as when the pharmacist recommends a medication therapy change. In some settings, pharmacists have been given the authority, in collaboration with the patient's physician (often referred to as a "collaborative practice agreement"), to make certain drug therapy changes under a preapproved protocol. In other settings,

the pharmacist must communicate his or her recommendation(s) to the physician; then, the patient follows up with a physician office visit to discuss the recommendation. Situations that may require an intervention or referral include a problem that requires further evaluation and/or diagnosis, additional disease management education beyond the scope of the pharmacist, or the need for patient monitoring for high-risk medications.

Documentation and Follow-Up

It is imperative for each step in the MTM process to be documented completely. As an old adage in pharmacy states, "If you didn't document it, you didn't do it." In the case of MTM services, documentation facilitates communication and compensation for MTM services, enhances continuity of care, ensures legal and regulatory compliance, protects against professional

Figure 9-2 Sample Personal Medication Record

MY MEDICATION RECORD side 1

Name:_____ Birth date: _____   LOGO

Include all of your medications on this record: prescription medications, nonprescription medications, herbal products, and other dietary supplements.
Always carry your medication record with you and show it to all your doctors, pharmacists and other healthcare providers.

Drug		Take for...	When do I take it?				Start Date	Stop Date	Doctor	Special Instructions
Name	Dose		Morning	Noon	Evening	Bedtime				
Glyburide	5mg	Diabetes	1		1		1/15/08		Johnson (000-0000)	Take with food

This sample Personal Medical Record (PMR) is provided
(or other user) should not, under any circumstances, solely
own risk. While intended to serve as a communication aid
advice or treatment. This PMR may not be appropriate for
Association assume no responsibility for the accuracy, cur

MY MEDICATION RECORD side 2

Name: _____ Birth date: _____ Phone:_____

Always carry your medication record with you and show it to all your doctors, pharmacists and other healthcare providers.

Emergency Contact Information

Name
Relationship
Phone Number

Primary Care Physician

Name
Phone Number

Pharmacy/Pharmacist

Name
Phone Number

Allergies

What allergies do I have? (Medicines, food, other)	What happened when I had the allergy or reaction?

Other Medicine Problems

Name of medicine that caused problem	What was the problem I had with the medicine?

When you are prescribed a new drug, ask your doctor or pharmacist:

- What am I taking?
- What is it for?
- When do I take it?
- Are there any side effects?
- Are there any special instructions?
- What if I miss a dose?

Notes:

Patient's Signature	Healthcare Provider's Signature	Date last updated
		Date last reviewed by healthcare provider

Source: American Pharmacists Association and the National Association of Chain Drug Stores Foundation. Medication therapy management in pharmacy practice: core elements of an MTM service model (version 2.0). *J Am Pharm Assoc.* 2008;48:341-353.

Figure 9-3 Sample Medication-Related Action Plan

MY MEDICATION-RELATED ACTION PLAN

Patient:	
Doctor (Phone):	
Pharmacy/Pharmacist (Phone):	
Date Prepared:	

The list below has important Action Steps to help you get the most from your medications.
Follow the checklist to help you work with your pharmacist and doctor to manage your medications
AND make notes of your actions next to each item on your list.

Action Steps ➡ What I need to do...	Notes ➡ What I did and when I did it...
☐	
☐	
☐	
☐	

My Next Appointment with My Pharmacist is on:_____(date) at _____ ☐ AM ☐ PM

Source: American Pharmacists Association and the National Association of Chain Drug Stores Foundation. Medication therapy management in pharmacy practice: core elements of an MTM service model (version 2.0). *J Am Pharm Assoc.* 2008;48:341-353.

liability, and demonstrates the value of pharmacist-provided services.

Comprehensive and Targeted Medication Reviews

CMRs and TMRs have additional rules in place regarding how often they should be offered to patients and what information should be documented. According to the 2020 Medication Therapy Management Program Guidance and Submission Instructions from the Centers for Medicare and Medicaid Services (CMS; available on the CMS website at https://www.cms.gov/Medicare/Prescription-Drug-Coverage/Prescription DrugCovContra/MTM), MTM plan sponsors must offer a minimum level of MTM services to each beneficiary enrolled in the program that includes all of the following:

1. Interventions for both beneficiaries and prescribers
2. An annual CMR with written summaries in CMS's standardized format
   - The beneficiary's CMR must include an interactive, person-to-person, or telehealth consultation performed by a pharmacist or other qualified provider in an individualized written summary in CMS's standard form.
3. Quarterly TMRs with follow-up interventions when necessary

A CMR is defined by CMS as "an interactive person-to-person or telehealth medication review and consultation conducted in real-time between the patient and/or other authorized individual, such as prescriber or caregiver, and the pharmacist or other qualified provider and is designed to improve patients' knowledge of their prescriptions, over-the-counter (OTC) medications, herbal therapies and dietary supplements, identify and address problems or concerns that patients may have, and empower patients to self-manage their medications and their health conditions."

The CMR is an essential step of the MTM process. It is a thorough medication review that should take 30 minutes or less to conduct. The completion rate of CMRs is an important metric, and beginning in 2016, the CMR completion rate affects a plan's Part D star rating. According to the 2019 guidance from CMS, it is expected that a CMR should meet the following professional service definition: A CMR is a systematic process of:

- Collecting patient-specific information
- Assessing medication therapies to identify medication-related problems
- Developing a prioritized list of medication-related problems and creating a plan to resolve them with the patient, caregiver, and/or prescriber

A standardized format and instructions for completing a CMR are available from CMS (https://www.cms.gov/Medicare/Prescription-Drug-Coverage/PrescriptionDrugCovContra/MTM) with a complete explanation of all required information in versions for English- and Spanish-speaking patients.

For ongoing monitoring, sponsors are required to perform TMRs for all beneficiaries enrolled in the MTM program with follow-up interventions when necessary. The TMRs must occur at least quarterly beginning immediately upon enrollment in the MTM program and may address specific or potential medication-related problems. In particular, TMRs may be performed to assess medication use, to monitor whether any unresolved issues need attention, to determine if new drug therapy problems have arisen, or to assess whether the beneficiary has experienced a transition in care. In contrast to the CMR, the TMR is focused on specific actual or potential medication-related problems.

A standardized format and instructions for completing a TMR are available from CMS (https://www.cms.gov/Medicare/Prescription-Drug-Coverage/PrescriptionDrugCovContra/MTM) with a complete explanation of all required information in versions for English- and Spanish-speaking patients. Table 9-2 lists potential roles the technician can play in MTM services.

Chronic Disease Management

In many cases, patients who most need in-depth patient care services are those with chronic diseases and at high risk for medication-related problems.

MTM Patient Identification and Recruitment

- Distribute and monitor patient communications about MTM services.
- Identify MTM opportunities through dispensing software, prescription issues, or conversations with patients.
- Connect pharmacists with patients or prescribers for service delivery.
- Follow up with additional communications as necessary until a response is received.
- Schedule appointments for patients and pharmacists.

MTM Patient Visit

- Collect medication and other information from the patient prior to their visit with the pharmacist.
- If a comprehensive medication review (CMR) is being performed, collect a complete medication list from the patient (over-the-counter medications, herbals, and prescription medications). Document these medications in the patient's Medication Profile or on the CMR intake form.
- Note new medications, questions, or concerns for the pharmacist to address during the appointment.
- Upon completion of the CMR, assist with updating the patient's profile and any follow-up documentation.
- Document, prepare, and submit the claim form, if applicable.
- Schedule follow-up appointments as needed for additional interventions identified during the CMR and remind pharmacists when it is time to follow up with patients or prescribers.

Adapted from information available at APhA MTM Central webpage found at www.pharmacist.com.

Outside of formal MTM services, pharmacies may also offer **disease management services** for some chronic conditions. In outpatient pharmacy settings, pharmacists are most commonly involved in the care of patients with diabetes, high cholesterol or "dyslipidemia," asthma, hypertension, and cardiovascular disease. Monitoring these conditions involves measuring blood glucose levels, lipid profiles, respiratory function, and blood pressure, as described in the following sections.

It is beyond the scope of this chapter to explain how to use all available devices for these 4 measurements, and new devices and meters are being marketed all the time. If you are involved in helping with disease state monitoring in your pharmacy, find out what devices are being used and make sure that the pharmacist shows you exactly how to use them.

Blood Glucose Levels

The amount of glucose, or sugar, present in the blood (blood glucose level) is generally measured directly from a blood sample obtained from a patient **fingerstick** (Figure 9-4). For the types of blood glucose measurements usually available in the pharmacy, drawing blood from a vein, known as **venipuncture**, is not needed. If you are helping to obtain the fingerstick or to analyze the blood for glucose, you must do so in accordance with the pharmacy's procedures and the blood glucose meter's instructions.

Lipid Profiles

Simple meters for measuring patients' **lipid levels** are also often available in pharmacies, which usually require a fingerstick sample of blood—often a larger volume of blood than is needed for measuring glucose. Lipid analyzers provide information about some or all of these blood components:

- Total cholesterol
- Triglycerides
- Low-density lipoproteins
- High-density lipoproteins

Ideally, the pharmacist needs all the values above to accurately assess a patient's clinical condition. However, for the purpose of screening patients and

Figure 9-4 Fingerstick

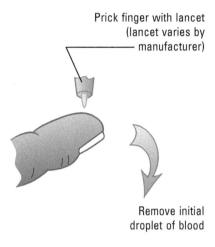

Prick finger with lancet
(lancet varies by
manufacturer)

Remove initial
droplet of blood

Take sample
from the next droplet

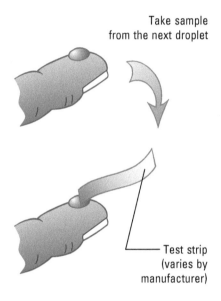

Test strip
(varies by
manufacturer)

Process of obtaining patient fingerstick for measuring blood components.

referring those with high cholesterol to physicians, the pharmacist needs only total cholesterol.

Respiratory Function

For patients with asthma, the most common means of measuring lung function outside a laboratory involves the **peak flow meter** (Figure 9-5), a device that is convenient for patients to use at home or in the pharmacy. The peak flow meter records peak expiratory flow (PEF), or the maximum amount of air the patient can blow out with one big breath. Measuring PEF with peak flow meters is easy, practical, and inexpensive, making these devices perfect for short-term monitoring, managing exacerbations, and long-term monitoring at home by the patient.

Because reference values vary widely for different available meters, the patient must be taught to compare daily values with his or her "personal best" PEF value obtained with the same meter. Each patient's personal best PEF can most accurately be estimated over a 2- to 3-week period, during which the patient records the PEF 2-4 times per day. Once the patient's condition is stabilized, the personal best value is usually achieved in the early afternoon. Occasionally, for reasons not well understood, patients will observe a much greater PEF value. Such "outlier" values should be used with caution in establishing a personal best PEF.

Blood Pressure

The most accurate device for measuring blood pressure is the **mercury sphygmomanometer**, which uses a cuff on the arm, a table-top unit with mercury, and a stethoscope. In addition, many easier-to-use—but not quite as accurate—devices are available (Figure 9-6).

Figure 9-5 Peak Flow Meter

Pharmacist counseling a patient on how to use a peak flow meter.

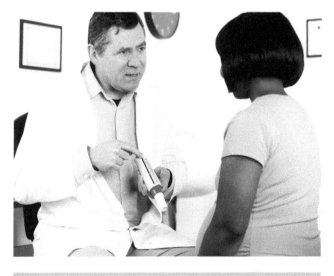

Figure 9-6 Blood Pressure–Measuring Devices

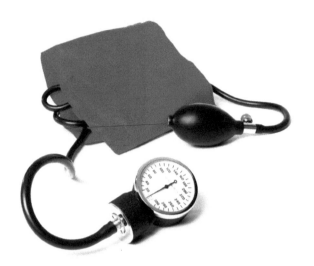

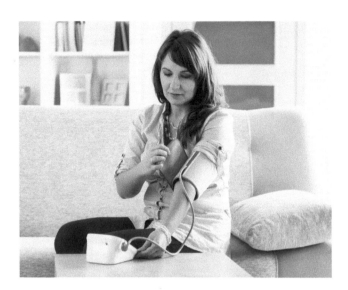

Whichever of these is used in your pharmacy, familiarize yourself with its proper operation, especially how to properly place the cuff on the arm.

Blood pressure is expressed as 2 numbers—one "over" the other. For example, a reading of 120/80 mm Hg is communicated verbally as "one-hundred and twenty over eighty millimeters of mercury." Both numbers represent important pressures generated in the blood vessels as the heart contracts and relaxes. The "top" number, known as systolic pressure, is the highest amount of pressure present in the blood vessels. It occurs at the moment when the heart contracts. The "bottom" number, the diastolic pressure, is the lowest blood pressure. It occurs when the heart relaxes.

These pressures occur because blood vessels are a closed system, just like water in a balloon. When the cuff is placed on the arm and pumped up, it stops the blood flowing in an artery just under the skin on the inside of the elbow. As the air is slowly let out of the cuff, the pressure at which the blood starts pulsing is the systolic pressure. Then, as air continues to go out of the cuff, the pressure at which the blood stops pulsing (and flows normally) is the diastolic pressure. Have someone take your blood pressure, and you will feel this "pulsing" between the 2 blood pressures.

Point-of-Care Testing

Point-of-care screening or testing for management of minor, nonchronic conditions is becoming an increasingly common component of pharmacist patient care services. Numerous states, including Washington, Kentucky, Idaho, and Florida, have passed "Test and Treat" or similar legislation allowing pharmacists to prescribe medication to treat strep/flu or minor skin conditions after administering a rapid diagnostic test. Similar to their role(s) in MTM or chronic disease management, technicians can assist with patient recruitment, scheduling, and workflow for patients undergoing diagnostic testing or screening. In point-of-care testing, the technician can also assist by:

- Obtaining needed approvals and maintaining records to administer diagnostic or screening tests in the pharmacy. Most of these tests are categorized as "CLIA waived." The **Clinical Laboratory Improvement Amendments of 1988 (CLIA)** created quality standards for different types of laboratory testing. The pharmacy must obtain a CLIA waiver and meet ongoing quality control and regulatory requirements for pharmacies to be able to offer these tests.

- Maintaining compliance with other regulatory standards, such as **Occupational Safety and Health Administration (OSHA)** bloodborne pathogens standards, plans for infection control, use of **personal protective equipment**, safety training, and equipment and procedures for handling and disposing of biohazardous waste in the pharmacy.

- Performing the test with the patient and documenting test results for the pharmacist's visit. This important function allows the pharmacist to see a larger number of patients because the pharmacy technician obtains objective information such as the laboratory value and the pharmacist can focus on clinical decision making.

Pharmacy-Based Immunization Delivery

In the past decades, pharmacists have become important sources of immunizations for the American people, especially against influenza. Pharmacists in all states and US territories are authorized to administer the influenza vaccine. Other vaccinations that can be administered by pharmacists on a state-by-state basis commonly include the pneumococcal shot; herpes zoster vaccine (which protects against shingles infection); the combination tetanus, diphtheria, and pertussis vaccine; and the human papillomavirus vaccine.

As a result of this expanded authority, pharmacies offering immunizations have proliferated, especially those providing flu shots in the fall. As a pharmacy technician, you may be called on to help register patients who visit the pharmacy to receive an immunization, ensure that the necessary information is available about the patient and his or her medical history, and see that patients remain in the pharmacy after their shot long enough to detect any adverse reactions. Discuss your role with the pharmacist so you know exactly what is expected of you and how to perform the tasks you are asked to help with. In the online Immunization Center (www.pharmacist.com /immunization-center), APhA provides a wealth of immunization information you can use in your pharmacy.

In 2017, Idaho became the first state to allow technicians to administer immunizations in the United States, and pharmacy technicians have since been authorized to immunize in several other states, including Rhode Island and Utah, while many other states have considered regulatory and policy changes. More recently, in October 2020, the US Department of Health and Human Services (HHS) released guidance that included a provision for qualified pharmacy technicians to administer "FDA-authorized or FDA-licensed COVID-19 vaccines to persons ages three or older and to administer FDA-authorized or FDA-licensed Advisory Committee on Immunization Practices (ACIP)-recommended vaccines to persons ages three through 18 according to ACIP's standard immunization schedule." The complete guidance is available from HHS at https://www.hhs.gov/sites /default/files/prep-act-guidance.pdf. Table 9-3 lists requirements that technicians and state-authorized pharmacy interns must satisfy to administer these immunizations. For legal and regulatory purposes, HHS states that "this authorization preempts any state and local law that prohibits or effectively prohibits those who satisfy these requirements from administering COVID-19 or routine childhood vaccines as set forth above. It does not preempt state and local laws that permit additional individuals to administer COVID-19 or routine childhood vaccines to additional persons."

In all states, technicians already have important roles that support pharmacy-based immunizations, such as assisting with the completion of vaccine administration record forms, accessing vaccination histories, managing inventory, entering

> Over the past decades, pharmacists and technicians have become important sources of immunizations for the American people.

> Many pharmacists have built extensive businesses in the field of durable medical equipment.

| Table 9-3 | Qualifications for Pharmacy Technicians to Administer COVID-19 Vaccines or Childhood Immunizations Under 2020 Guidance From the US Department of Health and Human Services |

To qualify under 42 U.S.C. § 247d-6d(i)(8)(B) when administering FDA-authorized or FDA-licensed COVID-19 vaccines to persons ages three or older or ACIP- recommended childhood vaccinations to persons ages three through 18, qualified pharmacy technicians must meet the following requirements:

- The vaccination must be ordered by the supervising qualified pharmacist.
- The supervising qualified pharmacist must be readily and immediately available to the immunizing qualified pharmacy technicians.
- The vaccine must be FDA-authorized or FDA-licensed.
- In the case of a COVID-19 vaccine, the vaccination must be ordered and administered according to ACIP's COVID-19 vaccine recommendation(s).
- In the case of a childhood vaccine, the vaccination must be ordered and administered according to ACIP's standard immunization schedule.
- The qualified pharmacy technician or State-authorized pharmacy intern must complete a practical training program that is approved by the Accreditation Council for Pharmacy Education (ACPE). This training program must include hands-on injection technique and the recognition and treatment of emergency reactions to vaccines.
- The qualified pharmacy technician or State-authorized pharmacy intern must have a current certificate in basic cardiopulmonary resuscitation.
- The qualified pharmacy technician must complete a minimum of two hours of ACPE-approved, immunization-related continuing pharmacy education during the relevant State licensing period(s).
- The supervising qualified pharmacist must comply with recordkeeping and reporting requirements of the jurisdiction in which he or she administers vaccines, including informing the patient's primary care provider when available and submitting the required immunization information to the state or local immunization information system (vaccine registry).
- The supervising qualified pharmacist is responsible for complying with requirements related to reporting adverse events.
- The supervising qualified pharmacist must review the vaccine registry or other vaccination records prior to ordering the vaccination to be administered by the qualified pharmacy technician or State-authorized pharmacy intern.
- The qualified pharmacy technician must, if the patient is 18 years of age or younger, inform the patient and the adult caregiver accompanying the patient of the importance of a well-child visit with a pediatrician or other licensed primary-care provider and refer patients as appropriate.
- The supervising qualified pharmacist must comply with any applicable requirements (or conditions of use) as set forth in the CDC's COVID-19 vaccination provider agreement and any other federal requirements that apply to the administration of COVID-19 vaccine(s).

Abbreviations: ACIP, Advisory Committee on Immunization Practices; FDA, Food and Drug Administration.
Available at https://www.hhs.gov/sites/default/files/prep-act-guidance.pdf. Last accessed December 9, 2020.

data, and handling billing. As their role in immunization becomes even larger, the work of technicians will continue to advance the level of medication safety and help pharmacists deliver optimum patient care.

Assisting With Medical Appliances and Devices

Many pharmacists have built extensive businesses in the field of **durable medical equipment** (DME). Ostomy products, canes, crutches, and home infusion and respiratory equipment are among the wide variety of products that fall into this category (Figures 9-7 and 9-8).

DME is attractive from a business standpoint because its cost is often reimbursable to the pharmacy under the federal government's Medicare Part A program. The Medicare program covers elderly and disabled Americans. When patients need the kinds of products listed above, Medicare Part A pays health care providers, including pharmacies, to provide them.

Figure 9-7	Durable Medical Equipment

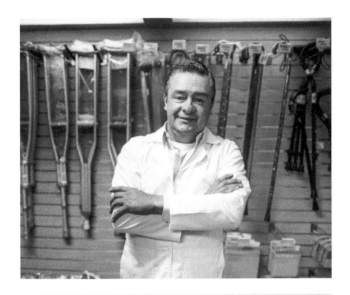

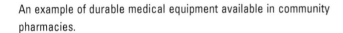

An example of durable medical equipment available in community pharmacies.

Figure 9-8	Providing Durable Medical Equipment Counseling

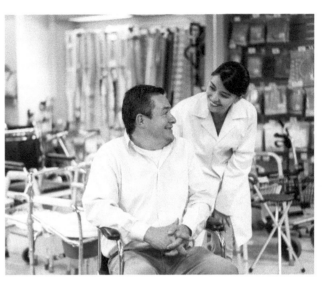

Here, a pharmacist in a community pharmacy counsels a patient about wheelchairs.

For you as a pharmacy technician, DME may be an important part of your job that includes:

- **Measuring patients** to fit them with devices such as ostomy products; canes, crutches, and walkers; and wheelchairs. Patients who need ostomy products have usually had cancer and, as a result, require alternative portals for excrement. The most common situation is colon cancer that requires surgical removal of the last part of the colon, including the anus. In this case, the remaining colon is rerouted to a position on the patient's side, where an ostomy bag can be attached to collect wastes.
- **Educating patients** about the device they are using. **Home infusion** equipment is used by patients to self-administer fluids, medications, or both on a long-term basis. These infusions generally run into the patient's veins (intravenous infusions), but some patients also receive peritoneal dialysis at home. In this case, large volumes of fluids are infused into the peritoneal cavity—the space around the patient's

large organs (stomach, liver, intestines). The fluid can draw out many of the wastes from the blood flowing through these organs, hence the term **dialysis**.

- **Making sterile products** for home administration to patients, a key area for pharmacy technician involvement in DME. The process by which you will make intravenous infusions, peritoneal dialysis fluids, and total parenteral nutrition (TPN) products is explained in Chapter 13, Sterile Compounding. TPN is a specialized type of infusion that contains nutrients for patients unable to eat foods or drink liquids. TPN contains high concentrations of sugars and amino acids along with vitamins, minerals, and trace elements. TPN solutions are often administered to patients continuously, and they are given through a special administration port placed into a large vein just before it reaches the heart (this is called a central line to differentiate it from normal intravenous sites, which are called peripheral lines). Fat emulsions are given with TPN several times each

| **Table 9-4** | Definition of Medication Reconciliation |

This definition was developed jointly by an expert panel convened by the American Pharmacists Association and the American Society of Health-System Pharmacists in 2007:

"Medication reconciliation is the comprehensive evaluation of a patient's medication regimen any time there is a change in therapy in an effort to avoid medication errors such as omissions, duplications, dosing errors, or drug interactions, as well as to observe compliance and adherence patterns. This process should include a comparison of the existing and previous medication regimens and should occur at every transition of care in which new medications are ordered, existing orders are rewritten or adjusted, or if the patient has added nonprescription medications to [his or her] self-care."

Source: Burns AL, Owens JA, Reilly C, Sheckelhoff D. Improving care transitions: optimizing medication reconciliation. *J Am Pharm Assoc.* 2012;52:e43-e52.

week to help the patient get the oils and fats needed in a healthy diet.

Medication Reconciliation

> Medication reconciliation involves compiling a complete and accurate list of a patient's medications and is conducted when patients move from one setting to another, such as from a hospital to a long-term care setting.

Similar to an MTR in the MTM process, medication reconciliation involves compiling a complete and accurate list of a patient's medications, including prescription, nonprescription, herbal, and supplements. A key difference, though, is that medication reconciliation is usually conducted at transitions of care, or when patients move from one setting to another, such as from a hospital to a long-term care setting (Table 9-4).

Medication reconciliation is an essential process in many settings to help ensure patient safety and minimize harm, and many medication errors or adverse drug events can be attributed to poor communication at transitions and interfaces of care. Pharmacists and technicians can play important roles in this process to help prevent medication errors and reduce health care costs.

As you assist the pharmacist in medication reconciliation, patient histories, or data collection, you may use a printed form or a computer data-entry screen to record the information. Be very careful to record the information accurately and in the correct space, because errors could compromise patient care or result in denial of payment by third-party payers. In addition, take care to always protect the confidentiality of the health-related information you have access to as a pharmacy technician.

Conclusion

By assisting the pharmacist with both dispensing and patient care activities, you can become a valuable and necessary part of the pharmacy. Pharmacy technicians are increasingly able to have a tremendous impact on patient outcomes through assisting the pharmacist as well as performing direct patient care services.

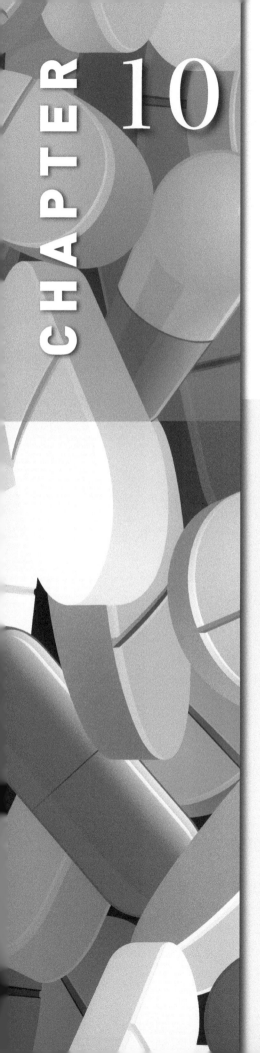

CHAPTER 10

Processing Prescriptions and Medication Orders

Most technicians spend the majority of their time preparing drugs for dispensing by the pharmacist. Chapter 10 covers, in detail, the process from the time a prescription is presented until the drug is delivered to the patient.

Introduction

Technicians generally spend most of their time preparing drugs for dispensing by the pharmacist. Chapter 10 describes, in detail, the process of receiving, entering, checking, preparing, and delivering a prescription or medication order.

A prescription usually refers to an order for a drug for an ambulatory patient. That is, the patient, or patient's representative, presents the prescription (Figure 10-1) to the pharmacy and the corresponding drug product is, in turn, delivered to the patient. In hospital, nursing home, and other institutional pharmacies, prescriber orders contain requests for medications, referred to as "medication orders" (Figure 10-2).

A prescription usually refers to an order for a drug for an ambulatory patient.

Figure 10-1 Example of a Prescription

Name Shorty Powell Date 11/16/10
Address
℞ Phenytoin Sodium Extended 100 mg tid #90
LABEL Refill 0-1-2-3-4-5-PRN
Generic Substitution Permitted M.D.

Prescriptions and Medication Orders

The parts of a prescription and medication order are described in Tables 10-1 and 10-2, respectively.

Prescriptions and medication orders may be written by various professionals, including physicians; nurses; pharmacists; respiratory, physical, or occupational therapists; social workers; or even clergy. They may be received in the pharmacy electronically by prescriber or pharmacist order entry, by fax, or as a paper hard copy. Whatever the mechanism, the pharmacist or technician must review them carefully to identify the drug orders on each page.

Because the hospital or institution already has information about patients and prescribers on file, medication orders may not have all of the information usually contained in a prescription. In the institutional setting, orders for Schedule II substances do not have to be separated and stored any differently from other medication orders, as nurses keep those medications in a locked cabinet or automated device on the patient care unit (although they may be stored this way in some cases and, if so, require additional paperwork and documentation). In addition, medication orders may come with special timing instructions such as "PRN," for medications ordered on an "as-needed" basis, or

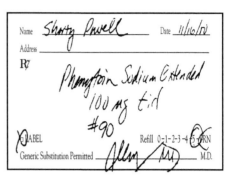

Figure 10-2 Example of a Medication Order

PHYSICIAN'S ORDERS
DATE-HOUR ALLERGIES
11/16 CBC + Electrolytes
1123 Thyroid panel STAT
After panel start
Levothyroxine 12.5 mcg QD

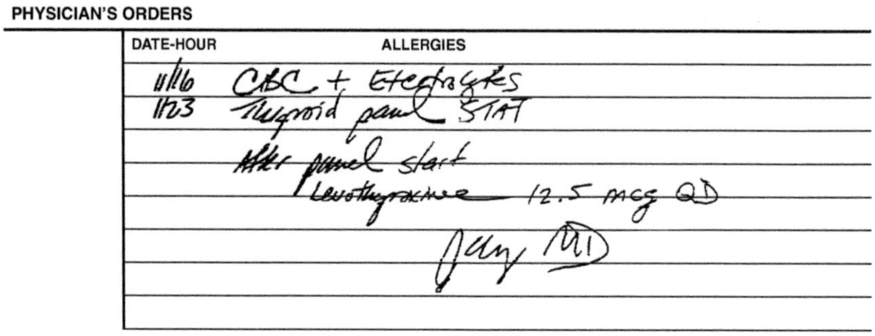

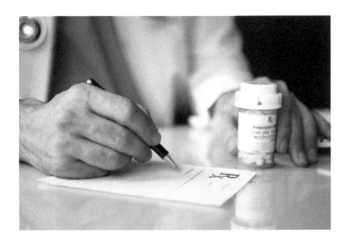

"STAT" orders, requiring medication to be filled within a short time frame (eg, 15 minutes) in an institutional setting.

Obtaining Information From Patients and Professionals

When information is missing from prescriptions or medication orders, you may need to talk with the patient, pharmacist, or prescriber. Although Chapter 8 discusses communication strategies with patients in more detail, a few general communication points are particularly relevant to the dispensing process.

Any contact that you as a technician have with the patient or prescriber should be within the guidelines established by your institution, pharmacy, or supervising pharmacist. Patients have a right to privacy with respect to their health, so you must take care as to when and how you talk with patients. In most pharmacies, technicians should assist with clarifying the spelling of patients' names or addresses, verifying the correct medication is dispensed, or engaging the pharmacist if the patient has questions, but be sure you know what other information you are responsible for obtaining.

Similarly, any contact that you have with the prescriber should be within the guidelines of your pharmacy or employer. Pharmacists may prefer—or even be required by law—to contact the prescriber directly about unclear critical information, such as the name of the drug; instructions on how to use it; whether a dose

> When information is missing from prescriptions or medication orders, you may need to talk with the patient, pharmacist, or prescriber.

Table 10-1 Parts of a Prescription

As shown in Figure 10-1, a prescription has the following parts:

- Patient name and, for controlled substances, a full address.
- Date the prescriber wrote the prescription—this is especially important because state laws often specify that prescriptions are valid for only a certain period of time after they are written.
- Rx symbol—standing for the Latin verb "recipe," meaning "you take."
- Name of the medication (the "inscription")—prescribers may use either generic or brand names. In the case of compounded prescriptions, the prescriber may list several ingredients that the pharmacist is to mix together.
- Directions to the pharmacist on what to dispense (the "subscription")—this usually consists of the number of tablets or capsules; a volume of a liquid; or 1 or more prepackaged medications from a manufacturer.
- Directions on how the medication is to be used (the "sig," which is short for "signa," Latin for "write")—prescribers use abbreviations, such as those presented in Chapter 2, to convey to the pharmacist how the patient should take the medication.
- Refills, special labeling, or other instructions—prescriptions may not be refilled without the prescriber's permission. Per federal law, prescriptions for Schedule II controlled substances cannot be refilled at all. Prescriptions for Schedule III through V substances may be refilled, with the prescriber's permission, up to 5 times over the 6-month period beginning on the day the prescription is written, not dispensed.
- Prescriber's signature and, for controlled substances, the Drug Enforcement Administration number (see Chapter 3).

Table 10-2	Parts of a Medication Order

As shown in Figure 10-2, a medication order has the following parts:

- Prescriber's information
- Date of order
- Patient information (eg, room number, medical record, or identification number)
- Name, strength, and dosage form of medication
- When to be administered (specific time of day)
- Duration of therapy
- Prescriber's signature

is correct; or whether the patient is allergic to a drug. In particular, if you think a prescription may be invalid or forged, work with the pharmacist in contacting the prescriber to verify it. See Chapter 3, Pharmacy Law and Regulation, for more information about forged prescriptions.

You may also need to get information on a patient's insurance or health coverage. Because this is confidential information, take care to obtain it in an appropriate manner. Errors in the beneficiaries' names, policy numbers, and other information can cause claims to be rejected, so record this information carefully. To be sure you can hear the patient, insurance and health coverage information should be collected in a quiet area.

Entering Prescriptions or Medication Orders Into the Computer

Once you receive a prescription or medication order, the next step in many cases is to enter this information into the pharmacy computer system. **Order entry** is the process of entering new prescriptions or medication orders into an existing patient profile, or record, or creating a new patient profile. Keep in mind that order entry may be accomplished by the prescribing physician or the pharmacist on the patient care unit in some institutions, or by prescribers using electronic prescribing systems. See Chapter 11, Pharmacy Computer and Information Systems, for more information

on pharmacy computer systems, patient profiles, and electronic health records.

If you are entering a prescription or medication order, make sure to verify the patient's name, medical record, or other identification number. Depending on whether you are entering a prescription or medication order, you will need to enter the date, drug name, dosage form, dispensing quantity, directions for use, and number of refills. If the patient has an existing profile or medical record, confirm that the patient information on the order matches that in the patient profile. If it does not, you will need to create a new profile. Compare the new order or prescription with the patient's profile. Stay alert for medication duplication, drug class duplication, or other potential problems. Notify the pharmacist if you detect an issue. Problems that may require a pharmacist's intervention include a potential adverse drug event, suspected drug nonadherence, or suspected drug interaction or duplication.

To avoid medication errors, be sure to read the name of the drug (and all other information) very carefully on the prescription or medication order. Many mistakes in pharmacy occur as a result of illegible instructions from prescribers or misreading of drug names by pharmacy personnel. If the name of the drug does not fit the directions for use, for instance, wrong number of doses per day or wrong route of administration, or if you are not 100% certain of what the prescriber has written, you or the pharmacist should contact the prescriber to clarify the name of the drug.

Pay close attention to **drug-utilization review (DUR)** or **drug-utilization evaluation (DUE)** warnings. These alerts warn pharmacy technicians and pharmacists about potential medication issues or problems, such as drug–drug interactions. An alert may appear when a prescription or medication order is entered, processed, or submitted electronically to a third party for billing. Let the pharmacist know if an alert pops up to help ensure patients are using medications safely and appropriately.

Order entry may also be the first point at which a technician or pharmacist is alerted to a potential prescription forgery. See Chapter 3, Pharmacy Law and Regulation, for more information on fraudulent prescriptions.

Processing Prescriptions and Medication Orders

Once you have obtained all necessary information and are satisfied that the prescription or medication order should be filled, you are ready to prepare the medication for the patient. The act of transferring a medication to the patient is central to the entire practice of pharmacy. When done correctly, patients obtain needed medication safely. An error in this system, however, can lead to patient harm or adverse events.

An old adage in pharmacy is that, in dispensing medications, you must get the right drug in the right dosage form to the right patient at the right time, labeled with the right directions and other instructions. Let's look at the process of ensuring these things happen correctly and avoiding medication errors while doing so.

Understanding Generic and Brand Names

Every bit of information on a prescription or medication order is important, but certainly the most important element is the name of the drug or drug product. As mentioned in Chapters 1 and 3, drugs may be prescribed by their generic or brand names, and generic drugs can generally be substituted for their brand counterparts if the 2 products are classified as being therapeutically equivalent. The generic name is the common name assigned to that chemical compound by the US Adopted Names Council; it may be used by any company that markets the drug. The brand name is a trademarked reference to the drug that only one company is entitled to use. This company is usually the innovator, or original creator, of that drug. Until its patent on the drug expires, the innovator is the only company entitled to market the drug. When a drug is available from only one company, it is called a single-source product. For example, Prevacid, shown in Figure 10-3, was a single-source product until the innovator's patent expired. When a drug is available from more than one company, it is called a multisource product. Notice in Figure 10-4 that all the products have the same generic name, glipizide, but the innovator product also has a trade name, Glucotrol. Occasionally, generic products also have a brand name. These are called branded generics, but they are still essentially generic alternatives to the original branded product.

In a community or ambulatory pharmacy, if a prescription is written for a brand-name drug but other (usually less expensive) generic products are available, you must follow the laws in your state concerning generic substitution (Figure 10-5). In several states, you must inform the patient of the availability of the lower-cost agents and let the patient decide which product he or she wants. If the prescriber has written "Brand Product Necessary" on the prescription or checked a box for "Dispense As Written," you must follow the prescriber's instructions and give the patient the brand-name product. In an inpatient setting, many institutions have a limited "formulary" or a predetermined list of preferred drugs that can be dispensed in that institution. In this setting, the therapeutic substitution is often automatic in the institutional pharmacy, and formulary restrictions are communicated to prescribers and pharmacists in an ongoing manner. Talk with the

> The act of transferring a medication to the patient is central to the entire practice of pharmacy.

Figure 10-3 Brand-Name Drug Packaging

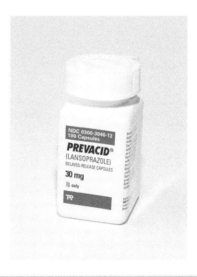

Prevacid was a single-source product until its patent expired.

Figure 10-4 Multisource Brand and Generic Products

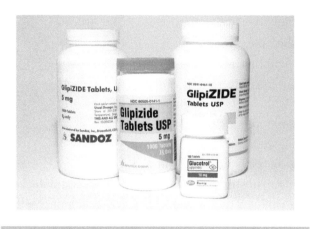

This photo shows the innovator product (Glucotrol) and generic alternatives.

pharmacists you work with about how to handle these situations in your pharmacy and your state.

Another situation that affects the drugs dispensed in community and ambulatory pharmacy settings occurs with some Medicaid or third-party plans. In the outpatient setting, when patients are covered by third-party payers, such as a state Medicaid system

Figure 10-5 Three Different Companies' Levothyroxine Products

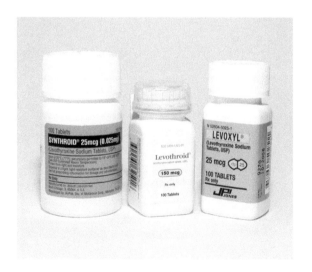

Depending on state laws, prescriber directions, patient preferences, and facts about bioequivalence as determined by the US Food and Drug Administration, the pharmacist may or may not want to substitute a generic alternative for the prescribed brand of medication.

or insurance company, the pharmacy is obligated by contract to fill some prescriptions with drugs that are similar to ones a prescriber may request but that are not the same chemically. This is called **therapeutic substitution** or drug-product selection. A phone call to the prescriber may be required to change the patient to the preferred product. Alternatively, the physician may choose to submit a **prior authorization** to seek coverage for the more expensive, nonpreferred medication. Again, talk with the pharmacist about what contracts the pharmacy has and what policies must be followed for patients covered in your practice setting.

Preparing the Medication Label

Another important step in filling the prescription or medication order is preparing the label that will be put on the vial or drug product. Because this is what the patient will read to know how to use the medication, the label must be clear in its instructions, prepared neatly, and affixed firmly to the final prescription packaging.

Under the pharmacy laws of your state, certain information must be put on the prescription label. While these laws vary, most states require the following on prescription labels:

- Pharmacy name and address
- A sequential number that enables the pharmacy to retrieve the prescription from the files

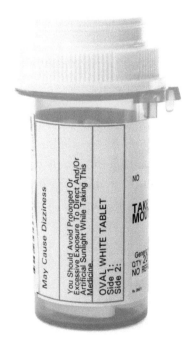

- Patient's name
- Date the prescription was filled
- Prescriber's name
- Directions for use of the medication
- The federal legend: "Caution: Federal law prohibits transfer of this drug to any person other than the patient for whom it was prescribed."

Many states also require the name of the medication and the strength dispensed. The brand name should be used only when the product dispensed is the brand-name drug; otherwise, the generic name should be used.

Similarly, requirements also exist for labels on medication orders. While these laws also vary, most states require the following:

- Name and location of patient
- Trade or generic name of drug
- Strength of drug
- Quantity of drug
- Expiration date of medication
- Lot number of medication

You must read the prescription or medication order to learn most of the above information, and you will usually need to interpret the Latin pharmaceutical abbreviations presented in Chapter 2, Pharmacy Calculations, Abbreviations, and Terminology, to do so. If you are not 100% certain of what the prescriber has written or requested, you or the pharmacist must contact him or her for clarification. In addition, if you are not completely sure that you remember what the Latin abbreviations stand for, ask for help from the pharmacist or other technicians.

The process of preparing the prescription label is generally automated. You must learn the codes that are used in your pharmacy's software to make the correct directions print on the label. Because small errors inputting these codes into the computer can cause serious mistakes on the label, be sure to read the label after it prints out to be certain that the directions are correct.

Obtaining and Checking Medications

Once you determine which drug product the prescriber has requested, you must retrieve it from the storage area and bring it back to the product preparation area. Before you get the product, you must know the name of the drug, the strength of the drug (for example, 25 mg or 50 mg), the dosage form requested (for example, tablets, liquids, eye drops, or ear drops), and the quantity you need.

During the dispensing process, 100% accuracy is needed. Most pharmacists strive to achieve this level of perfection by checking the prescription or medication order 3 times: once when they get the product from the shelf, once when they begin to measure the product, and once after they affix the prescription label to the vial.

> **During the dispensing process, 100% accuracy is needed.**

In the process of getting products from the storage shelves or bins, many mistakes can occur when pharmacy personnel rely on viewing the color of a package or the shape of a box rather than on reading the name of the drug product. The correct dosage form is just as important as the right drug. For instance, if you accidentally give a patient ear drops and they are placed in the eyes, the patient could suffer eyesight damage. Be certain that you know what the prescriber is asking for and that you have pulled the right product, whether it's a cream or ointment, syrup or elixir, tablet or capsule, or short- or long-acting product (Figure 10-6).

> **The correct dosage form is just as important as the right drug.**

Tip: One quick way to verify that you are pulling the intended product is to check the National Drug Code (NDC) number on the pharmacy label against the NDC on the stock bottle. Because this coding system includes different numbers for different drugs and package sizes, NDC numbers are often the first clue if a similar, but incorrect, product has been pulled by mistake. You will learn more about NDC numbers in Chapter 4, Inventory Control and Management.

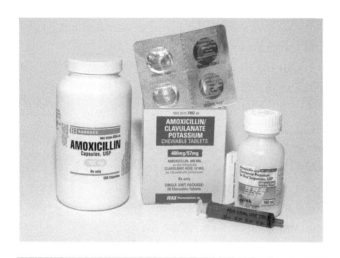

Figure 10-7 Counting Trays

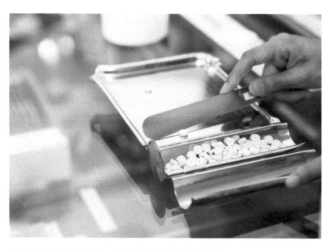

Counting trays, which have come to symbolize pharmacy in recent years, are used to obtain the correct numbers of tablets or capsules.

Finally, the right strength is critical. Some drugs—such as levothyroxine or warfarin—have narrow therapeutic indexes, meaning that the right dose in one patient may be toxic in the next patient. The blood thinner warfarin is a high-alert, narrow therapeutic index drug—accidentally dispensing 10-mg tablets in place of 1-mg tablets would lead to a 10-fold dose increase and the possibility for a serious and potentially fatal bleeding event. Again, be sure that you have retrieved the exact strength the prescriber is asking for, whether it's 100 mcg or 100 mg, 0.1 mg or 1 mg, 1% or 10%, or 125 mg/5 mL or 250 mg/5 mL.

These measuring devices have specific properties that you will need to be familiar with. For example, if you take a graduated cylinder and put some water in it, you will notice how the liquid curves, with the higher edges on the sides and the lower level in the middle. When reading

Measuring Drug Products

Measuring solid oral drug products is generally simple—for tablets and capsules, you just need to count out the appropriate number. For this purpose, most pharmacies have counting trays (Figure 10-7), and many have automated counting devices that can save you time (Figure 10-8). Be sure that these devices are kept clean; otherwise, one patient's medication can contaminate the next patient's drug. In the case of agents that many people are allergic to, like penicillin, this amount of contamination has sometimes been associated with serious reactions.

When measuring liquids, you need clean graduated cylinders or other appropriate equipment (Figure 10-9).

Figure 10-8 Automated Tablet Counters

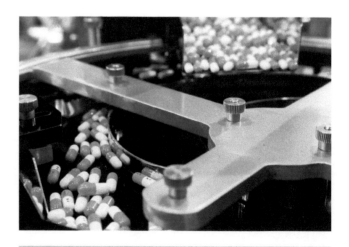

Automated tablet counters are used in many pharmacies to quickly and accurately obtain the needed numbers of tablets and capsules for individual patient prescriptions.

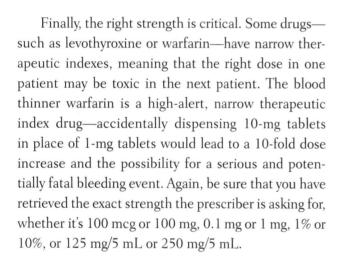

Figure 10-9 Equipment for Measuring and Grinding

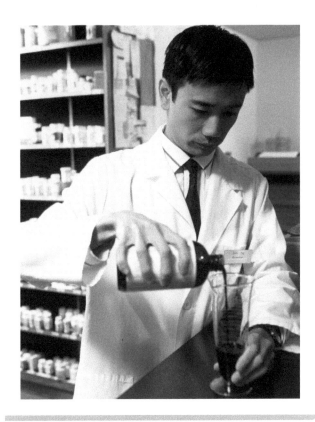

Graduated cylinders, funnels, beakers, and mortars and pestles are used during prescription filling in the pharmacy for tasks such as measuring liquids and grinding solids into powders.

the amount of liquid in any measuring device, you always read at the bottom of this curve, which is called the **meniscus**.

Many antibiotics come from the manufacturer as powders in a bottle. You must add the appropriate amount of water, usually distilled or sterile water, to the bottle and shake it well to prepare a suspension of the antibiotic. Also check the bottom of the container, where powder sometimes sticks during storage, to be sure you have completely mixed all of the powder. Be sure to read the directions for reconstitution and storage on each antibiotic container and follow them carefully. Antibiotic suspensions are usually refrigerated by the patient to maintain stability of the antibiotic for the 10 or more days of drug administration. Be clear on whether the bottle must be refrigerated. The patient must also understand the importance of shaking the bottle immediately before pouring a dose.

In Chapters 12 (Nonsterile and Bulk Compounding) and 13 (Sterile Compounding), we will discuss many other important aspects of measuring drugs and drug products, including the use of scales and syringes.

Packaging the Prescription and Affixing the Label

Once the label is prepared and the drug product has been counted or measured, you are ready to place the drug in the container the patient will receive. Drugs must be stored in airtight containers so that the moisture, light, and air will not cause them to lose potency before the patient finishes taking the prescription. For this reason, special prescription vials are used. These vials, usually brown or amber, also limit the amount of light that the drug product is exposed to, as some drugs can be degraded by light (Figures 10-10 and 10-11).

Under federal law, you must use vials with **child-resistant** containers unless the patient requests easy-open tops. When you are preparing prescriptions for arthritis medications or for older patients who are unlikely to have children at home, ask them which kind of closure they want. If they ask for easy-open tops, be sure to advise patients to store their medicines in a safe

Figure 10-10 Prescription Vials

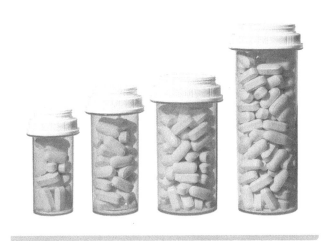

Examples of prescription vials used for solid oral dosage forms (tablets and capsules).

Figure 10-11 Prescription Bottle

Figure 10-12 Unit-of-Use Packaging

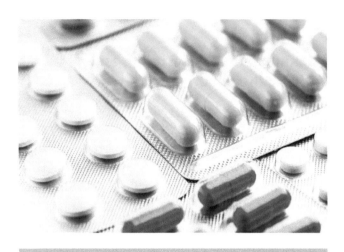

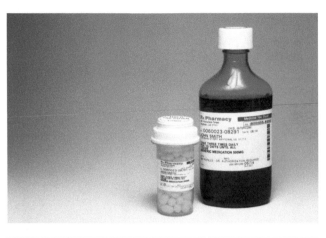

Example of a prescription bottle used for oral liquid dosage forms (syrups, elixirs, suspensions, and solutions) as compared with a bottle for tablets.

Unit-of-use packaging is increasingly available from pharmaceutical companies.

place. Child-resistant containers have greatly reduced poisonings in children, but many incidents still occur when children visit the homes of older adults, such as grandparents.

The same guiding principles apply to vials for oral liquids. These vials are airtight, light-resistant containers that help to protect the stability of drug products. When measuring the liquid in these vials, the meniscus should be at the correct line on the side of the vial. Use the smallest possible vial with child-resistant closures, unless the patient asks for easy-open containers.

Many drug products today come in packages that are appropriate for dispensing directly to the patient. An example of such packaging is oral contraceptives (birth control pills), which usually come in 21- or 28-day supplies with the days of the week or numbers marked so that patients can remember if they have taken their medicine. This is called **unit-of-use** or **unit-dose** packaging because it is prepared by the manufacturer in the most commonly dispensed unit. It is used increasingly for various types of prescription drugs (Figure 10-12). Pharmacies may also prepare individualized packaging for use in nursing homes or to help patients at home remember which medicines to take at which times of day. In inpatient settings, you may dispense medication orders in unit-of-use packaging directly to the patient care floor or through an automated dispensing cabinet. In outpatient pharmacies, many drugs that must be dispensed with a medication guide (see Chapter 3) are supplied by the manufacturer in 30-day supply bottles with an affixed Medication Guide so that each prescription can be easily dispensed in the manufacturer's bottle with the required Medication Guide for the patient.

Once you have put the prescription product in the appropriate container or packaging, you are ready to affix the **prescription label** (Figure 10-13). Before or after you affix the label, stop for a moment to double-check the drug product, the directions on the label, the name of the patient, and the name of the prescriber. Be sure that everything is correct before you pass the prescription or medication order on to the pharmacist for the final check.

For unit-of-use packages, the prescription label will be placed somewhere on the container. Some pharmacists prefer to place products such as eye or ear drops in larger bottles so that the full prescription label

> Many drug products today come in packages that are appropriate for dispensing directly to the patient.

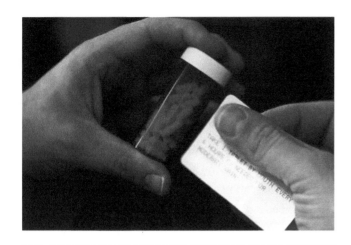

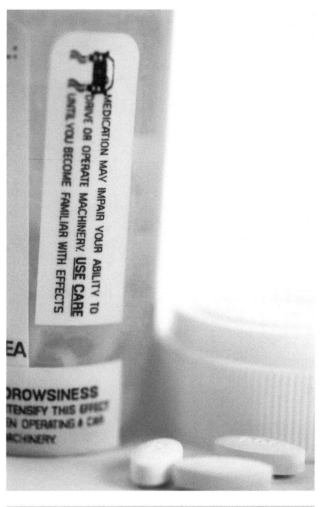

can be affixed. In addition, bottles of some tablets such as nitroglycerin are too small for a label, but the tablets must be kept in the original container to maintain product stability. Put the original container inside a larger prescription vial, and affix the label to the larger vial. For inpatient settings, in which individual doses may be dispensed to patients or to the patient's floor or unit to cover a shorter period of time, follow policies and procedures specific to the pharmacy setting.

Most pharmacies have historically put **auxiliary labels** on prescription vials (Figure 10-14), although these have been displaced in many cases by special messages that are printed directly on the label by pharmacy computer software. If your pharmacy uses auxiliary labels, such as "May cause drowsiness" or "For external use only," be sure to place the correct ones on the prescription vial after you have put the label on. When adding auxiliary labels to the prescription vial or packaging, take care not to cover any part of the label or other area with important information, such as the product's expiration date or lot number.

Providing Information to Patients

Pharmacists are responsible not only for telling patients what medications are and what they are used for (Figure 10-15) but also for undertaking a full range of patient education activities. To assist in this role,

nearly all prescriptions are dispensed with written information detailing what the drug is, how it works, and what side effects the patient should watch for. This information sometimes prints out of the computer system with the label, while at other times, it comes in the package with the drug product. These information requirements generally do not apply in the same manner in institutional settings, even with most Medication Guides, since patients have access to health care providers directly to get information or ask questions when their medications are administered.

When you prepare the prescription or medication order, place any necessary information, including a Medication Guide if required, with the completed

Figure 10-15 Pharmacist Counseling Patient

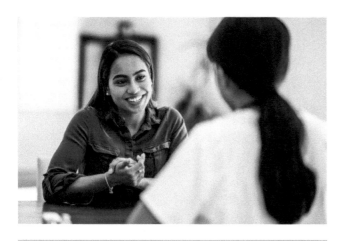

When you are sure that you have put the right drug in the right strength and dosage form in the right container for the right patient, you are ready to send the prescription or medication order to the pharmacist for a final check.

product so that it can be delivered to the appropriate area or given to the patient and explained to them by the pharmacist.

Performing the Final Check

When you are sure that you have put the right drug in the right strength and dosage form in the right container for the right patient, you are ready to send the prescription or medication order to the pharmacist for a final check. With the availability of pharmacy computer

systems and devices, scanners, and barcode technology, this check is often linked to the computer system. The pharmacist can verify your work by reviewing it on the computer screen: a scanned copy of the written order, a picture of the correct tablet or capsule, and the instructions you entered into the computer. Barcoding technology often allows an additional check to verify that the right drug product and patient are linked to the prescription or medication order at various steps in the dispensing process.

Using older systems, the pharmacist can check the actual written prescription, the label you prepared, and which bottle you used to obtain the medication. Once the pharmacist is satisfied that everything is correct, he or she will dispense, or authorize the transfer of, the drug product to the patient. Under the pharmacy laws of most states, this act of dispensing the medication must be performed by a registered pharmacist. Advanced pharmacy technicians are allowed to check the work of other technicians in some states under certain conditions. Studies show that technicians' performance meets or exceeds accuracy rates for pharmacists doing a visual check for dispensing activities such as restocking automated dispensing machines or filling batches of unit-dose medications.

Conclusion

In this chapter, the process of preparing a prescription for dispensing to the patient is summarized. However, 2 factors can complicate this process. One is the role the pharmacist plays in making sure that the drug the prescriber has requested is the best choice for a specific patient. The other, which has been mentioned, is the use of pharmacy computer systems and other types of automation in the process of drug dispensing and distribution.

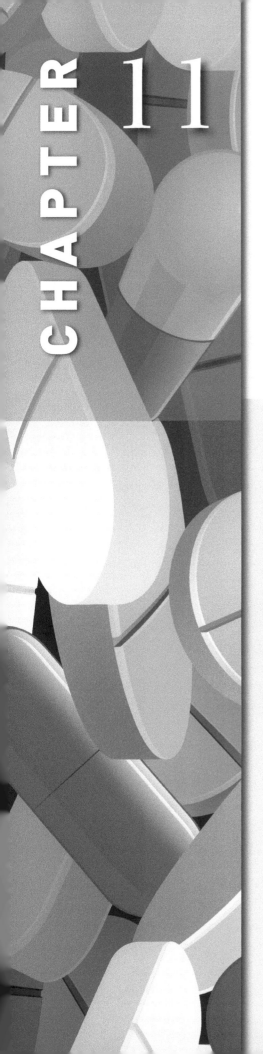

CHAPTER 11

Pharmacy Computer and Information Systems

Adonice Khoury, PharmD, BCPS

The field of pharmacy computers and information systems is progressing so fast that presenting timely information on specific programs and systems is not possible in a textbook. The details of specific electronic health information programs are best found in the training manuals of the respective programs. This chapter reviews the importance of information systems in contemporary pharmacy practice and describes some of the ways in which these systems can support complex clinical, documentation, and communication functions. Computer systems and automation also help to streamline dispensing and patient care processes in the pharmacy.

Introduction

Pharmacy computer systems facilitate workflow efficiency in prescription processing and the financial aspects of pharmacy operations. Everything from patients' prescriptions to drug inventories and patient education materials is maintained on computer. In most hospitals and many busy community pharmacies, automated dispensing machines and robotic devices assist in drug-dispensing activities every day. With advancing technology, pharmacy technicians will have more job opportunities in these fields.

> Pharmacy is probably the most computerized part of the health care world.

This chapter describes the basic types of pharmacy information systems that support documentation, communication, dispensing, and patient care activities. To understand specifics of the information and automation systems used in your practice setting, you will need to learn about them on the job or take advantage of special training classes.

Pharmacy Information Systems

As a pharmacy technician, you will play an important role in a larger health care system. Just as pharmacy has advanced and become more complex, so has the overall health care system in the United States. On a small scale, this complexity is reflected in the number of treatment options available. For a patient who has recently suffered a stroke or heart attack, treatment options may include surgery, rehabilitative therapy, medications for prevention and treatment, and comprehensive dietary and lifestyle changes. On a larger scale, the need for implementation of the various treatment options has necessitated an expansion of type and number of health care facilities. Thus, the information tied to a single patient for any given condition has expanded. Accordingly, pharmacy information systems that maintain patient records and health information have grown more integrated and complex to keep pace with these advances.

Pharmacy information systems are computer systems that a pharmacy uses to manage all the

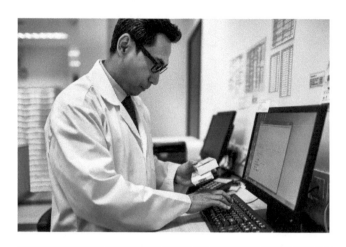

Figure 11-1 Pharmacy Computer Order Entry Screen

information required to care for patients. Although such systems may appear straightforward at first glance (Figure 11-1), they accommodate some of the most important clinical, documentation, and communication functions in the pharmacy, such as:

- Clinical screening for drug interactions
- Prescription order entry
- Prescription and inventory management
- Patient profiles
- Reports of medication use
- Interactions with other systems related to payment, regulatory compliance, and so on

These systems have led to many improvements in data management and patient safety, including faster processing of orders and prescriptions, reduced medication errors, and improved adherence to medication-use policies or drug formularies (see Chapter 4) within an institution. Table 11-1 includes terminology related to pharmacy information systems and their most common functions.

Clinical Screening

When information is entered into the patient profile, the pharmacy clinical information system stores the records and applies the information to future prescriptions filled in the pharmacy. Whether in the

Table 11-1	Pharmacy Information System Terminology

TERM	DEFINITION
Computerized physician order entry (CPOE)	Physicians or other providers enter medication orders directly into the computer system on the patient care unit or floor instead of transmitting a written or verbal order to the pharmacy for order entry.
Electronic medical record (EMR)	An electronic or digital version of a patient's chart that allows providers to track patient data, identify ongoing patient needs, monitor specific laboratory or other parameters over time, and handle many other components of a patient's care within a single pharmacy or institution.
Electronic health record (EHR)	Similar to an EMR, but often provides additional information about the patient's history outside of a single institution or provider. In some cases, patients may have access to their EHR information when they see providers in different institutions or practices.
Clinical information system	A computerized pharmacy information system that also provides information on the clinical care of patients, such as electronic medication administration records, laboratory and other patient data, and diagnoses.
Clinical decision support (CDS)	Electronic tools to help pharmacists, physicians, and other providers or individuals involved in health care make informed decisions about treatment or other options. CDS systems may include drug-interaction alerts with alternative treatments, predetermined order sets for high-risk medications, links to clinical guidelines, and many other resources.
Electronic prescribing (e-prescribing, e-Rx)	Computer-based generation and transmission of a prescription directly from the prescriber, usually to an outpatient or mail-order pharmacy. In contrast to CPOE, which generally occurs within a single closed system, e-prescribing transmits a prescription electronically between separate systems (eg, from the provider's office to the pharmacy), taking the place of paper, faxes, or telephone orders. E-prescribing can reduce medication errors because it removes subjective factors such as illegible handwriting, but it may also introduce new types of errors, such as a prescriber selecting the wrong medication from a drop-down menu.
Health Level 7 (HL7)	HL7 is one of several standard-setting organizations whose mission is to provide interoperability standards for EHR systems.
Medication administration record (MAR)	MARs are usually handwritten or printed from an electronic pharmacy information system.
Electronic medication administration record (eMAR)	A version of the MAR viewable online and not printed.
Personal health record (PHR)	An electronic record of health-related information about an individual that conforms to nationally recognized interoperability standards and that can be drawn from multiple sources while being managed, shared, and controlled by the individual.

community or hospital setting, each time a new prescription or medication order is entered for a specific patient, the pharmacy computer system screens the patient's information to aid the pharmacist in ensuring the appropriateness of the new medication. The information screened includes the patient's medication list, drug allergy information, current or former smoking or alcohol use history, pregnancy status, age, height, weight, kidney function, dietary restrictions, and much more. Some pharmacy information systems also allow you to document previous medication adverse events or patient risk factors. When entering information into the computer, be complete and accurate to ensure that all data are correct and properly updated.

Prescription Records and Management

At minimum, a patient's prescription record will include basic information about the patient's current and past prescriptions (Table 11-2). Although specific details depend on which computer system your pharmacy uses, nearly all pharmacy systems use prescription records in the dispensing process. Many also interface prescription records with inventory to verify if a specific product is in stock or to track the stage of dispensing that any given prescription or medication order is in at the time. As a pharmacy technician, understanding the prescription records and management components of your pharmacy's information system will be a key to your success in the pharmacy.

Inventory Management

Given the number of drugs and pharmaceutical products on the market, it would be nearly impossible to keep track of pharmacy inventory (see Chapter 4) without computerized systems. Pharmacy computer systems are often used to maintain accurate counts of current inventory, display an alert when products go below a preset quantity, identify appropriate suppliers for product replacement, or automatically reorder products.

Table 11-2	Prescription Records in a Database

A prescription record in a database includes the following fields:

- Date
- Patient name and address (often stored in a separate patient database)
- Drug name and dosage (often stored in a separate drug database)
- Quantity
- Directions for use
- Refills
- Prescriber name and address (also often stored in a separate prescriber database)
- Patient education and counseling information (stored in the drug or a related database)
- Patient prescription history (stored in the prescription database or some other related database)

Patient Profiles

Although the patient profile serves as the electronic repository of the patient's drug and medical history, it has grown to serve many more functions. In a community chain pharmacy, patient profiles are often integrated among different pharmacy locations to facilitate data sharing and prescription transfers. In a health system, the patient profile may integrate with information in other areas of the patient chart and may interface with the larger clinical information system in a health system. This integration and interfacing allow the pharmacist access to important disease state and monitoring information when verifying medication orders.

Reports

As pharmacy systems have become larger and more complex, managing patient and drug-related information in the advanced computer database has become necessary. The pharmacy information system allows pharmacists and administrators to generate reports that can assist with overall patient care and management of the pharmacy or institution. Key reports, which allow administrators to identify trends or problems that might otherwise be missed, may include the following:

- Inventory activity
- Drug usage
- Overrides
- User access
- Controlled substances
- Drug diversion

For example, if a major drug–drug interaction warning is nearly always overridden, patients may be at risk of adverse events. Identifying high usage rates of a very expensive drug when an equal but more cost-effective option is available within a health system can help target an intervention that could lower system-wide costs.

Computerized Systems for Pharmacy Dispensing

Pharmacists have been using computer technology for prescription ordering, processing, and dispensing since the late 1970s. Although **computerized physician**

order entry (CPOE) and **electronic prescribing (e-prescribing)** are rapidly becoming the industry standard, pharmacists and technicians are still closely tied to the prescription or medication order entry process. CPOE screens use codes for drug names and dosage strengths as well as instructions for use. Although it may take time to become accustomed to these codes, their use greatly increases the rate at which pharmacists and technicians can enter prescription information into the computer system.

Computer-related technology is also now used routinely to improve accuracy and efficiency of the dispensing processes. Health systems, mail-order pharmacies, high-volume community pharmacies, and pharmacies utilizing centralized fill procedures at remote locations depend on computer-related technology to dispense medications to patients in a safe and timely manner. The types of computer-related technology in routine use include the following:

- **Automated prescription-dispensing systems**—For community pharmacies, automated prescription-dispensing systems may fill one-half or more of the daily workload in the pharmacy department. The process begins when the technician enters an order into the prescription software system and the actual prescription is scanned into the system. Using drug products that have been placed into bins—usually by pharmacy technicians—robotic or automated devices interpret the prescription order, prepare a label, place medication into a vial or other container, and transfer the prescription label onto the container. The pharmacist then checks the entire process and uses computer-generated patient-counseling materials to make sure the patient knows how to take the medication properly.

- **Automated cart-fill machines**—A similar type of machine used in hospital and nursing home operations is the automated cart-fill machine. In institutions, medications are often transferred from the pharmacy to the patient care areas using carts. These carts have drawers, called **cassettes**, which are also referred to as cubies or pockets. Each cassette contains the medications ordered by the physician for 1 patient for a given period of time (usually 24 hours in a hospital but up to 30 days for a long-term care facility such as a nursing home). The automated cart-fill machine picks the drugs that are on each patient's computerized profile from medication bins filled by pharmacy technicians. It then places the correct number of medications into the patient's cassette. These automated systems rely on barcodes to be certain that the right medication is being prepared based on each prescription order.

- **Automated dispensing machines**—Another type of technology in use in institutions is the automated dispensing machine. Although often referred to as "the Pyxis®," which is the name of one brand of these machines, other common brands are used including AcuDose® or Omnicell®. These dispensing machines are placed in patient care areas so nurses can obtain medications for patients in a timely manner. The dispensing machine interfaces with the system containing the patient's medication profile, which allows the nurse to select medications available in the machine ordered for the patient. Nurses may also be granted access to medications in the machine that are not on the patient's profile (often for emergency use) via an override function. Pharmacy technicians have the important responsibility of refilling each medication in the machine once the machine's inventory drops below a prespecified par level.

Figure 11-2 Example of Automated Dispensing Machines and Robotic Equipment

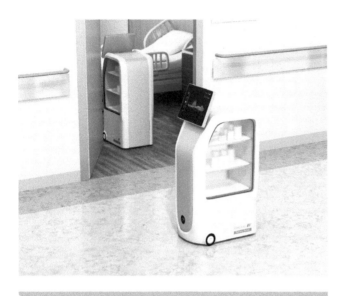

The machines have limited storage, so they usually are loaded with common fast-moving medications and medications for emergency use. One beneficial use of these devices is storing controlled substances—that is, those medications that have abuse potential (see Chapter 3, Pharmacy Law and Regulation). Because controlled substances cannot be placed in the regular medication carts, dispensing machines are used to restrict access to controlled substances. Additional procedures are usually required when the nurse obtains a controlled substance from the automated dispensing machine. The nurse can be required to document the name of the patient who is to receive each dose; count and document the supply with each dispensing; document the wasting of unused controlled substance at the end of each work shift; and request a second witness to cosign the dispensing, wasting, or override of the controlled substance.

> Two needs of MTM services match perfectly with the capabilities of computer programs: documentation and billing.

- **Robots for product delivery**—Primarily in very large hospitals, automated systems can be used for delivering medications to patient care areas (Figure 11-2). These robotic machines roll through the halls, get on and off elevators, and talk to people that they sense nearby. On the nursing unit, they deliver patient medications to nurses, recording who accepted transfer of the medications. The robots can be very useful in hospitals that do not have other, less expensive delivery mechanisms, such as pneumatic tube systems. Pneumatic tubes are used in many hospitals to bring medication orders to the pharmacy and to send medications to the patient care areas.

As automated systems continue to develop, they will present more opportunities and challenges to pharmacists and technicians. Computerized technology will become more sophisticated and will start performing tasks that humans now do. As a pharmacy technician in the years ahead, you will likely find yourself needing to become familiar and proficient in the use and management of the specific automated systems in your setting.

Computerized Systems for Medication Therapy Management Activities

Just as information technology is an essential feature of pharmacy-dispensing processes, computers are increasingly important in medication therapy management (MTM) services. In several key areas, pharmacists are using technology to manage clinical tasks and information. Two needs of MTM services match perfectly with the capabilities of computer programs: documentation and billing.

Documentation involves recording information about the patient and the interventions made by the pharmacist and other pharmacy personnel. This record keeping is essential for 2 reasons. First, to be paid by third-party payers, the pharmacist must have a record of the work performed. Second, if something goes wrong and the patient later becomes ill or dies, the pharmacist may need information that can be presented in a court of law to show that the interventions made were necessary and appropriate.

Billing, which is covered in more detail in Chapter 14, Pharmacy Billing and Reimbursement, is the process of obtaining payment from insurance companies, the government, or health plans. Pharmacy owners sign contracts with third-party payers, and the contract requires the pharmacy to keep records of the prescriptions dispensed and other interventions. The records must be made available to the third-party payer on demand so the payer can be sure the pharmacy has, in fact, done what it was paid for. These records are critically important to avoid contract cancellation or criminal charges that the pharmacy has defrauded the third-party payer.

For patient care, many types of information are recorded in computer software programs:

- Care plans (what problems the pharmacist has found and how they are to be treated)
- Disease management (interventions unique to various diseases)
- Therapeutic outcomes (the effects of interventions on the patient's clinical condition as well as quality of life)
- Progress notes (documentation of the pharmacist's observations in each visit with the patient)
- Billing information (when and how payment was requested)

If you are asked to enter patient care information into the computer, you will need to complete training for the systems used in your workplace.

Computer-Related Issues in Pharmacy Practice

Information today is a very powerful and valuable commodity. As people are concerned about companies sharing or selling information about their credit card transactions, they may also be troubled to learn that their pharmacy provides information to outside parties. This practice has become a part of a broader discussion of confidentiality with respect to health care information. Confidentiality is discussed in more detail in Chapter 3, Pharmacy Law and Regulation,

and Chapter 8, Interacting With Patients, but a brief mention is warranted here with respect to computers.

The data available in pharmacy computer systems are of interest to several outside parties, but federal law requires data **confidentiality**. If patients cannot share private information with their pharmacists without fear that other people or outside companies will learn about it, then they are not likely to tell the pharmacist everything necessary for pharmacists to provide quality care. Pharmacies have sometimes encountered public outcry or lawsuits when they have engaged in the following practices:

> If patients cannot share private information with their pharmacists without fear that other people or outside companies will learn about it, then they are not likely to tell the pharmacist everything necessary for pharmacists to provide quality pharmaceutical care.

- Using pharmaceutical industry grants to pay outside companies to send prescription refill reminders to patients
- Providing names and addresses of patients who have had prescriptions filled for certain drugs to the manufacturers of those or competing drugs, and providing the names of prescribing physicians to manufacturers

Another important computer-related issue in pharmacy practice is the need to have backup policies and procedures in the event that a computer system is malfunctioning or is having scheduled maintenance. Sometimes referred to as **computer downtime procedures**, these contingency plans specify the necessary steps that the pharmacy must follow to avoid interruption in continuity of workflow and patient care. Computer downtime procedures are usually developed for both unplanned and planned downtimes and are specific for each affected computer and automated system used in the pharmacy. It is essential for you, as a pharmacy technician, to become familiar with the existing computer downtime procedures used in your workplace. Likewise, there may be opportunities for you to be involved in the development of computer downtime procedures as your workplace adopts new technologies.

Conclusion

Pharmacy information and computer systems have become workhorses of the pharmacy to manage all the complex aspects of patient care in our health care system. Even so, you must never forget the "people" side of pharmacy practice. Everything you do is aimed at producing a positive impact on patient care and health outcomes. In your role as a pharmacy technician, you will interact with patients—who are in all respects the reason the pharmacy was established and continues to operate—and with the health professionals who take care of these patients.

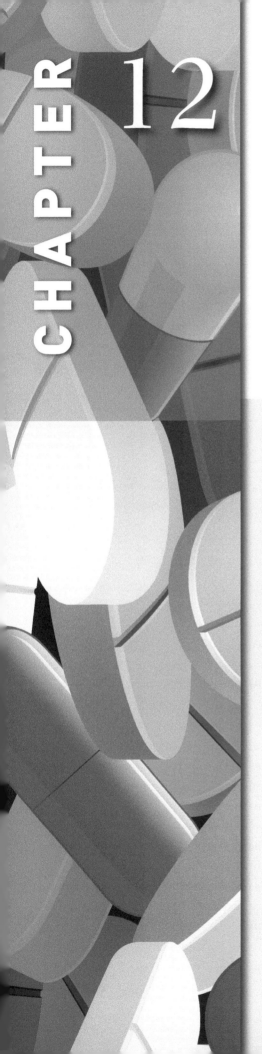

CHAPTER 12

Nonsterile and Bulk Compounding

Chapter 12 briefly defines the process of compounding special prescriptions for patients, including an overview of United States Pharmacopeia standards for nonsterile compounding. It then presents bulk compounding, along with regulatory distinctions between bulk compounding and manufacturing.

Introduction

Most medications needed on a daily basis in pharmacy practice are available in manufactured dosage forms. But pharmacists still frequently use their knowledge of medications and chemistry and their skills in the art of pharmacy to make special preparations for patients—ones that would otherwise be unavailable. The process of mixing ingredients to prepare a special medication for a patient is called **compounding**. As a pharmacy technician, you may be called on to assist the pharmacist in compounding prescriptions for patients. Nonsterile compounding occurs in all practice settings, including community, hospital, managed care, home care, and long-term care pharmacies, but is currently more common in independent and hospital pharmacies.

> Compounding is the process of mixing ingredients to prepare a special potion for a patient.

Nonsterile products are intended to be used by mouth or externally (on the outside of the body). Examples include capsules, oral liquids, creams, ointments, emulsions, and pastes. Because these medications are placed into or on the body in places where natural defenses can stop any microorganisms that might be present, they do not need to be sterile or free from bacteria, fungi, and viruses. This chapter describes standards and processes for preparation of these nonsterile products. In addition, it details the preparation of large quantities of compounded products, called bulk compounding, along with specialized packaging machines that are used in pharmacy.

Standards for nonsterile compounding are set by the US Pharmacopeia (USP) Chapter <795> (https://www.usp.org/compounding/general-chapter-795). Regulatory bodies, such as The Joint Commission and each state's board of pharmacy, have the responsibility of assuring compliance with the USP standards pursuant to the General Notices, 2.30 Legal Recognition. USP <795> has the force of law because USP is recognized as a standards-setting organization in federal statutes and regulations. It is also endorsed by The Joint Commission and incorporated into the National Association of Boards of Pharmacy's Model State Pharmacy Act and Rules. USP Chapter <795> is an essential regulatory and guidance document for any pharmacy that is involved with compounding.

USP published revisions to General Chapter <795> for nonsterile compounding in 2019, which had last been updated in 2014. After publication, USP received appeals on certain provisions in Chapter <795>, and it was remanded to an expert committee for additional consideration. At the time of writing of this text, the currently official version of General Chapter <795> (last revised in 2014) remains official until further notice. Always access the most up-to-date version of any standard before applying it in practice. Current USP standards for nonsterile compounding are available on the USP website (https://www.usp.org/compounding/general-chapter-795).

Standards for Nonsterile Compounding

USP defines 3 categories of nonsterile compounding (see https://www.usp.org/compounding/general-chapter-795):

- **Simple compounding**—reconstitution or manipulation of a commercial product (eg, adding water to a product as directed by the manufacturer) or use of a USP Compounding Monograph that includes specific information on all components, compounding procedures, and stability data. Examples include a reconstituted antibiotic suspension, captopril oral solution, and ketoprofen topical gel.
- **Moderate compounding**—making preparations that require special calculations or procedures to determine quantities or dosage units or compounding a preparation for which stability information is not available. Examples include morphine sulfate suppositories and diphenhydramine hydrochloride troches.
- **Complex compounding**—preparing specialized drug products that require special training, equipment, or facilities. Examples include transdermal dosage forms and modified-release preparations.

| **Table 12-1** | Tips for Safety and Accuracy in Nonsterile Compounding |

- Only compound 1 preparation at a time to avoid errors or cross contamination.
- Inspect your compounded products at each step to ensure appropriate mixing, quality, purity, and other desired characteristics.
- Always prepare compounded products in pharmacy space that is specifically designated for compounding prescriptions.
- Prepare nonsterile compounds in an area separate from that in which sterile compounds are prepared (see Chapter 13, Sterile Compounding).
- Use purified water when formulas require the inclusion of water in a compound and when rinsing equipment and utensils.
- Be sure to dispose of any hazardous waste products (eg, carcinogens) according to federal and state regulations. Ask your pharmacist if you are unsure how to dispose of any compounding waste products.
- Always follow record-keeping and documentation requirements for your pharmacy and those required by your state board of pharmacy. Ask your pharmacist if you need more information on these requirements.
- Keep any compounding records for the same amount of time that you maintain prescription records in your state.
- Clean equipment carefully to avoid cross contamination. This occurs when a surface or container is contaminated by a drug that is potentially hazardous to a patient (eg, penicillin in an allergic patient) and then subsequently used for another patient.

Source: United States Pharmacopeia and National Formulary (USP34-NF 29). *Pharmaceutical Compounding—Nonsterile Preparations.* Rockville, MD: United States Pharmacopeial Convention; 2011:330-336.

USP Chapter <795> places an emphasis on patient safety and preparation accuracy in the compounding processes (Table 12-1). This chapter reviews common terms and procedures used in nonsterile compounding but is not intended to replace USP Chapter <795>. Practice standards are updated frequently. You should always access the most up-to-date version of any standard before applying it in practice. Current USP standards for nonsterile compounding are available on the USP website (https://www.usp.org/compounding/general-chapter-795).

Additional guidance has been provided by regulatory authorities for compounding activities during the COVID-19 pandemic. Always verify that compounding procedures are consistent with your institutional and regulatory guidance on nonsterile compounding during the pandemic. More information is available from:

- Food and Drug Administration (https://www.fda.gov/drugs/emergency-preparedness-drugs/coronavirus-covid-19-drugs)
- American Pharmacists Association (https://www.pharmacist.com/coronavirus/compounding)
- USP (https://go.usp.org/Compounding_EC_Resources)
- Professional Compounding Centers of America (https://www.pccarx.com/covid19)

Equipment and Materials Used in Nonsterile Compounding

Compounding a prescription is a lot like baking a cake. You need to work in a clean, organized area; you work from a recipe or set of instructions; you need to gather all the right ingredients; you must accurately measure those ingredients and mix them in the correct order and manner; and you want the appearance of your final product to be pleasing. While the ingredients of prescriptions are very different, all these elements of baking apply to compounding.

For compounding, you need to learn how to use several basic types of equipment.

Weighing Equipment

By law, your pharmacy must have a **prescription balance**. This is a scale used to weigh small quantities of solid or very thick semisolid pharmaceutical ingredients (Figure 12-1). When measuring solids on a balance, you will use weighing papers (a type of waxed paper) or cups to keep ingredients from soiling or staining the pans on the scale. Other procedures used on scales vary, depending on the model and type. Ask your pharmacist to give you instructions on how to use the balance in your pharmacy.

Figure 12-1 Prescription Balance

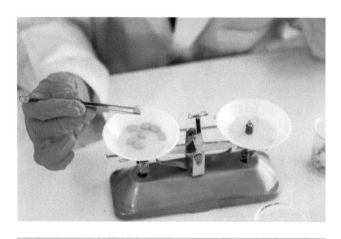

Here, you see a prescription balance being used to weigh ingredients for compounding a prescription.

Figure 12-2 Graduated Cylinders

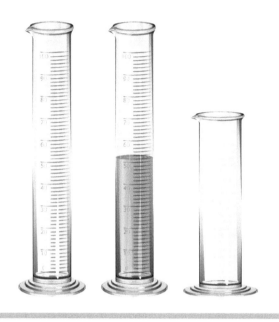

Select a graduated cylinder that has a capacity equal to or just exceeding the volume to be measured.

The most common scale present in pharmacies is a Class III balance. If you need to weigh quantities of less than 120 mg, this scale is not sufficiently accurate. Talk with the pharmacist to determine if a different type of scale is available for such small amounts.

Scales must be calibrated periodically. This means that known quantities should be measured on the scale to be sure the scale is accurate. Records should be kept of these calibrations as well as other equipment maintenance.

Measuring Equipment

Your pharmacy should also be stocked with an appropriate supply of equipment for measuring liquids. For most nonsterile products, you will use a **graduated cylinder** to measure liquids. Several different sizes of these graduates should be available, such as 10 mL, 25 mL, 50 mL, 100 mL, and 1000 mL (Figure 12-2). To ensure greater measurement accuracy, you should select a graduated cylinder that has a capacity equal to or just exceeding the volume to be measured. For instance, you would not measure 8 mL in a 100-mL graduate; rather, you should use a 10-mL graduate. For measuring amounts of 0.1 mL to 5 mL, you may use syringes (without a needle attached) or pipettes/

micropipettes. For measuring very small amounts of liquids (<0.1 mL), use micropipettes.

Compounding Equipment

The pharmacy must also have an adequate supply of **mortars and pestles** (with both pieces made of glass or Wedgwood/porcelain; Figure 12-3), stainless steel and plastic spatulas of different sizes, an ointment slab or pill tile, funnels, filter paper, beakers, glass stirring rods, a heat source (hot plate or microwave oven), a refrigerator, and a freezer. These are used in various steps of the compounding process, as directed.

The pharmacist will generally stock the compounding area with chemicals that meet requirements of USP, National Formulary (NF), or Food Chemicals Codex (FCC) substances. Ideally, these ingredients should be manufactured in a facility registered with the Food and Drug Administration (FDA). USP, NF, and FCC list the standards the chemical must meet for strength, quality, and purity. FDA inspects the plants in which the chemicals were made for compliance with "Good Manufacturing

Figure 12-3 Mortar and Pestle

Figure 12-4 Trituration

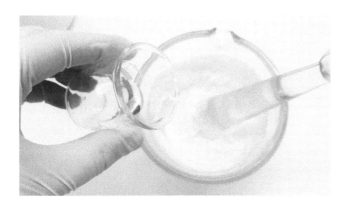

A mortar and pestle, like the glass one shown here, are used in compounding. A mortar and pestle can also be made of porcelain; in this case, it is called a Wedgwood mortar and pestle.

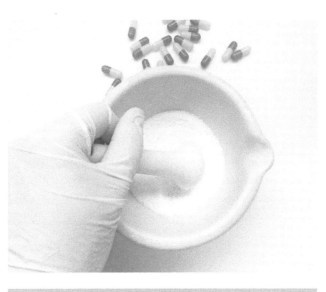

Here, a solid drug is triturated into a smaller particle size in a glass mortar and pestle.

Practice" standards, ensuring that the chemicals are suitable for use in people.

Techniques Used in Nonsterile Compounding

Many pharmaceutical ingredients can be mixed without any concerns about compatibility. However, certain ingredients must be mixed carefully or in a special way to prevent problems in compounding. Pharmacists spend a considerable amount of time in pharmacy school learning the principles and techniques used in these situations. While these principles and techniques cannot be detailed in this text, the following are brief descriptions of the basic techniques used most commonly to mix pharmaceutical ingredients.

Trituration

Trituration is a grinding of a drug solid using a mortar and pestle to reduce the particle size or to mix 2 or more solids (Figure 12-4). This technique is generally used to:

- Create a finer powder to make dissolution easier
- Keep a cream or ointment from feeling gritty
- Ensure thorough mixing of solid ingredients

Levigation

Levigation entails dispersing a drug solid into a small amount of mineral oil, glycerin, or other liquid before incorporating the paste into an ointment (often by trituration). This technique is used to keep the ointment from feeling gritty.

Geometric Dilution

Geometric dilution is a technique used to ensure consistent mixing of a small amount of a potent drug with a large amount of a nonpotent or inactive compound. The potent drug is triturated with an approximately equal amount of the other substance. That mixture is then combined with an approximately equal amount of the other substance and so forth, until all of the second substance is incorporated.

> Many pharmaceutical ingredients can be mixed without any concerns about compatibility. However, certain ingredients must be mixed carefully or in a special way to prevent problems.

Increasing Dissolution

Sometimes it is necessary to increase dissolution. When preparing a solution, the **solute** (usually a solid drug) must be dissolved in the **solvent** (just like dissolving sugar or salt in water). Many drugs, being organic, carbon-based compounds, are not very soluble in water-based vehicles. In these instances, only a small amount of the drug will dissolve, or the substance dissolves very slowly. Various techniques can sometimes be used to increase the amount or rate of dissolution, such as heating the solvent or the mixture, reducing the particle size of the solute (by trituration or levigation), using a solubilizing agent that coats the solute and makes it dissolve more easily, or agitating the mixture by shaking or other means.

Checking for Problems or Instability

After the prescription has been compounded, inspect it for problems or signs of instability. These include particles in products that should be clear solutions, separation of ingredients in an emulsion or ointment, or discoloration on the outside of capsules. Based on your past experience or knowledge of what the product should look like, consult with the pharmacist if anything is not correct when you have finished mixing the ingredients. A properly prepared prescription should be "pharmaceutically elegant"—it should have the appropriate color, texture, smell, and feel when applied or used.

> A properly prepared prescription should be "pharmaceutically elegant" with the appropriate color, texture, smell, and feel when applied or used.

Handling Product Spills

If at any time during the preparation of a compound, an ingredient or product spills on a person or on any surface, it is important to consult the **Safety Data Sheet (SDS)** for appropriate handling instructions. SDSs are written documents that give specific instructions

for working with certain chemicals, including emergency procedures, manufacturer information, and physical and chemical substance properties. These should be easily accessible in the pharmacy for all chemicals you are compounding in case of a product spill or other mishap.

Choosing an Appropriate Container

Once you have completed the compounded product and verified that it appears to be correct and stable, you should place it in an appropriate container. Considerations in choosing a container include the following:

- Containers should meet USP requirements and should be child-resistant unless the patient requests a non–child-resistant closure.
- To avoid medication errors, oral liquids should not be placed in syringes that can be used for injection (oral syringes—ones that will not accommodate a needle—are preferred).
- The container should not physically or chemically interact with the product.
- Amber or light-resistant containers should be used when the product is sensitive to light.
- The container should be of an appropriate size—the product should fill most or all of the container, and the container should hold all of the product.

Labeling the Final Product

The final product must be labeled in accordance with state and federal laws. In addition to the elements required on labels of all prescriptions, the compounded **product label** should state the following:

- The generic or chemical name of all active ingredients
- Names of vehicles (the liquid used to make a solution or the ointment base used in compounding a topical product) if the vehicle differs among products (as when one vehicle contains sugar and another is sugar free)

- Strength and/or quantity
- Pharmacy lot number (if applicable; see next section on bulk compounding)
- Beyond-use date (see below)
- Special storage and handling requirements, if any
- A label indicating that "this is a compounded preparation"

Some commonly used products may have acquired short names (for example, a pediatrician's product for diaper rash may be known locally by that physician's name, as in Smith's Diaper Cream). Labeling of product with such names is discouraged because the contents cannot be easily determined if a poisoning occurs. In addition, in instances where a commercially available product has been used as the source of active ingredient in the prescription, the use of trade names is discouraged because the brand-name product has been altered in compounding the prescription.

Assigning Beyond-Use Dates

The beyond-use date is the date after which a compounded preparation should not be used. Unlike a standard expiration date, it is not usually determined by the manufacturer but from the date when the preparation is compounded. The beyond-use date is usually not very far into the future because compounded prescriptions are meant for immediate dispensing and use by the patient. The beyond-use date is assigned by the pharmacist after considering factors such as the following:

- **Chemical stability**—how long the chemicals as mixed are stable in each other's presence.
- **Physical stability**—how long the product as mixed will remain in the proper form.
- **Microbial contamination**—whether there is a risk of microbial growth in the product.

Follow these general guidelines from USP Chapter <795> when assigning beyond-use dates, making sure to keep in mind that the beyond-use date is never

later than the expiration date on the labeled container of any single ingredient:

- **Nonaqueous formulations**—beyond-use date is no later than the amount of time left until the earliest expiration date of any active ingredient, or 6 months, whichever is longer.
- **Water-containing oral formulations**—beyond-use date is no later than 14 days when stored at controlled cold temperatures.
- **Water-containing topical, dermal, mucosal liquid, or semisolid preparations**—beyond-use date is no later than 30 days.

Keeping Records

An important element of compounding is keeping records of the chemicals and processes used to make each prescription (Table 12-2). USP Chapter <795> specifies that pharmacies must have a Master Formulation Record and Compounding Record for all nonsterile compounds, and these must be retained in the pharmacy for the same period of time that is required for any prescription under state law. Your pharmacy may have additional specific documentation requirements—always follow these to the letter when preparing compounded products.

These records are critical in situations where a patient has an adverse reaction to a compounded product or when one of the ingredients is recalled by its manufacturer.

Table 12-2	Record of Chemicals in Compounded Prescriptions

The record of the chemicals used in making each prescription usually includes the following:
- Who prepared the product
- Names, manufacturer, lot numbers, and quantities of all ingredients used
- Order of missing and special processes used
- Storage information
- Pharmacy lot number when a supply of product is made for several patients

Master Formulation Record

A Master Formulation Record is the master "recipe" file used for each compound and must be on record for every nonsterile product compounded in the pharmacy. USP Chapter <795> lists specific components that are required in a master formulation record, including ingredients, required calculations, equipment, mixing instructions, labeling and packaging instructions, and quality control procedures.

Compounding Record

A Compounding Record provides documentation for each individual product or prescription that is compounded in the pharmacy and must be completed each time a compound is made. USP Chapter <795> lists specific components required in a compounding record, including the names and quantities of all ingredients, total quantity compounded, name of compounder, date compounded, prescription number, and beyond-use date.

Bulk Compounding

When one or more prescribers in an area use the same compounded prescription repeatedly, pharmacists will sometimes make batches of the product to use when prescriptions are received. This process is called bulk compounding. It saves time for both the pharmacy and the patient, because many compounded prescriptions are complicated and patients typically would have to wait for them to be made.

During bulk compounding, an appropriate amount of product should be prepared based on the stability of the product and how often it is prescribed. After preparation, batches of product should be assayed for consistent potency (when applicable), tested for bacterial or other microbial growth (when applicable), and inspected routinely during storage for product instability, contamination, or breakdown.

> During bulk compounding, an appropriate amount of product should be prepared based on the stability of the product and how often it is prescribed.

Repackaging

Many pharmacies are now repackaging commercially available drug products to fit into their automated dispensing machines and specialized drug delivery systems. You may be involved in placing individual doses of medication into various types of strip packaging, pouch or blister cards, or oral syringes.

While the specifics of repackaging will depend on the type of equipment used in your pharmacy, the principles are the same as with compounding and bulk compounding:

- **Preparation**—Gather the correct drug products and supplies needed and organize them in a clean, neat work area.
- **Procedure**—Follow procedures carefully for the repackaging equipment in your pharmacy.
- **Quality control**—Check the repackaged product to be sure that everything is correct and that the drug product has not been damaged during the process.
- **Record keeping**—Meticulously record lot numbers of products used and other details in case questions arise, patients have adverse effects, or manufacturers recall the product.

Repackaging oral liquids usually involves oral syringes or cups. Never use syringes that can be used for injection to repackage oral liquids—rarely, nurses, patients, and others have mistakenly injected these liquids. Also, because it is impossible to tell what is in a liquid once it is repackaged, be extremely careful that you have the correct drug product and are placing the correct volume into the syringe or cup.

Conclusion

For some patients, the preparation of specially compounded prescription products is crucial to preventing or treating disease. By carefully preparing pharmaceutically elegant compounded products, you can make an important difference in these patients' lives.

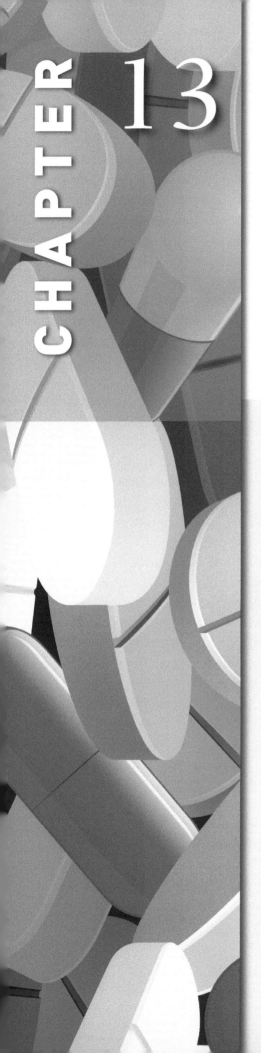

CHAPTER 13

Sterile Compounding

Janet Schmittgen, PharmD

Chapter 13 highlights the basics of preparing compounded sterile products. It presents topics such as United States Pharmacopeia sterile compounding standards, sterile admixture, laminar flow, and aseptic technique to help the pharmacy technician be comfortable with these subject areas. Chapter 13 also introduces hazardous drug products and radiopharmaceuticals.

Introduction

Many pharmacy technicians spend the majority of their time preparing sterile pharmaceutical products. This is a specialized type of compounding, and the same principles and considerations apply to sterile products as were described in Chapter 12 for nonsterile preparations. The main difference is that you must make a special effort to avoid contamination of sterile products with microorganisms such as bacteria and fungi.

> Many pharmacy technicians spend the majority of their time preparing sterile pharmaceutical products that are injected into patients.

This chapter presents an overview of **sterile product preparation** for those technicians who have not yet trained or worked in this part of pharmacy practice. If you are already working in this area, you will need to consult more detailed manuals, training videos, and/or educational materials to increase your skills and knowledge about compounded sterile preparations (CSPs).

Some pharmacy technicians are hired directly into sterile product—or **intravenous admixture**—positions. Others are promoted into such roles after becoming familiar with medications and pharmacy practice through on-the-job experience with compounding. Some specialized pharmacies produce radiopharmaceuticals. These are prepared similarly to other sterile products, and some technicians work in this setting. Chapter 6, Role and Advancement of the Pharmacy Technician in Pharmacy Practice, details how technicians can become certified in Compounded Sterile Preparation Technique through the Pharmacy Technician Certification Board (https://www.ptcb.org/) and summarizes certification exam domains and content. The National Pharmacy Technician Association (https://www.pharmacytechnician.org) and the American Society of Health-System Pharmacists (https://www.ashp.org/) also offer sterile product preparation certificate programs.

Preparation of Compounded Sterile Products and Infection Control

Standards for sterile compounding are set by the United States Pharmacopeia (USP) Chapter <797> (https://www.usp.org/compounding/general-chapter-797). Regulatory bodies, such as The Joint Commission and each state's board of pharmacy, have the responsibility of assuring compliance with the USP standards pursuant to the General Notices, 2.30 Legal Recognition. USP <797> has the force of law because USP is recognized as a standards-setting organization in federal statutes and regulations. It is also endorsed by The Joint Commission and incorporated into the National Association of Boards of Pharmacy's Model State Pharmacy Act and Rules. USP Chapter <797> is an essential regulatory and guidance document for any pharmacy that is compounding sterile products.

USP published revisions to General Chapter <797> for sterile compounding in 2019, which had previously been last updated in 2008. After publication, USP received appeals on certain provisions in Chapter <797>, and it was remanded to an expert committee for additional consideration. At the time of writing of this text, the currently official version of General Chapter <797> (last revised in 2008) remains official until further notice. Always access the most up-to-date version of any standard before applying it in practice. Current USP standards for sterile compounding are available on the USP website (https://www.usp.org/compounding/general-chapter-797).

USP <797> defines **sterile compounding** as the process of combining, admixing, diluting, pooling, reconstituting, repackaging, or otherwise altering a drug or bulk drug substance to create a sterile medication. Compounding personnel are responsible for following these guidelines and procedures when processing CSPs to minimize the potential for patient harm that may result from microbial contamination or excessive bacterial endotoxins. **Microorganisms** (fungi, bacteria, and viruses) can be transmitted if CSPs are not prepared using techniques that reduce

Figure 13-1 Examples of Microbes

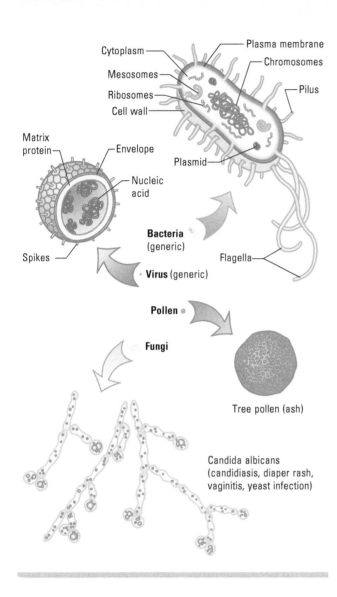

Cytoplasm — Plasma membrane
— Chromosomes
Mesosomes —
Ribosomes — — Pilus
Cell wall —

Matrix protein — — Envelope
— Nucleic acid
— Plasmid

Spikes — Flagella —

Bacteria (generic)

Virus (generic)

Pollen

Fungi

Tree pollen (ash)

Candida albicans
(candidiasis, diaper rash, vaginitis, yeast infection)

the risk of contamination. As shown in Figure 13-1, microbes include the following organisms, ranked by size from largest to smallest:

- Fungi
- Bacteria
- Viruses

Fungi are the largest of these microorganisms. Bread mold is an example of a fungus. When fungi are present in intravenous (IV) fluids, they may cause a mold-like growth in the solution, or they may simply make the fluid look cloudy. However, many millions of fungi and other microbes can be present in each milliliter of fluid without any visible changes.

Bacteria are microorganisms that are found in the environment, on our skin, clothing, cosmetics, and surfaces that we touch. Bacteria are one of the most common contaminants of CSPs. Bacteria can multiply in a rapid manner. When bacteria are present in large enough quantities (about 10 million to 100 million organisms per milliliter), the CSP will look cloudy or turbid.

Viruses are the smallest microbe. They are so small that they can pass through pharmaceutical filters. Viruses require a living host to grow, so they do not grow in IV fluids even though they may cause infection in the patient when the fluid is administered. Viruses do not cause the solution to appear turbid, and they cannot be detected by commonly used methods of checking IV fluids for contamination. Thus, the patient's only defense against viruses is for viruses never to be introduced into the fluid in the first place.

Injectable Products

CSPs that are placed into patients' veins are often referred to as **intravenous or IV fluids** (Figure 13-2). Some fluids for IV administration come in small containers called piggyback bags, which usually contain at least 50-100 mL of fluid. Larger bags containing 500-1000 mL are used for administration of maintenance fluids. Other types of CSPs can be infused into arteries, administered into the fluid that surrounds the brain and spine, placed into the peritoneal cavity that surrounds the gastrointestinal organs of the gut, or placed into the eyes or joints of the body. CSPs are also used as baths for live organs and tissues after they are harvested from donors but before they are placed into recipients.

> To avoid introducing microbial organisms into CSPs, pharmacists and technicians use aseptic technique.

Figure 13-2 Intravenous Lines

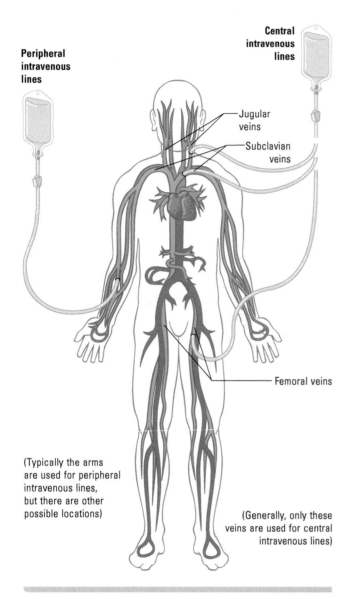

Peripheral intravenous lines

Central intravenous lines

Jugular veins

Subclavian veins

Femoral veins

(Typically the arms are used for peripheral intravenous lines, but there are other possible locations)

(Generally, only these veins are used for central intravenous lines)

Parenteral Solutions

Parenteral solutions are generally packaged in bags or bottles. Parenteral solutions of less than 250 mL are considered **small-volume parenteral (SVP) solutions** and are used primarily for administering injectable drugs to patients. For instance, a physician might order the antibiotic, cefazolin 1 g IV every 8 hours for a patient with an infection. The pharmacy would prepare this amount of drug in 50-100 mL of a small-volume product, usually either 5% dextrose (a sugar solution) or 0.9% sodium chloride (a salt solution). These solutions would then be infused directly into the patient's veins.

SVPs are increasingly provided by manufacturers in a ready-to-infuse form. Some of these products are premixed solutions that are stored frozen until ready for use, while others keep the drug separated from the fluid until the time of dispensing or administration. Some newer products allow the drug and solution to be mixed in a closed system. This is advantageous because the manipulation can safely occur in any location, even in the patient's home if needed.

When larger amounts of parenteral fluids are required, such as when volume replacement is needed, a **large-volume parenteral (LVP) solution** should be used. These are usually given to patients continuously, for example, as a 5% dextrose injection administered at a rate of 125 mL/h. In this case, the solution would keep running into the patient's veins during all hours of the day and night. The patient would receive a total volume of 3 L/day of 5% dextrose solution (125 mL/h × 24 hours).

SVP and LVP fluids may be packaged in several different types of glass bottles, plastic bags, or plastic semirigid bottles. Individual hospitals, health systems, or community pharmacies often use products from a single company or supplier. You should become familiar with the SVP and LVP fluids used in your practice setting, including the various sizes and container types.

Just as with nonsterile compounds, CSPs must be assigned a beyond-use date (BUD), or the date or time after which a CSP may not be stored or transported. A CSP's BUD identifies the time by which the preparation, once it is mixed, must be used before it is at risk for physical or chemical degradation, microbial contamination and proliferation, and impact on the integrity of the container-closure system. The 2019 revisions to USP Chapter <797> included updates to the BUDs for CSPs. In general, the storage periods in the official (2008) chapter are similar and sometimes longer than the BUDs in the revised (2019) chapter. Table 13-1 describes USP levels of risk and allowed BUDs according to the official 2008 USP <797>, and Table 13-2 compares drug storage periods

Table 13-1 Definitions and Examples of USP Chapter <797> Levels of Risk

CLASSIFICATION	CONDITIONS	EXAMPLES	ALLOWED BEYOND-USE DATING
Immediate Use	• CSPs for emergency or immediate patient administration, as in cardiopulmonary resuscitation or emergency room use. • Not intended for storage or batch compounding. • Continuous compounding process must not be greater than 1 hour. • Administration to patient no later than 1 hour after compounding process is started, and if administration has not begun by this time, CSP should be discarded.	• Transfer of sterile, nonhazardous drugs • Preparation of diagnostic radiopharmaceuticals	1 hour following the start of preparing the CSP
Low Risk	• CSPs are compounded within a physical area (eg, hood) that restricts particle counts to 3520 particles per cubic meter or less (referred to as ISO Class 5, previously named Class 100). • Manipulations are limited to transfer, measuring, and mixing of no more than 3 manufactured products. • Involves no more than 2 entries into any 1 sterile container or package (eg, bag).	• Preparing admixtures using vials, ampuls, bottles, and bags whose contents are already sterile • Reconstitution of single-dose vials of antibiotics • Preparation of hydration solutions	• Room temperature: 48 hours • Refrigeration: 14 days • Frozen: 45 days • Time periods can be extended if sterility tests show CSPs are not contaminated.
Low Risk With <12-Hour Beyond-Use Date	• CSPs prepared in an ISO Class 5 device or room (eg, hood or biological safety cabinet) restricted to sterile compounding that is separated from other noncompounding areas. • Must be administered within 12 hours of commencing compounding, or as recommended in package insert, whichever is sooner.	• Simple admixtures prepared using closed system transfer methods	• - 12 hours or less
Medium Risk	• Multiple individual or small doses of sterile products combined or pooled to prepare a CSP that will be administered either to multiple patients or to 1 patient on multiple occasions. • Compounding process includes complex aseptic manipulations other than the single-volume transfer, and the compounding process requires unusually long duration.	• CSPs, such as TPN, made from multiple sterile products • Pooled admixtures • Batch-compounded preparations that do not require bacteriostatic components	• Room temperature: 30 hours • Refrigeration: 9 days • Frozen: 45 days • Time periods can be extended if sterility tests show CSPs are not contaminated.

(table continues on next page)

Table 13-1 (continued)

CLASSIFICATION	CONDITIONS	EXAMPLES	ALLOWED BEYOND-USE DATING
High Risk	• CSPs include nonsterile ingredients, including manufactured products for nonsterile routes of administration (eg, oral), or a nonsterile device employed before the finished CSP is sterilized; or • CSP is made from sterile ingredients, components, devices, and mixtures that have been exposed to air quality inferior to ISO Class 5, including storage in such environments of opened or partially used packages of manufactured sterile products that do not contain antimicrobial preservatives. • CSP should be prepared in an ISO Class 5 environment. • CSPs include open system transfers.	• Dissolving nonsterile bulk drug and nutrient powders in solutions that are sterilized later • Measuring and/or mixing sterile ingredients in nonsterile containers before sterilization • Assuming that bulk packages contain correct amounts of labeled active ingredients without verification that the product has not been adulterated or contaminated between uses	• Room temperature: 24 hours • Refrigeration: 3 days • Frozen: 45 days • Time periods can be extended if sterility tests show CSPs are not contaminated.

Abbreviations: CSP, compounded sterile preparation; ISO, International Organization for Standardization; TPN, total parenteral nutrition.
Source: United States Pharmacopeia and National Formulary. *Pharmaceutical Compounding—Sterile Preparations.* Rockville, MD: United States Pharmacopeial Convention; 2008.

Table 13-2 Drug Storage Periods and BUDs in the Official and Revised USP Chapters

OFFICIAL <797> (LAST REVISED IN 2008)	REVISED <797> (PUBLISHED JUNE 1, 2019)
Low risk in segregated compounding area • 12 hours at CRT	Category 1 • ≤12 hours at CRT • ≤24 hours in a refrigerator
Low risk • 48 hours at CRT • 14 days in a refrigerator • 45 days in a freezer	Category 2 Aseptically processed, no sterility, only sterile starting composite • 4 days at CRT • 10 days in a refrigerator • 45 days in a freezer
Medium risk • 30 hours at CRT • 9 days in a refrigerator • 45 days in a freezer	Aseptically processed, no sterility, one or more nonsterile starting component(s) • 1 day at CRT • 4 days in a refrigerator • 45 days in a freezer
High risk • 24 hours CRT • 3 days refrigerator • 45 days frozen	

Abbreviations: BUD, beyond-use date; CRT, controlled room temperature.
Source: Adapted from US Pharmacopeia. USP compounding standards and beyond-use dates. Available at: https://www.usp.org/sites/default/files/usp/document/our-work/compounding/usp-bud-factsheet.pdf. Accessed December 11, 2020.

and BUDs in the official (2008) and revised (2019) USP Chapters <797>.

Nutritional Solutions

In addition to SVPs used for drug delivery and LVPs used for volume replacement, pharmacies commonly produce specialized solutions. **Total parenteral nutrition (TPN)** is an important type of specialized solution that provides nutrition without the use of the gastrointestinal tract. TPNs are used in clinical situations in which patients cannot take any food or products by mouth, such as when surgery has been performed on the gastrointestinal tract and it needs to rest so that it can heal (Figure 13-3).

TPN solutions have high concentrations of glucose (up to 35%), amino acids, and sometimes fats. TPN solutions may also contain multivitamins, trace elements, electrolytes, and insulin. These solutions are so concentrated that they would be toxic if they were infused into a small vein. For this reason, most

TPN solutions are administered through IV lines inserted into a larger vein just before it reaches the heart (called central lines). However, some less concentrated TPN solutions are infused into smaller veins in the arms (peripheral lines). Every time that a needle is inserted into a patient to administer an IV solution, there is an increased risk for infection because the skin—the body's first line of defense—is broken. This is true for peripheral lines, but it is even more critical for central lines because they are used for long time periods (weeks or months).

When TPN solutions are made in the pharmacy, the pharmacist or technician mixes concentrated glucose solutions, amino acid solutions, and sterile water to create the proper final amounts. Various electrolytes are added to the TPN solution, including sodium, potassium, magnesium, and calcium. Electrolyte parenteral solutions are supplied in various salt forms: calcium is available as calcium gluconate or calcium chloride. Because calcium can form insoluble salts with some ingredients (such as phosphate), it must be added in a specific manner to prevent problems. Usually calcium gluconate is used to decrease the risk of precipitation or formation of insoluble particles in the solution. Smaller amounts of vitamins, trace elements (such as chromium, copper, zinc, iodine, selenium, and manganese), and other ingredients may also be added to the TPN solution according to the physician's instructions. Adults generally need about 2-3 L per day of TPN solutions.

To assist in the preparation of TPN solutions, many pharmacies have an automated compounding device that can be programmed to mix the proper amounts of glucose, amino acids, and other solutions. TPN compounding systems are computer-based devices that assist with calculations and help to ensure proper compounding of TPNs and avoid precipitation of the solution. Some compounding systems can also add electrolytes, vitamins, and other ingredients based on

> In addition to SVPs used for drug delivery and LVPs used for volume replacement, pharmacies commonly produce specialized solutions.

| **Figure 13-3** | Senior Man With a TPN Connection in His Chest |

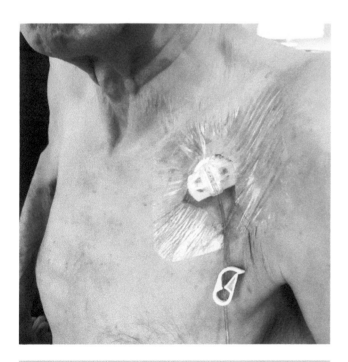

A senior man with a total parenteral nutrition (TPN) connected in his chest. The tube is connected to provide nutrition and medication when needed.

your instructions. Keep 2 factors in mind when using an automated compounding device:

1. The system must be properly calibrated—or adjusted—before you begin, and the proper solutions inlet tubing must be connected to the correct port as it goes through the compounding machine.
2. Any error you make in entering the ingredients into a compounding system will result in the wrong product. Small errors in TPN solutions can harm the patient or cause clinical problems. To avoid errors, many pharmacies require all TPN orders, calculations, and entries be verified by 2 individuals. Even if your pharmacy does not require this check, it is a good idea to ask a pharmacist or another knowledgeable technician to check your work when making TPN solutions.

> To help prevent problems, many pharmacies require that 2 people check all TPN orders, calculations, and entries.

Enteral nutrition is a liquid emulsion (similar in appearance to a milk shake) that is given through a tube inserted through the mouth or nose into the patient's stomach or small intestine. If at all possible, enteral nutrition solutions are used rather than TPN because they keep the patient's gastrointestinal tract active and avoid the need for an IV route of administration. Some pharmacies handle enteral nutrition products, but they are also provided by dietitians, or in some institutions, the dietary department.

Sterile Compounding Standards

USP Chapter <797> provides the minimum practice and quality standards designed to prevent patient harm, including death, that could result from one of the following:

- Microbial contamination
- Excessive bacterial endotoxins
- Variability in the intended strength of correct ingredients

- Unintended physical and chemical incompatibilities or contaminants
- Ingredients of inappropriate quality

To increase the likelihood that patients receive unadulterated CSPs containing the right ingredients and fluids, USP Chapter <797> spells out the minimum requirements for sterile compounding policies and procedures; personnel training and evaluation; environmental quality and control; equipment used in CSP production; procedures for compounding immediate-use CSPs; processes for compounding with single-dose and multiple-dose containers; verification of automated procedures such as the TPN compounding devices described in the previous section; checks of finished products, storage and beyond-use dating, quality control, packaging, and transport/shipping of CSPs; patient or caregiver training; patient monitoring and adverse event reporting; and quality assurance programs. While discussion of all of these aspects is beyond the scope of this chapter, some basic aspects are described here.

Compounding personnel must complete training and demonstrate competency every 12 months in the following areas: hand hygiene, garbing, cleaning and disinfection, calculations, measuring, mixing, aseptic technique, achieving/maintaining sterility and apyrogenicity, use of equipment, documentation of compounding process, principles of high-efficiency particulate air (HEPA)-filtered unidirectional airflow in an International Organization for Standardization (ISO) Class 5 area, proper use of primary engineering controls (PECs), and principles of movement of materials and personnel within the compounding area.

Physical Facilities for Sterile Compounding

Physical facilities and engineering controls are designed and maintained to minimize the risk of airborne microbial contamination in sterile compounding areas. The physical environment set forth in USP Chapter <797> can be as simple as a laminar airflow cabinet or biological safety cabinet or as complex as a cleanroom, buffer area, and anteroom. Laminar airflow hoods blow the air across the work surface in

Figure 13-4 Laminar Flow Hood

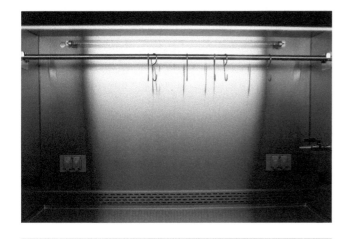

an even—or laminar—manner. Figure 13-4 depicts a laminar flow hood in a hospital pharmacy.

Many hospital pharmacies and facilities that make CSPs have built **cleanroom suites** to meet these requirements. Cleanroom suites provide an area that meets specific air quality standards or ISO classifications of particulate matter in room air in each area of the sterile compounding facility. The **anteroom** is the area where handwashing, garbing, and staging the compounding components take place. This area can generate higher levels of particulate matter, and it must meet the requirements for ISO 8 classification. The **buffer room** is accessed through the anteroom and must maintain ISO 7 classification standards. Only staff authorized to work in the cleanroom and materials needed to make CSPs should be brought into the buffer zone. The buffer room includes where the PEC is located and may contain carts and computer equipment. The PEC device or zone provides ISO 5 standard air quality.

Air is supplied into the cleanroom suite through the ceiling of the buffer room and anteroom using HEPA filters that prevent microorganisms and particulate matter from entering the area. Air quality must be tested, monitored, and documented in all of these zones. USP Chapter <797> defines how to create cleanroom suites with surfaces and fixtures that can easily be cleaned and disinfected to minimize the possibility for microorganisms and contaminants to accumulate.

It also gives clear and specific requirements for cleaning, disinfecting, and applying sporicidal agents to PECs and surfaces in areas of compounding. Cleaning should be performed from clean to dirty areas. Each facility will have specific written standard operating procedures (SOPs) for cleaning and disinfecting with state-required processes and facility-approved cleaning agents.

Personnel Cleansing and Garbing

Personnel must follow procedures to ensure that CSPs are prepared under proper conditions to minimize microbial contamination in the cleanroom. This includes personal hygiene practices such as handwashing, limiting the use of cosmetics or hair products, limiting jewelry, and always abiding by aseptic technique practices. Personnel who make CSPs should practice appropriate handwashing technique and always wear gloves when compounding CSPs to help decrease the number of particles shed from skin cells since these can be a source of microbes. Personal protective equipment (PPE) can help prevent microorganisms from being introduced and help contain particles that can be shed from skin cells. Any person who enters the sterile compounding area must wear certain items of PPE (Figure 13-5) to help prevent microorganisms on clothing from being introduced into the sterile

Figure 13-5 Example of Personal Protective Equipment

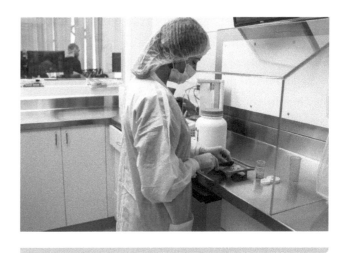

compounding area. Garbing refers to the procedure for donning and doffing PPE such as shoe covers, hat, masks, beard covers, gowns, and gloves. Each facility has a policy for the proper order of garbing.

USP Chapter <797> provides detailed guidelines for appropriate personal grooming for individuals working in clean areas. Personnel working in CSP preparation areas must keep their nails natural and trimmed neatly (artificial nails and extenders are prohibited) and should remove all cosmetics (since they can shed flakes and particles); outside garments (such as bandannas, coats, hats, and jackets); and all hand, wrist, and other visible jewelry or piercings (such as earrings and lip or eyebrow piercings) that can interfere with the effectiveness of PPE before entering the buffer or segregated compounding area. Food, drinks, candy, and chewing gum are not permitted in any of the clean areas.

Standard Operating Procedures for Sterile Compounding

Detailed SOPs for the cleanroom are provided in USP Chapter <797>. Within a **laminar airflow workbench (LAFW)**, the sterile air is usually flowing in one direction from the back toward the front, where the operator stands. It is important that this airflow is maintained and not obstructed when compounding CSPs. The interior surfaces of the LAFW should be cleaned using an approved cleaning agent daily and when surface contamination is known or suspected. The LAFW should be disinfected with an agent such as sterile 70% isopropyl alcohol at the beginning of each shift, every 30 minutes during ongoing compounding activities, and after spills when surface contamination is known or suspected. Alcohol wipes are used to disinfect the tops of vials or the entry ports on containers before they are punctured with needles. When using sterile 70% isopropyl alcohol, it is important to wet the surfaces or containers with the isopropyl alcohol and allow it to dry. Sporicidal agents are generally used on a monthly basis. Cleaning procedures should be documented according to the facility's SOPs.

Aseptic technique is a process or method used during the compounding of CSPs to keep objects and areas free of microorganisms to help minimize the risk

of infection to patients. When working in an LAFW, it is important to maintain unobstructed HEPA-filtered airflow. The airflow is unidirectional from back to front to help prevent contamination of the sterile compounding environment. All supplies, such as IV bags, syringes, needles, and vials, that are introduced into the sterile compounding area should be placed in the LAFW in an organized order so that each object is not blocking the airflow to these critical sites. After removing the protective packaging, handle the syringes and needles in such a way that you never place your hands or nonsterile equipment between them and the flow of sterile air. It is critical to keep the product free from contamination; never put your hands or nonsterile equipment between the flow of air and the product. By using aseptic technique properly, you can minimize the chances of introducing microbes into the sterile product.

Labels for CSPs should generally include the following information:

- Active ingredient(s) and amounts or concentrations
- Total amount or volume
- BUD
- Appropriate route(s) of administration
- Storage conditions if other than room temperature
- Other information for safe use

Disposal of Sterile Compounding Waste

Materials used in making CSPs must generally be discarded as **biomedical waste**. Pharmacies should manage the environmental impact of pharmaceutical waste in accordance with federal and state laws and regulations. A waste stream describes the specific type of waste generated by a pharmacy and its disposal procedures. For example, chemotherapy medications (discussed more in the next section) should be destroyed in the appropriate hazardous waste stream.

Safety Data Sheets (SDSs), supplied by the **Occupational Safety and Health Administration** (available at: https://www.osha.gov/), provide guidance on disposal information and personal protection for spills of potentially hazardous drugs and/or waste.

The SDS includes information such as the properties of each chemical; the physical, health, and environmental health hazards; protective measures; and safety precautions for handling, storing, and transporting the chemical. SDS disposal procedures for used supplies should also be considered. Use sharps containers to dispose of used needles, syringes, ampuls, and vials. Biohazard containers or receptacles are used for disposing of any clothing that comes in contact with body fluid or hazardous substances, such as gloves, gowns, or masks. Follow the procedures in your pharmacy or institution to comply with applicable laws and regulations when disposing of pharmaceutical materials and supplies used for sterile compounding.

Quality Assurance and Infection Control

As with bulk compounding, you must make a special effort with sterile products to be certain that they have the correct ingredients, that the products are free from contamination, and that no precipitate (substances that are not dissolved into the solution) or particulate matter is in the container. **Quality assurance** steps to check the final preparation of the sterile products include:

- Visual examination of the solution using a bright light placed behind the product. This helps to see particulate matter or precipitates that may result when 2 ingredients are incompatible with one another.
- Sampling of the contents of products to measure key ingredients, such as a drug, sodium, potassium, chloride, or glucose (sugar).
- Sampling of the contents of selected products for microbial contamination (sterility testing).

The application of the quality assurance method is described further in Chapter 7, Pharmacy Quality Assurance and Medication Safety. Additional measures may also be in place in your hospital to prevent infection and eliminate sources of microbes, such as physical precautions that require you to use special protective equipment when entering patients' rooms if they have certain infections or if they are easily susceptible to infection.

Special Considerations: Hazardous Drugs

USP Chapter <797> classifies drugs as hazardous if they are **carcinogens** (studies in animals or humans indicate that exposures have a potential for causing cancer), are **teratogens** (cause developmental or reproductive toxicity or birth defects), or can harm organs or genes. Some hazardous drugs can impair fertility, particularly in women but also potentially in men. Chemotherapy treatments for cancer are a specialized type of parenteral products classified as hazardous products by USP Chapter <797>. Chemotherapy drugs often require special handling or dilution when compounding.

USP Chapter <800> includes a section on handling hazardous drugs to help ensure the safety of pharmacists and technicians during the compounding of hazardous drugs. Additionally, the **National Institute for Occupational Safety and Health (NIOSH)** provides similar guidance for health care workers. This guidance and a complete list of drugs classified as hazardous are maintained by NIOSH and freely available on its website (www.cdc.gov/NIOSH).

Technicians preparing CSPs with hazardous drugs need special training and testing in the storage, handling, and disposal of these drugs. Although the complete requirements for these are beyond the scope of

> Follow the procedures in your pharmacy or institution to comply with applicable laws and regulations in disposing of pharmaceutical materials and supplies used in sterile compounding.

> Pharmacists or technicians handling chemotherapy or other hazardous drugs must take special precautions to keep the product off their own bodies and out of their mouths, throats, and lungs.

Figure 13-6 Chemotherapy Preparation

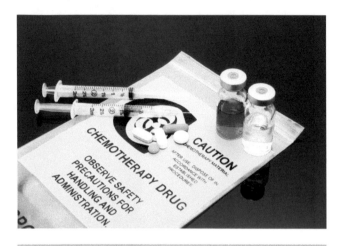

Chemotherapy drugs in oral and injection forms.

this textbook, a few important points will help you to understand policies that may be in place in your pharmacy for handling hazardous drugs. Ask your pharmacist if you have questions about current procedures or need additional training for compounding or preparing hazardous drugs.

It is important for the pharmacist or technician who is handling chemotherapy or other hazardous drugs (Figure 13-6) to take special precautions to keep the product off their own bodies (to prevent absorption through the skin) and out of their mouths, throats, and lungs (to prevent absorption through the mucous membranes). Most pharmacies, institutions, and home care settings follow these 4 rules to prevent exposure to hazardous agents by workers (including pharmacy, nursing, delivery, and other personnel), patients, patients' families, and visitors:

1. Protect and secure packages of hazardous drugs.
2. Inform and educate any involved personnel about hazardous drugs and train them in safe handling procedures relevant to their responsibilities.
3. Do not let drugs escape from containers when they are manipulated.
4. Eliminate the possibility of inadvertent ingestion or inhalation and direct skin or eye contact with the drugs.

Some strategies that pharmacies use to protect workers from accidental contamination with hazardous agents include the following:

- Warning labels are applied to packages containing chemotherapy drugs, and shipping boxes from manufacturers contain warning symbols.
- Rather than using laminar airflow hoods, biological safety cabinets are used to manipulate chemotherapy products (Table 13-3). These cabinets use a vertical flow of air and are ventilated to provide protection from exposure to airborne drugs.

PPE, defined in Table 13-3 and described in more detail in the following bullets, should be worn at all times when working with hazardous substances to shield pharmacists and technicians from harm if exposed to hazardous materials. USP Chapter <800> describes how to wear and dispose of this PPE if used with hazardous drugs.

- Pharmacists and technicians should always wear 2 sets of gloves (double gloving) that are chemo rated, and one or both sets of gloves should be discarded between products or batches or if the gloves are torn or punctured.
- A disposable gown should be worn to protect the body and clothes from contamination.
- Masks should be worn to prevent contamination of the respiratory tract, particularly if a biological safety cabinet is not being used. However, these masks provide no protection against powdered or liquid aerosols (very fine sprays) of these drugs. Compounding certain hazardous drugs may require a respirator to be worn to protect from exposure.
- A plastic face shield or splash goggles should be worn if eye contact with the drugs is possible.
- Syringes and needles should have Luer-lock fittings to minimize the possibility of separation during product preparation. In addition, other devices may be used in your work setting, including safety needles, vented needles, filters, and filter needles. Some closed system transfer devices may also be used for these purposes. Be sure that you thoroughly understand such equipment before you use it.

Table 13-3   Selected USP Chapter <797> Definitions, Abbreviations, and Terminology

Term	Definition
Biological safety cabinet (BSC)	A ventilated cabinet for CSPs, personnel, product, and environmental protection. This cabinet has an open front with inward airflow for personnel protection, downward high-efficiency particulate air (HEPA)-filtered laminar airflow for product protection, and HEPA-filtered exhausted air for environmental protection.
Buffer area	An area where the primary engineering control (PEC) is physically located. Activities that occur in this area include the preparation and staging of components and supplies used when compounding CSPs.
Closed system vial transfer device (CSTD)	A vial transfer system that allows no venting or exposure of hazardous substances to the environment.
Compounding aseptic isolator (CAI)	A form of isolator specifically designed for compounding pharmaceutical ingredients or preparations. A CAI maintains an aseptic compounding environment within the isolator throughout the compounding processes.
Compounding aseptic containment isolator (CACI)	A type of CAI that is designed to provide worker protection from exposure to undesirable levels of airborne drug throughout the compounding processes.
Critical area	An ISO Class 5 (see Table 13-1) environment.
Critical site	A location that includes any component or fluid pathway surfaces (eg, vial) or openings (eg, opened ampuls) exposed and at risk of direct contact with air, moisture, or touch contamination. Risk of microbial particulate contamination of the critical site increases with the size of the openings and exposure time.
Personal protective equipment (PPE)	Appropriate garb to wear when compounding or preparing hazardous drugs in a BSC or CACI and when using CSTD devices. PPE should include gowns, face masks, eye protection, hair covers, shoe covers or dedicated shoes, double gloving with sterile chemo-type gloves, and compliance with manufacturers' recommendations when using a CACI.
Segregated compounding area	A designated space—either a demarcated area or room—that meets physical requirements for, and is restricted to, preparing low-risk-level CSPs with 12-hour or less BUD (see Table 13-1).
Sterilization by filtration	Passage of a fluid or solution through a sterilizing grade membrane to produce a sterile effluent.
Terminal sterilization	The application of a lethal process (eg, steam under pressure or autoclaving) to sealed containers for the purpose of achieving a predetermined sterility assurance level of usually less than 10^{-6}, or a probability of less than 1 in 1 million of a nonsterile unit.

Source: United States Pharmacopeia and National Formulary. *Pharmaceutical Compounding—Sterile Preparations.* Rockville, MD: United States Pharmacopeial Convention; 2008.

■ Needles should not be recapped after use to minimize needlestick injuries to workers. Syringes and needles should be disposed of as hazardous materials in accordance with the policies in your workplace, which must comply with federal, state, and sometimes local laws and regulations (see previous section, Disposal of Sterile Compounding Waste).

Table 13-4 summarizes standardized resources for sterile compounding provided by professional associations and government agencies for additional resources.

> A few pharmacies specialize in handling radio-pharmaceuticals, which are medications that contain radioactive compounds.

Special Considerations: Radiopharmaceuticals

A few pharmacies specialize in handling radiopharmaceuticals, which are medications that contain **radioactive** compounds. These pharmacies are also called **nuclear pharmacies**.

Understanding radioactivity and nuclear pharmacy requires recalling a few definitions from chemistry:

■ **Atoms** are the smallest particles in nature that still retain the characteristics of the substance from which they came. Atoms are made up of 3 subatomic particles: protons, neutrons, and electrons.

■ **Protons** are subatomic particles found in the nucleus (middle) of an atom. The number of protons defines what substance the atom is, such

Table 13-4	Online Resources for Sterile Compounding

ONLINE RESOURCE	WEBSITE ADDRESS
United States Pharmacopeia (USP) and National Formulary • Standards for compounding sterile products • Standards for handling hazardous drugs • Standards for preparing radiopharmaceuticals	https://www.usp.org/compounding/compounding-general-chapters
American Society of Health-System Pharmacists • Discussion guides on USP compounding chapters • Guidelines on compounding sterile preparations • Guidelines on handling hazardous drugs	https://www.ashp.org/
National Institute for Occupational Safety and Health • Recommendations for preventing occupational exposure to antineoplastic and other hazardous drugs	https://www.cdc.gov/niosh/index.htm
Institute for Safe Medication Practices Guidelines for Safe Preparation of Compounded Sterile Preparations Provides consensus statements for core processes in compounded sterile preparations (CSPs), including: • Policies and procedures for CSPs • Order entry and verification • Drug inventory storage • Assembling products and supplies for preparation • Preparation of source/bulk containers • Quality control/final verification • Product labeling	https://www.ismp.org/guidelines/sterile-compounding

as carbon, oxygen, or hydrogen. For instance, an atom with 6 protons is carbon, an atom with 8 protons is oxygen, and an atom with 1 proton is hydrogen. Protons have a positive charge.

■ **Electrons** are very small subatomic particles that circle around the nucleus. You might think of the sun as the nucleus, with the planets circling the sun like electrons. Electrons are so small that their weight is not considered when determining the mass of an atom. Because electrons carry a negative charge, a proton and an electron together are neutral.

■ **Neutrons,** as their name implies, are neutral—they do not have a charge. They are located in the nucleus of the atom with the protons. An atom can have any number of neutrons without changing into another kind of atom, as long as the number of protons remains the same. For instance, carbon normally has 6 protons, 6 neutrons, and 6 electrons, and its total molecular weight is 12 (6 protons + 6 neutrons; the electrons do not count).

As long as the atom in the above example keeps the 6 protons, it will be carbon. It can have 6, 7, or 8 neutrons and still be carbon as long as it has 6 protons. When it has 7 neutrons, its molecular weight is 13, and the atom is called "carbon-13." When it has 8 neutrons, its molecular weight is 14, and it is called "carbon-14." All 3 of these are called **isotopes** of carbon.

Some isotopes are not stable because of the arrangement of the protons and neutrons in the very tight nucleus. These isotopes will decay over time and spontaneously transform into a more stable form. They decay by emitting **particles** from the neutrons, protons, or both. There are 3 types of particles: alpha particles, beta particles, and gamma particles. These particles can be detected by special instruments (such as Geiger counters or scintillation counters) and photographic films that are sensitive to specific radiation (such as X-ray film).

■ **Alpha particles**—the emission of 2 protons and 2 neutrons from the nucleus into the environment. This changes the substance from one element to another (the element with 2 fewer protons).

■ **Beta particles**—a neutron that changes into a proton and an electron; the proton stays in the nucleus, and the electron is emitted into the environment. This changes the substance into the element with 1 more proton.

■ **Gamma particles**—high-energy radiation that does not affect protons, neutrons, or electrons. This type of radiation, which approaches the power of X-rays, usually occurs with alpha and beta radiation.

To return to the carbon example above, carbon-14 is not as stable as the other isotopes of carbon. It will gradually, over thousands of years, return to a more stable form. It does so by emitting a beta particle and thereby changing into nitrogen-14. These emissions occur along very precise timelines that are described as the **half-life** of the isotope, meaning the amount of time required for one-half of the atoms to change from the unstable to the stable state. For carbon-14, the half-life is 5730 years. In the process of carbon dating, the half-life of carbon-14 is used to estimate the age of archaeological relics unearthed on the sites of ancient cities and civilizations.

In **nuclear medicine**, the various properties of radioactive elements and compounds are used to detect, assess, and treat disease in people. Some examples of clinically useful radioisotopes include the following:

■ **Iodine-131** is used to assess thyroid function and to treat thyroid overactivity and cancer.

■ **Technetium-99m** (Figure 13-7) is used in imaging many parts of the body. The "m" after the 99 stands for "metastable," which indicates that it does not change into another element after decay. It remains technetium-99 by emitting only gamma radiation. The half-life of this agent is only 6 hours, making it very useful in clinical imaging because it does not expose the patient to prolonged radiation.

■ **Cobalt-60** is used in radiation therapy for cancer.

Because many of the radioisotopes used in medicine have short half-lives, nuclear pharmacists must generate the isotope and provide the preparation to the nuclear medicine department just before various

Figure 13-7 Computed Tomography Scan for Clinical Imaging

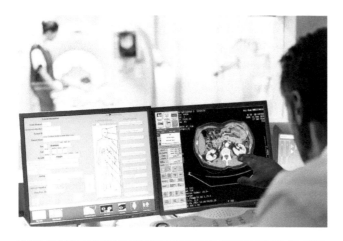

Technetium (Tc-99m) is commonly used in a number of medical diagnostic imaging scans.

imaging studies or treatments are to be performed. Radioisotope (also called radionuclide) generation is a daily procedure in the nuclear pharmacy. In situations where no nuclear pharmacy is available, nuclear medicine departments prepare radionuclides using commercially available kits.

All aspects of sterile compounding apply to nuclear pharmacy practice. In addition, other quality control considerations must be kept in mind, including checks required by the federal Nuclear Regulatory Commission (NRC):

- **Radionuclide purity** is the proportion of radioactivity that comes from the correct radioisotope. For instance, if the preparation is labeled as iodine-131, how much of the radioactivity present is actually generated by iodine-131?

- **Radiochemical purity** is the portion of the labeled radionuclide that is in the stated chemical form. For instance, if chromium-51 is in a solution of sodium chromate, how much of the radioactive chromium is in this chemical complex?

- **Specific activity** is the amount of radioactivity per unit weight of the compound. This is expressed in millicuries (mCi), a unit of radioactivity per milligram of compound. Generally, this number should be as high as possible, but there are situations where more nonradioactive compound needs to be present for the radioactive compound to reach its active site.

- **Radioactivity concentration** is the amount of radioactivity (in mCi) per milliliter of solution. Again, high radioactivity concentrations are preferred.

Conclusion

Pharmacy technicians who have the necessary knowledge and skills make valuable contributions through their work in sterile product preparation. If the ideas and information in this chapter appeal to you, seek out more information from pharmacists you work with or professional associations such as PTCB and other resources for advanced pharmacy technician training in sterile compounding.

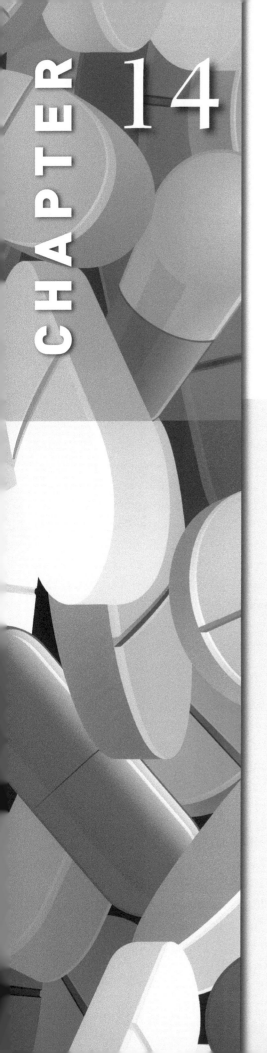

CHAPTER 14

Pharmacy Billing and Reimbursement

Chapter 14 highlights the key facts that pharmacy technicians need to know in assisting with billing for reimbursement. It includes descriptions of payment mechanisms, types of payers and intermediaries, and the importance of using the right billing method.

Introduction

Until the establishment of the Medicaid and Medicare programs in the 1960s, pharmacists charged individual patients for the prescription drugs they received. Since that time, however, the payment of pharmacies by government agencies, insurance companies, and health plans has become increasingly important. Today, most prescriptions are paid for by these outside entities, which are collectively known as third-party payers. With the launch of Medicare Part D in 2006 (see Chapter 3), nearly every prescription is covered by some type of third-party plan.

This chapter describes the types of payers and special nuances about each one. You can use this information to better understand those tasks you are asked to complete that help ensure your pharmacy gets paid for the products and services it provides.

> Most prescriptions are paid for by outside entities, which are collectively known as third-party payers.

Understanding the Methods of Payment

Pharmacists are generally paid for prescriptions in 1 of 3 ways:

- Direct payment by the patient
- Reimbursement from a government program, usually either Medicaid (for indigent patients), Medicare (for the elderly and the disabled), or Tricare (for uniformed service members, retirees, and their families)
- Reimbursement from a nongovernment payer, such as a managed care plan, insurance company, or employer

Patients whose health care or insurance plans do not cover prescription drugs must pay the pharmacy directly. Direct payment was once the most common method of payment but has dramatically declined over the past decades as health plans and Medicare have added prescription drug coverage.

This decline in direct payments can sometimes be troublesome for community pharmacies. Patients who are paying for their own prescriptions are able to choose the pharmacy of their choice and make their selection based on the quality of professional services they receive. However, some community pharmacies are not included in third-party networks, and patients may be forced to end long-standing relationships with their pharmacists when their prescription drug benefits are not available in that pharmacy.

As discussed in Chapter 3, Pharmacy Law and Regulation, the federal Centers for Medicare and Medicaid Services (CMS) manages the Medicare and Medicaid programs. The Medicare program covers primarily acute care for the elderly and patients under age 65 with disabilities, while the Medicaid program covers the indigent (people of all ages who have low—usually poverty level—income and few assets) or individuals with special health conditions. There are 4 primary parts to Medicare coverage: **Medicare Part A** provides inpatient/hospital coverage, **Medicare Part B** provides outpatient/medical coverage, **Medicare Part C** provides an alternate way to receive Medicare benefits, and **Medicare Part D** provides prescription drug coverage. Specifically, Medicare pays for prescription drugs if they are used in an acute care institution (hospital) or if they are used in conjunction with certain medical devices such as indwelling catheters. Medicaid pays for prescription drugs (including those dispensed from community pharmacies) and other care in nursing homes or hospitals. Medicare Part D covers outpatient prescription drugs for the elderly and the disabled (Figure 14-1), and Part B covers certain injectable drugs. These programs provide some $1 trillion in reimbursements to health care providers (hospitals, physicians, pharmacies, and other types of health providers) each year.

Even though the Medicare and Medicaid systems are administered by CMS, they work very differently from one another. As described in Chapter 3, Medicare Part D is administered through dozens of private **prescription drug plans (PDPs)**. Every PDP has its own formulary, and Medicare beneficiaries can choose any PDP operating in their geographic area (usually a state). Pharmacists' interactions are generally with these intermediaries when it comes to obtaining reimbursement

Figure 14-1 Medicare Part D at a Glance

2020 EDITION

Medicare Part D
AT A GLANCE

PART D COVERAGE

Part D is an optional prescription drug coverage benefit offered to everyone who has Medicare

46.3M
Total Part D Enrollees

25.7M
Stand-Alone Prescription Drug Plan Enrollees

20.6M
Medicare Advantage Prescription Drug Plan Enrollees

74.7%
of total Medicare enrollees also have Part D prescription drug coverage

Current as of December 2019

TYPE OF MEDICARE COVERAGE

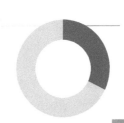

62.4%
are in the **Medicare Fee-For-Service (FFS)** program

37.6%
are in the **Medicare Advantage (MA)** program

2020 Average Estimated Medicare Advantage Premiums: $23
Lowest in 13 years

-14%

2019   2020

2020 Average Estimated Part D Basic Premiums: $30
Lowest in 7 years

-5.7%

2019   2020

MEDICARE PART D DEFINED STANDARD BENEFIT FOR 2020

Beneficiary   Plans   Manufacturers   Medicare

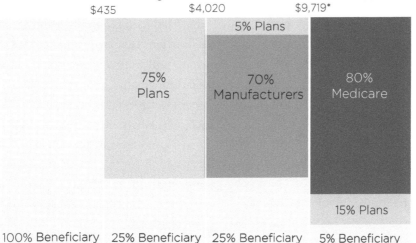

Deductible

Initial Coverage Limit
$4,020

Coverage Gap

Catastrophic Phase
$9,719*

$435

5% Plans

75% Plans

70% Manufacturers

80% Medicare

15% Plans

100% Beneficiary   25% Beneficiary   25% Beneficiary   5% Beneficiary

*$9,719 is the estimated total covered Part D spending for applicable beneficiaries to reach catastrophic; the out-of-pocket threshold to reach catastrophic for 2020 is $6,350

Source: Centers for Medicare & Medicaid Services. Available at: https://www.cms.gov/files/document/insulin-costs-beneficiaries-infographic.pdf.

for prescriptions and getting approval for nonformulary medications. Pharmacies must contract with these intermediaries, and either party can decline to contract with the other. Thus, the owner or managers of your pharmacy may have decided not to participate in all plans available in your state or geographic region, or some PDPs may have declined to contract with your pharmacy (perhaps because few enrollees live in your area, the plan managers believed they had enough pharmacies available in the city or town, or the 2 parties simply could not agree on the terms of the agreement).

Medicaid works quite differently. Even though about one-half of the money for Medicaid comes from CMS, the rest is provided by state governments, which are directly responsible for their own Medicaid programs. These programs vary from state to state. Nearly all pharmacies are recognized Medicaid providers, making it an open network (rather than a closed network, which might be limited to a small number of pharmacies in a city or town). For a pharmacy to be recognized, its owner or manager must enter into a contract with the state Medicaid agency. The state agency will likely have many requirements. For example:

- All Medicaid patients must be served without discrimination.
- The prices charged Medicaid must be equal to or lower than the best prices given to any other payer or patient of the pharmacy.
- All Medicaid patients must be offered the opportunity to be counseled about their medications by the pharmacist.

- The pharmacy must review Medicaid prescriptions and identify improper or incorrect prescribing patterns and work with physicians to improve them.

To be paid by third-party payers, including Medicare PDPs and Medicaid, the pharmacy must transmit claims electronically for the prescriptions dispensed. Any error in the computer—whether patient name or plan number, National Drug Code number, or incorrect quantity or directions—will result in either an incorrect payment to the pharmacy or a rejected claim. When entering any prescription into the computer, you must be very careful to input all the information correctly to avoid problems with both patients and reimbursement.

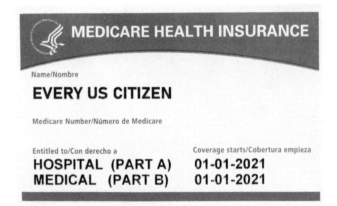

Third-party payers generally reimburse pharmacies for the cost of the drug plus a professional dispensing fee. In determining the cost of the drug, most state Medicaid programs differentiate between those medications that are available from multiple manufacturers (multisource products) and those that are available through only 1 company (single-source products). For a multisource product—regardless of how much the pharmacy paid and whether the name brand or generic product was dispensed—Medicaid will generally pay only for the less expensive generic product. In some states, the Medicaid program has a list of frequently used multisource drug products for which it has established maximum allowable costs. For these products, Medicaid will pay only for the least costly of the generic products.

Medicare pays for hospitalized patients (inpatients) based on a set amount for various **diagnosis-related**

> When entering any prescription into the computer, you must be very careful to input all the information correctly to avoid problems with reimbursement.

> Third-party payers generally reimburse pharmacies for the cost of the drug plus a professional dispensing fee.

groups (**DRGs**). For instance, for a Medicare beneficiary with uncomplicated pneumonia, Medicare might pay $4000 to the hospital regardless of how long the patient stays in the institution or what drugs or procedures are performed. The incentive in such a system is for hospitals to provide more efficient care. However, some critics have denounced this prospective payment system as encouraging hospitals to discharge elderly patients "sicker and quicker." In addition, in the past, CMS has monitored whether specialty hospitals are declining to accept transfers of patients with complicated illnesses from community hospitals, thereby allowing the specialty hospitals to profit from the less sick patients within a given DRG and causing financial problems at the community hospitals—and placing the very patients who need more specialized care in danger.

If a Medicare patient receives unusually expensive care during a hospitalization, the institution may qualify for direct reimbursement outside the DRG system. Cost of care for these outliers is sometimes driven up by expensive medications, especially those derived from biotechnology research. When this is the case, pharmacy personnel are sometimes involved in determining those costs.

As detailed in Chapter 3, an area of much concern is **fraud, waste, and abuse** in the Medicaid and Medicare systems. This can occur when health care providers (such as physicians, dentists, nurses, or pharmacists) bill the government for products or services that were not provided to patients. Specific problems that have occurred in a pharmacy include the following:

- Billing for nonexistent prescriptions and for medications not dispensed
- "Partial filling," in which the pharmacy gives the patient part of the quantity called for in a legitimate prescription (asking the patient to come back later to get the rest) and bills Medicaid for the full quantity—but doesn't return part of the reimbursement if the patient never returns
- Billing for name-brand products when generic alternatives are actually dispensed

These problems are usually uncovered by either computer detection of unusual dispensing patterns in a given pharmacy or by "whistleblowers"—people who come forward with information about activity they believe to be fraudulent. During investigation of the problem, state Medicaid or other government officials likely will visit the pharmacy for an in-store audit. You might be asked to help them find records for prescriptions they are checking on. During such audits, it is important that the pharmacy provide as much documentation of the validity of prescriptions as possible, which can be the last step before criminal prosecutions.

It is important to note that Medicaid also conducts in-store audits as part of routine compliance checking. Do not assume that an audit means someone suspects a problem.

Reimbursement by Nongovernment Third-Party Payers

The Medicaid reimbursement model described above is fairly simple in most cases. In a given state, there is usually 1 payer, 1 set of rules, and 1 set of beneficiaries. The pharmacy receives the prescription order and dispenses the medication, and someone pays for it.

But when you add in the PDPs and other nongovernment third-party payers, the situation becomes more complex. Patients are covered under many different policies and plans, each with its own rules and coverage limits (Table 14-1). Drugs may be covered under one plan (if they are on that plan's formulary or preferred drug list)

> An area of much concern is fraud, waste, and abuse in the Medicaid and Medicare systems.

> Patients are covered under many different policies and plans, each with its own rules and coverage limits.

> Because health care is such an expensive employee benefit, it gets a lot of attention from human resource personnel.

Table 14-1 Commercial Payer Models

Conventional indemnity plan	Allows the participant the choice of any provider without effect on reimbursement. Claims reimbursed as expenses are incurred.
PPO (preferred provider organization)	Coverage is provided through a network of selected health care providers. Enrollees may go outside network but incur larger cost.
HMO (health maintenance organization)	The entity assumes financial risks associated with providing medical services and for health care delivery, usually in return for a fixed, prepaid fee.
	Reimbursement is provided only to contracted or employed HMO providers.
	Out-of-network coverage is only provided in an emergency.
POS (point-of-service)	An HMO/PPO hybrid that resemble HMOs for in-network services.
	Plan requires a referral from an in-network provider to an out-of-network provider to receive improved coverage for the out-of-network provider.
Medigap supplemental plans	Pays Medicare deductibles, copayments, and other expenses.

Adapted from Kliethermes MA. Understanding healthcare billing basics. *Pharm Today.* 2017;23(7):57-68.

> **Employers may contract with managed care plans or organizations to provide health care benefits to covered workers and their families (collectively called covered lives).**

but may not be on the list of another plan (even one from the same company). The amount the patient must pay, or the **copayment**, differs between plans and for different types of medications (brand-name or generic products, formulary or nonformulary status).

Most patients whose prescription medications are covered under nongovernment third-party payers are employees who receive prescription coverage as part of their benefits package at work. Several different entities are involved in such prescription drug benefits:

■ **Employers**—Most large employers have active human resource departments that manage employee benefits programs. While it is unlikely that you would contact the employer directly about a specific prescription, pharmacists and pharmacy owners sometimes meet with human resource personnel to talk about problems their policies are causing for the employees or to offer additional services to a group of employees. Employers are very receptive to interventions that can increase employees' productivity by making them healthier or decreasing absences from work.

■ **Insurance companies**—Some employees may choose from a range of insurance companies contracting with their employer for coverage. In addition, most small employers and individuals who must purchase their own policies contract with insurance companies for

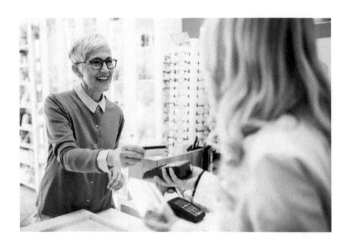

health care coverage. These companies may have their own networks set up for care, or they may contract with some or all of the types of organizations listed below.

- **Managed care plans**—Employers may contract with managed care plans or organizations to provide health care benefits to covered workers and their families (collectively called covered lives). The employer pays a set amount into the plan each month per person or family, meaning that the income available to the managed care plan is a fixed amount per individual. For this reason, managed care plans base many of their financial analyses and projections on how much they are spending per person for each component of health care (for example, drugs, hospital care, doctor visits). These calculations can be per member per month (PMPM) or per member per year (PMPY). These plans are increasingly asking pharmacies to share in their risk by paying a fixed amount, such as $10 PMPM, regardless of the number of prescriptions dispensed.

- **In-house pharmacies**—Some managed care organizations are health maintenance organizations (HMOs) that hire their own providers (physicians, nurses, pharmacists, technicians) and purchase their own facilities (care centers, hospitals, pharmacies). A prominent example of this type of staff-model HMO in many large US cities is Kaiser Permanente. In such plans, patients have a strong financial incentive to obtain their medications at these pharmacies—copayments are lower at in-house pharmacies than at outside pharmacies.

- **Third-party administrators**—Outside the staff-model HMO, other managed care plans contract for some or all of the services they offer. For the prescription drug benefit, these plans either contract with a third-party administrator (TPA) or a pharmacy benefits management company (see next bullet discussion). TPAs are companies that issue drug cards to beneficiaries, organize networks of pharmacy providers, and pay those pharmacies for the prescriptions they dispense to beneficiaries.

These networks may be open (all pharmacies can become members) or closed (not all pharmacies are able to join). TPAs are paid a set fee per paid claim by the managed care plan. As a result, the more prescriptions the TPA dispenses, the more the TPA is paid. Likewise, the TPA pays each pharmacy for the cost of the drug plus a dispensing fee, with increased prescriptions meaning increased revenues to the pharmacy.

- **Pharmacy benefits managers**—Reimbursement for prescriptions is often handled through an intermediary company, such as Caremark or Express Scripts. These companies—known as pharmacy benefits managers (PBMs)—are very important parts of the current payment system in community pharmacy. PBMs differ from TPAs in that they are more involved in clinical activities and programs such as patterns of drug use among prescribers, pharmacies, and groups of patients; establishment and enforcement of preferred drugs in formulary listings; disease management; prior authorization of selected or expensive drugs; and establishment of prescribing guidelines. PBMs are typically involved in payments for Medicare Part D prescriptions, acting as intermediaries between the PDPs and pharmacies. While some PBMs are paid by plans for each prescription processed, they are increasingly paid a set amount PMPM. For instance, a plan

> Reimbursement for prescriptions is often handled through an intermediary company, such as Caremark or Express Scripts. These companies—known as pharmacy benefits managers or PBMs—are very important parts of the current payment system in community pharmacy.

might pay a fee of $10 PMPM to the PBM for all drugs needed by members of the plan. This puts the PBM at risk with the plan, especially because most pharmacies are still reimbursed for each prescription processed. This capitated arrangement—payment of a fixed amount of money per person—gives the PBM an incentive to ensure efficiency in care and to reduce the use of unnecessary drugs or expensive agents for which less expensive alternatives would work just as well as the prescribed drug. PBMs may also require patients to get long-term supplies of medications for chronic diseases from PBM-owned mail service pharmacies, which dispense a 3- or 6-month supply of medication from a centralized dispensing location and send it to the patient via the US mail or an overnight delivery service.

Depending on the kind of pharmacy you work in, you may see these entities from very different perspectives. But regardless of where you are, you can be sure that third-party payers are an essential component of pharmacy and the overall health care system.

Interacting With Third-Party Payers

The basis for getting paid by Medicaid, TPAs, and PBMs is the prescription claim for a specific beneficiary. The vast majority of claims are processed in real time according to electronic data interchange standards set by the National Council for Prescription Drug Programs (NCPDP). This is called a point-of-service claims adjudication system or, more commonly, electronic claims processing, and it enables the pharmacy to perform the following functions at the time a prescription is dispensed:

- Verify eligibility of the beneficiary for prescription benefits
- Determine that the medication is covered
- Alert the pharmacist or technician that prior authorization is needed for restricted medications

- Determine the maximum quantity that may be dispensed and whether there is a maximum allowable cost for multisource products
- Ensure that refills are not being filled too early
- Check for possible drug–drug interactions
- Confirm the amount of copayment
- Submit the claim for payment

If all of the information has been entered correctly and verified by the claims processor, the pharmacy will then be paid for the prescription through a process known as **claims adjudication**. Payment is usually made by electronic transfer into the pharmacy's designated bank account on a daily, weekly, or other periodic basis.

When there is a problem, you or the pharmacist may need to call the TPA or PBM for assistance. In some cases, a claim is rejected electronically with a message that the prescribed medication is "nonformulary" or requires a **prior authorization**. As with health-system formularies, which are discussed more in Chapter 5, TPAs and PBMs may have a tiered—or preferred—formulary when there are multiple drugs that can be used to treat the same condition. A patient may be required to first try a less expensive alternative medication before the TPA or PBM will cover the more expensive option. Patient copayments are generally higher for nonformulary agents and agents in higher tiers of the formulary.

Within some e-prescribing systems, the prescriber has access to this formulary information so that he or she can consider these options at the time of prescribing. If the prescriber feels strongly that the patient needs the more expensive medication for their care, a prior authorization request sent from the prescriber to the TPA or PBM may be needed.

For these and many other reimbursement snags that arise in the claim adjudication process, you will be required to follow up by phone with the TPA or PBM and/or the prescribing physician to help ensure the patient gets their medication. Although these phone interactions can sometimes be frustrating and time consuming, keep in mind that you are filling an important role by serving as the patient's advocate to help the patient access much needed drug therapy at an affordable price.

Billing for Patient Care Services

If your pharmacist is involved in administration of immunizations, conducting point-of-care diagnostic testing, medication therapy management (MTM), chronic disease management, or other types of patient care services (see Chapter 9, Patient Care Services and the Pharmacy Technician), you will also need to be familiar with billing for these clinical activities. This type of billing involves detailing the services that have been provided, along with any point-of-care laboratory tests performed in the pharmacy.

The process of billing for patient care services differs from claim submission for prescription drugs for 2 important reasons: patient care services are usually billed to the patient's major medical provider rather than their prescription drug provider, and reimbursement is sought for provision of a service (eg, development of an MTM medication action plan) or administration of a drug (eg, a vaccine) rather than for dispensing of a drug product.

In many pharmacies, the most common and straightforward patient care service that you might bill for is the administration of a vaccine by the pharmacy technician or the pharmacist. Vaccines may be covered under the patient's pharmacy benefit, their medical benefit, or both, or may be billed to Medicare. Immunizations are an exception to one of the rules listed above. While the cost of medication is usually *not* billed as part of other patient care activities, it may be included for immunizations. This is because the patient is receiving a drug product (the vaccine dose) and a patient care service (patient assessment, vaccine administration, and appropriate counseling). In most cases, immunization billing is handled in the pharmacy electronically in a manner similar to that of prescription billing, but you will also need the patient's major medical card to submit the claim for the administration fee that accompanies each dose that is administered. While pharmacy claims are adjudicated electronically in real time, claims for medical services such as immunizations are of higher value and may receive a denial of service days or weeks after a claim has been submitted. Claims for medical benefits

such as immunizations are submitted in batches, using the American National Standards Institute X12 837 batch standard or CMS 1500 form. In these cases, the pharmacy must be contracted directly with the payer to be eligible to bill under the medical benefit. Specifically, for Medicare Part B, the pharmacy must be enrolled as a mass immunizer and submit a CMS 855B application. Once this application is completed, the pharmacy can bill influenza and pneumococcal vaccines under Medicare Part B with a Provider Transaction Access Number (PTAN) that they receive from Medicare. Ask your pharmacist if you have questions about policies and procedures in your pharmacy when billing for immunization services.

> In many pharmacies, the most common and straightforward patient care service that you might bill for is administration of an immunization by the pharmacist or technician.

If your pharmacy provides more in-depth patient care services, such as disease-specific patient counseling (eg, hormone replacement consultation, point-of-care diagnostic testing) or medication management services, the billing process may be more complex. Receiving compensation for medication management or other patient care services is becoming increasingly common. To bill for these patient care services, you need to be familiar with the following terms and forms:

- **Current Procedural Terminology (CPT) codes**—CPT codes are used to describe clinical interactions with patients. These codes vary according to (1) whether the patient is a new or an established patient, (2) the complexity of the clinical situation, and (3) the amount of time the pharmacist spends with the patient. CPT codes most often used by pharmacists are referred to as "incident-to" codes because they are used in conjunction with a physician or another prescriber, and the

Table 14-2 — Current Procedural Terminology (CPT) Codes

CATEGORY 1

Evaluation and management (E&M): 99201-99499
   Example: 99211 ("incident-to" code)
Anesthesia: 00100-01999; 99100-99150
Surgery: 10000-69990
Radiology: 70000-79999
Pathology and laboratory: 80000-89398
Medicine: 90281-99099; 99151-99199; 99500-99607
   Example: 99605-99607 for medication therapy
management services

CATEGORY 2

Supplementary tracking codes used for performance measurement, consisting of 4-digit numeric codes with an F at the end.

CATEGORY 3

Emerging technology temporary codes that have a T after the code, designating that they are temporary.

Adapted from: Kliethermes MA. Understanding healthcare billing basics. *Pharm Today.* 2017;23(7):57-68.

pharmacist is caring for the patient incident to the prescriber's care. Table 14-2 lists the Category 1 CPT codes that are routinely used in health care billing.

■ **National Provider Identifier (NPI)**—Beginning in 2007, pharmacists and other health care providers were required to begin using an NPI, a 10-digit provider identification number, in billing transactions. Patient care services may be billed under the organization's or the individual's NPI, depending on the pharmacy setting and rules.

■ **International Classification of Diseases, 10th Revision (ICD-10) Codes**—The ICD-10 codes are a set of standard numbers used for designating patients' diseases. Because the physician makes the diagnosis of patients' conditions, the pharmacist must simply obtain the correct ICD-10 code from the physician to use on the reimbursement forms. However, an error in entering this code will cause rejection of the claim.

■ **Healthcare Common Procedure Coding System (HCPCS)**—These codes are used for billing for medical devices, such as walkers, wheelchairs, syringes, and medication administration sets. These codes consist of a letter and 4 numbers. Codes beginning with the letters A-R and T-V describe supplies and medications and are the same throughout the United States. Codes that start with the letters S or W-Z are established by local Medicare carriers for claims for physician services, such as laboratory tests or surgical procedures.

■ **CMS 1500 forms**—This form was historically the most commonly used form for billing patient care services. Pharmacists used the various boxes on the form to convey to the third-party administrator or payer the kinds of services that were provided to the patient.

Conclusion

Reimbursement is the important last step in the process of dispensing prescriptions. Without adequate cash flow from Medicare Part D, Medicaid, and other third-party payers, few pharmacies would survive in today's environment.

Index

Page numbers followed by *f* indicate figures and those followed by *t* indicate tables.

billing, 209–218
  computers for, 183
  for immunization, 208
  for Medicaid, 212
  for Medicare, 210–212, 211f, 217
  for patient-care services, 217–218,
    218t
Billing and Reimbursement Certificate, of
    PTCB, 117
bioavailability, 21–22
biohazard disposal, 161, 203
biological safety cabinet (BSC)
  in CSPT, 118t
  for sterile compounding, 205t
blood, 11–13
blood glucose levels, 158
blood pressure
  disease management services for,
    159–160, 160f
  hypertension and, 19
  renal regulation of, 17
blood vessels, 11–13, 12f
bonding (insurance), 111
bone and joint agents, 41t–42t
bone marrow, 5, 13, 14f
bones, 5, 6f
borrowing, from other pharmacies, 101
branded generics, 169–170
brand name medications, 26
  billing for, 213
  in CSPT, 118t
  generic medications and, 169–170,
    169f, 170f
breasts, 17
bronchi, 13, 15f
buffer room (area), 201
  for sterile compounding, 205t
bulk compounding, 192
Bureau of Labor Statistics, 120
burglary, 110
Bush, George W., 84

C

calcium channel blockers, 37t
calculations, 60–67
  household equivalents, 67, 67t
  percentage, 63–65
  in PTCE, 116t
  ratio and proportion, 60–61
  ratio strengths, 65–66
  temperature conversion, 66
  units of measures in, 60t, 61–63, 61t,
    62t
cancer. See chemotherapy
Canopy Medical Translator, 149

capillaries, 13
capsules, 24t
carbohydrates, 3
carbon dioxide, respiratory exchange of,
    13
cardiac agents, 37t–38t
cardiac muscle, 9
cardiovascular system, 11–13, 12f
care plans, computers for, 183
cartilage, 5
cells, 3, 4f
cellular physiology, 2–4
Celsius scale, 66
Centers for Medicare and Medicaid
    Services (CMS). See also
    Medicaid; Medicare
  billing to, 210
  1500 forms of, 218
  MTM and, 156
central intravenous line, 163
centrally acting pain medications, 29t–30t
central nervous system (CNS), 9
  agents for, 27t–32t
cephalosporins, 43t
certification, 114–120, 115f
certified pharmacy technicians (CPhTs),
    114–120
chemical physiology, 2–4
chemical stability, of nonsterile
    compounding, 191
chemotherapy
  common drugs and drug categories in,
    48t–54t
  sterile compounding of, 203–206, 204f
child-resistant containers, 174
cholesterol
  dyslipidemia and, 158–159
  lowering agents, 38t–39t
chromosomes, 3
class I recalls, 79
class II recalls, 79
class III recalls, 79
Class III balance, 188
cleanroom suites, 201
clinical decision support (CDS), 179t
clinical information system, 178, 179t
Clinical Laboratory Improvement
    Amendments of 1988 (CLIA),
    point-of-care screening and testing
    and, 160
clinical screening, computers for, 178–180
clinical trials, 74
closed-ended questions, 141
closed system vial transfer device (CSTD),
    for sterile compounding, 205t

cobalt-60, 207
Code of Ethics, of APhA, 120, 121t
Code of Ethics for Pharmacy Technicians,
    120, 122f
colon (large intestine), 15, 15f
Combat Methamphetamine Act of 2005,
    91
communication
  with angry or uncooperative patients,
    145, 145f
  confidentiality in, 148
  with dying patients, 143–145
  with English as a second language,
    148–149
  about medication orders, 175–176,
    176f
  with patients, 139–149
  about prescriptions, 175–176, 176f
  principles and definition of, 140–141,
    140f
  on product availability, 137
  on social media, 147–148
  with stressed patients, 145
community pharmacies
  brand name medications in, 169
  household equivalents in, 67
  therapeutic substitution in, 170
Community Pharmacy Accreditation, by
    NABP, 93
complex compounding, 186
compounded sterile preparation
    technician (CSPT), 117,
    118t–119t
compounding, percentage calculations in,
    63–65
compounding aseptic containment isolator
    (CACI), for sterile compounding,
    205t
compounding aseptic isolator (CAI), for
    sterile compounding, 205t
Compounding Record, 192
Comprehensive Drug Abuse Prevention
    and Control Act of 1970, 86
comprehensive medication review (CMR),
    152, 157, 158f
computer downtime procedures, 183–184
computerized physician order entry
    (CPOE), 179t, 180–181
computers, 177–184
  for dispensing, 180–182, 182f
  for inventory control/management, 180
  medication orders in, 168
  for MTM, 182–183
  order entry on, 168, 178f
  for patient profiles, 180

efferent nerves, 9
efficiency, quality assurance with, 134
electrolytes, in TPN, 198
electronic health record (EHR), 179*t*
electronic medical record (EMR), 179*t*
electronic prescribing, 179*t*
electrons, 2–3
   in radiopharmaceuticals, 207
elements, 2–3
   common, in human body, 3*t*
   radioactive, 3
elimination (excretion), 22–23, 22*f*
elixirs, 24*t*
Elixir Sulfanilamide tragedy, 74
Emergency Use Authorization, 78
employers, prescription benefits from, 214
emulsions, 24*t*
encoding, 140
endocrine system, 9–11, 11*f*
endocrinologic agents, 34*t*–36*t*
endotoxins, in CSPT, 119*t*
English as a second language, 148–149
enteral nutrition, sterile compounding for, 200
enzymes, 3, 22
epidemiology, 20
epilepsy, 30*t*–31*t*
epinephrine, 9–11
erythrocytes (red blood cells), 13
esophagus, 15, 15*f*
estrogen, 11, 36*t*
ethics, codes of, 120, 121*t*
event reporting, in PTCE, 116
excretion, 22–23, 22*f*
expiration date, 99
   in PTCE, 116*t*
   for returned drugs, 104

F

facilities
   for pharmacies, 93–95
   for sterile compounding, 200–201, 201*f*
Fahrenheit scale, 66
fallopian tubes, 17, 18*f*
fats (lipids), 3
   in TPN, 198
Federal Food and Drug Act of 1906, 74
feedback, 140
female reproductive system, 17, 18*f*
1500 forms (CMS), 218
fingerstick, 158, 159*f*
Food, Drug, and Cosmetic Act of 1938, 74
food, drug interactions with, 57

Food and Drug Administration (FDA)
   COVID-19 and, 75, 78, 161
   dietary supplement regulations of, 78–79
   drug approval process of, 74–78, 75*f*–76*f*
   drug withdrawals and recalls by, 78–79
   Emergency Use Authorization by, 78
   generic name requirements of, 26
   history of, 74
   on immunizations, 161
   labeler code assigned by, 98
   legend drugs of, 74, 92
   MedWatch of, 134, 136*f*–137*f*
   on nonsterile compounding, 188
   Nutrition Facts label of, 81*f*–83*f*
   in PTCE, 116*t*
   recalls by, 78–79, 108
   Risk Evaluation and Mitigation Strategies of, 80, 84
   on shortages of drugs, 109
   state boards of pharmacy and, 92
   on storage of ph107armaceutical products, 107
   therapeutic equivalence ratings of, 78
Food and Drug Administration Amendments Act of 2007, 80
Food Chemicals Codex (FCC), 188
forged prescriptions, 89
Form 41 (DEA), 89
Form 106 (DEA), 89
Form 222 (DEA), 87, 88*f*, 89, 103
Form 224 (DEA), 87
formularies, 85, 105–106
   for preferred drugs, 169
fraud, in Medicaid and Medicare, 86, 213
fungi, 195, 195*f*

G

gallbladder, 15*f*, 16
gamma particles, 207
garbing, for sterile compounding, 201–202
gas exchange, 13
gastroenterologic system, 13–16, 15*f*
   agents, 34*t*
gastrointestinal tract, 13–15, 15*f*
generic medications, 26, 78
   availability of products for, 169
   branded name medications and, 169–170, 169*f*, 170*f*
   in CSPT, 118*t*
   in PTCE, 116*t*
genes, 3
gene therapy, 19

genetic predisposition, 19
genetics, 3, 19–20
genitourinary agents, 40*t*–41*t*
geometric dilution, for nonsterile compounding, 189
glands, 9–11, 11*f*
gloves, 201, 202, 204, 205*t*
glucagon, 11, 15
glucocorticoids, 9–11
glucose
   blood levels of, 158
   in TPN, 198
goggles, 204
Good Manufacturing Practices, 188–189
gout, 42*t*
government agencies for reimbursement. *See* Medicaid; Medicare
gowns, 202, 203, 205*t*
gray-market, 109

H

hair, 5, 5*f*
half-life, 207
Hazardous Drug Management Certificate, of PTCB, 119
hazardous drugs, sterile compounding of, 203–206, 204*f*, 205*t*
Healthcare Common Procedure Coding System (HCPCS), 218
Health Insurance Portability and Accountability Act (HIPAA), 91
   social media and, 148
Health Level 7 (HL7), 179*t*
health maintenance organizations (HMOs), 215
hearing, 9, 11*f*
heart, 11–13, 12*f*
hematopoietic agents, 54*t*
herbal remedies, 57
high-alert medications
   in CSPT, 118*t*
   medication errors with, 131, 131*f*–132*f*
high-efficiency particulate air (HEPA) filtration
   in CSPT, 118*t*
   for sterile compounding, 200, 201, 202
histamine-2 H1 antagonists, 34*t*
HIV/AIDS, 46*t*–48*t*
home infusion equipment, 163–164
homeostasis, 17
hormones, 9–11, 35*t*–36*t*
   for chemotherapy, 52*t*
household equivalents, 67, 67*t*
human anatomy, normal, 2–17
Human Genome Project, 19